*Language
Disorders
of
Children*

Under the advisory editorship of
Hayes A. Newby

Language
Disorders
of
Children: The Bases and Diagnoses

Mildred Freburg Berry

APPLETON-CENTURY-CROFTS
EDUCATIONAL DIVISION
New York MEREDITH CORPORATION

Library of Congress Card No.: 69-10876

PRINTED IN THE UNITED STATES OF AMERICA

390-08875-7

To James and Kim

Preface

Perhaps the most significant development in language disorders has been the contribution in the last two decades of interdisciplinary studies to the wide field of communication. The union of psychology, linguistics, biochemistry, physics, neurophysiology, and neuropathology in common research has stretched the boundaries of our province and stimulated our own study. Interdisciplinary study, aided by computer science, has developed a broad spectrum of linguistic knowledge and problems that are basic to our understanding of oral language.

My purpose in writing this book has been to focus the results of these studies and of those within our discipline on the language disabilities of children. I have tried to present relevant facts, concepts, and theories in lucid form and to apply them specifically to the bases and diagnoses of language disorders. I have tried to present them as completely and accurately as possible, avoiding turgidity and undue terseness. "Language may conceal as well as express thought, but it does not have to confuse it," someone has said. It is not my intention to muddy the meaning. My "purpose plain" in writing this book is to undergird theories and practices of language disorders with knowledge borrowed both from the laboratory and the library. The references are voluminous but with good reason. The student may wish for ampler discussion of certain concepts and theories. If the reader wishes he may find my borrowings in their original state and make his own application to the specific area of language disorder under consideration.

The student will find little statistical ritual in the sections devoted to evaluations of language problems. There is scant reference to Pearson product-moment, analysis of variance, chi-square techniques, or Kuder-Richardson Formula 21. Evaluations and tests, both projective and objective, are presented but they are ancillary to diagnostic teaching. Diagnostic teaching may be slower but it is far more productive than statistical ritual in tracking down deficits. Testing, it seems to me, too frequently results in incomplete silhouettes rather than full portraits. The children with whom we work cannot be drawn in black-white profiles.

This is not a handbook of therapy, yet if the principles underlying all evaluative processes, including diagnostic teaching, are understood, the student also may have reliable guidelines for therapy. The book may accordingly serve as a basic text for students electing their first course in language disorders.

In diagnostic teaching of the language-handicapped child I have given considerable attention to several sensory-motor fields. Tactile-kinesthetic (haptic) pathways may be equally powerful or superior in potential to audition in the perception of *certain aspects* of language, notably its morphemic and syntactic-lexical elements. We discuss deficits and distortions affecting perceptual focus, categorization and retention of verbal sequences, inner language, and oral expression. In view of my particular persuasion, the student should not be dismayed by the limited attention paid to the stimulation and learning of speech sounds in isolation, and the considerable space devoted to activities in which the child must comprehend the continuum of language as an integral part of learning situations both inside and outside the classroom.

For the teacher this is not a sit-and-drill approach. Diagnostic teaching demands more of him in brain and brawn than the conventional modes that have been used in our discipline. "Thinking is so rare a sport because it is so rarely tried," said Winston Churchill. Here is an opportunity to *think* and to *act*. This area of education is not for the faint heart. Anyone who has worked, even briefly, in this field has often found himself going "up the down staircase." Yet he is not likely to remain in this field of work unless he can find in every child a way of securing response to an organized, imaginative, child-centered program of diagnostic teaching. If he has no match with which to light a candle, he need not curse the darkness.

Neither is this a field of work for the blithe spirit who generally dismisses all problems with an insouciant remark: "That's the way the world wags, my friend." In the field of language disorders, however, one intervenes by dint of his own resources to change the "world's wagging," to find for children in his charge a way to change the pattern, or to seek at least a feasible, if not totally satisfactory, pattern of accommodation to irreversible awards of fortune. Here is a truism worthy of repetition: The field of language disorders needs dynamic students, resolute in purpose, definite in plan, but labile in approach; energetic, forthright, and persistent in teaching; always ready to engage upon the adventure and the search.

I am indebted to my friends and coworkers in the field, here and abroad, who have argued the premises of this book with me at institutes and workshops, and who have generously permitted me to quote from their publications. Grateful acknowledgment also must be paid to the stimulating discussions of my students in several universities, notably the Universities of Wisconsin, Toronto, and Texas Woman's University. Children's clinics in Oslo, Copenhagen, and Ankara, where I served as Fulbright lecturer, have given me the opportunity to test theories and practices. Thanks are due to my former student, Ruth Talbott, who made the preliminary sketches of illustrations.

To LaVera Tillman, Librarian, Winnebago County (Ill.) Medical Library and to the reference librarians of the John Crerar Library (Chicago) I am in debt for checking countless references and providing me with photostat copies of innumerable articles. And to my rare and patient friends, Margaret Dahlgren and Mary Wilt, who typed the manuscript and assisted in countless details of the final preparation, I shall always owe much more than I can express.

Finally I wish to acknowledge the encouragement and assistance of the late Andrew T. Weaver in planning this work. He was more than an advisory editor, counseling wisely, befriending generously, and unfailingly sustaining the spirit.

Mildred Freburg Berry
Rockford, Illinois

Contents

II *Language and Learning*

III *Evaluation of the Linguistically Handicapped Child*

IV Children With Disorders of Verbal Communication

Appendices

*Language
Disorders
of
Children*

Introduction

> The world is full of wonderful things
> But none more so than man,
>
>   .   .   .
>
> Speech he has made his own, and thought
> That travels swift as the wind,
> And how to live in harmony with others.
>
> —Sophocles, *Antigone*

Dolphins, crows, and chimpanzees may have the gift of tongues; they do not have the gift of symbolic formulation of meaning—and that makes all the difference. Although they can be taught a type of speech, words are symbolic only to the human primate who hears them, not to the animal. These animals also have their own signal systems of communication but they are not symbolic signals. The American crow will react to the calls of other species, for example, to its French relatives, but *only* if it has been exposed to the general features of the crow calls by previous association with crows from other sections.[1] Jane Goodall's chimpanzees also employ highly conventionalized signals and emotional gestures (disgust, appeasement) and control the behavior of other chimpanzees by vocalizations. "They have a tremendous variety of calls, each one induced by a different emotion," but Miss Goodall concedes that the calls do not constitute a language, albeit they are a means of communication.[2]

Human Oral Language. The design of the system of human oral communication consists, according to Hockett's brilliant analysis, of

[1] H. and M. Frings, The language of crows. *Sci Amer* (November 1959), 201: 119.
[2] J. Goodall, My life among wild chimpanzees. *Nat Geog Mag* (August 1963), 124: 272–308.

1

thirteen features that are common to all languages of the world (Figure 0).[3] The design includes many steps that are self-explanatory. The sixth design feature, *specialization,* "refers to the fact that bodily effort and spreading sound waves of speech serve no function except as signals." The eighth design feature calls for *arbitrary ties* between meaningful message elements. Hence *whale* is a small word for a large object; *microorganism* is the obverse. *Displacement* (feature 10), an almost unique characteristic of human language, makes it possible for man to talk "about things that are remote in space or time (or both) from where the talking is going on." *Productivity* (feature 11) means the capacity, also peculiar to man, "to say things that have never been said or heard before and yet to be understood by other speakers of the language." In other words, man can construct speech by putting together pieces from other previously learned speech patterns. *Traditional transmission* (feature 12) simply means that "human genes carry the capacity to acquire a language, and probably also a strong drive toward such acquisition, but the detailed conventions of any one language are transmitted extragenetically by learning and teaching." [4]

Scope of the Subject. Language disorders represent an area that, like outer space, seems to have no boundaries; they have infinite parameters. There are reasons for the wide scope of the subject. Verbal communication is as complex as the human being who engages in the art of language. One cannot track language down, as a rabbit to its lair, because it has many tracks. These tracks extend into physics, physiology, neurology, chemistry, psychology, linguistics, phonetics, and education. Language is the universal cross-reference. One must be informed, for example, about the physical phenomena associated with the perception of speech. He must reckon with the influence of the endocrines on emotional stability. He must understand the integrative action of the reticular and limbic systems in coding language, the chemical shifts in synaptic potentials, the psychological bases of coding, of attention and memory, the morphemological approach to sound sequences, the morphological principles of language learning, and the marshalling of large sequences for oral expression. He must know how to study the problems of the individual handicapped by verbal communication disorders. If he would work in language disorders, he must borrow from many related fields. We have borrowed too little in the past. Much of our knowledge and many of our teaching methods are hapless and worthless because they have emerged from *terra incognita.* The unmapped territory now has been partially charted for us mainly by workers in other domains. If today's student is to assume leadership in this new territory, he must pursue language disorders to their scientific, artistic, and social taproots.

[3] C. F. Hockett, The origin of speech. *Sci Amer* (September 1960), 203: 89–97.
[4] *Ibid.,* p. 91.

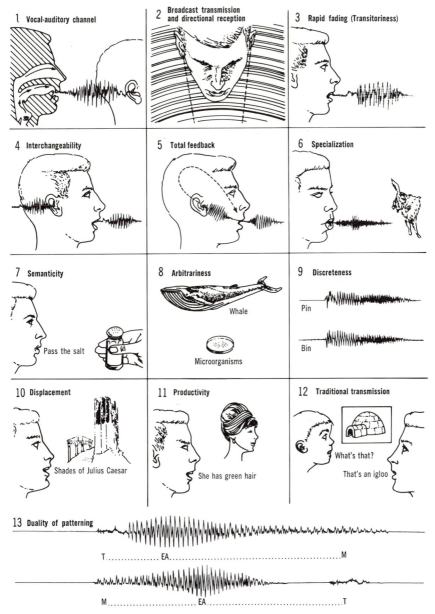

Figure 0. *Symbolization of design features of communication. Thirteen design features of animal communication, discussed in detail by Hockett, are symbolized in the figure. The patterns of the words* pin *and* bin *(9) and* team *and* meat *(13) were recorded at Bell Telephone Laboratories.*

SOURCE: C. F. Hockett, The origin of speech. *Sci Amer* (1960), 203 (3): 91. Copyright

The assignment is not easy. The impatient or shallow student may find the way too arduous, for the road does wind uphill most of the way. The scholar will find it an exciting, vexatious, disquieting experience. For a time he may feel as if he were walking through an "homogenized ambience" but, certainly, with study the atmosphere will clear and the outlines, solid structures, and main thoroughfares will emerge to occupy the foreground of his thinking. He does not ask if this knowledge is usable, practical. The scholar bends all knowledge to his use. He knows that one does not get nearer the ideal state of things—truth—by proclaiming meager beginnings as final principles and by owing to the facts what one saves on theory.

Thus the lengthy discussions of the psychoneurological, psycholinguistic, and psychosocial dimensions of language behavior are well justified. Equipped with knowledge of these, the student should be ready to tackle the diagnostic study and teaching of children who find language learning difficult. No categorical lists of "cause and cure" will be found. The bias for longitudinal studies during diagnostic teaching stems from years "in the vineyard." The student will find greater profit in studying the profiles of children who are handicapped by disabilities in language than by discursive chapters on symptoms and etiology. No profile will exactly fit the child who sits at a given moment with the student of language disorders. If the student remembers, however, all the possible variables—neurophysiological, psychological, linguistic, educational— hopefully he will be competent to tackle the problems of *this child* and *then* design a program of diagnostic teaching especially for him.

New Evidence for Old Ideas. Other workers in the field may take issue with some neurological and psychological premises upon which diagnostic study and teaching are based. Many views are old but are upheld by new evidence.

1. If language learning is to be economical, it cannot be taught on a phonetic basis. The teaching of sounds in isolation is not supported by results of research in language learning or of our practice of this method.
2. Tactile-kinesthetic (or haptic) modalities must be regarded as coequal with the auditory modality in language learning. The exclusive or major emphasis upon auditory stimulation and feedback runs counter to results of research by physicists and psycholinguists on the nature of language acquisition.
3. We must give much greater attention to the knowledge of psycholinguists who have provided us with substantial information on the development of language in the child and of the comprehension of linguistic morphology. Their analyses of the morphemic and syntactical elements should be useful to us in understanding and training the child handicapped in oral language.

4. We cannot support neurological concepts of strict cortical localization, neural hierarchies of control, and point-to-point transmission of impulses, of afferent-efferent hegemonies, or cortical reception-association-perception pathways. These must give way to sounder concepts of neural functioning. The new concepts, however, are not predicated upon haphazard sluiceways and chance neuronic connections but upon a concept of neuronal assemblies united in patterns of operation through their synaptic potentials and similarity in electronic charge or power. The plasticity and power of the synapse are the agent.

5. The phenomena of coding, perception, attention, and recall must also be understood in terms of their neurological correlates of function, if correlates can be found. As far as it is possible, they should be equated with semantic principles and terminology. Without this knowledge, the language clinician's position is tenuous.

These concepts cannot be completely unfamiliar, even to the undergraduate student who has survived his courses in the biological and physical sciences. In this book he is enjoined to apply them to the problems of the child with language disabilities.

Who Has a Language Disorder? Language vs. Speech. Many disturbances of speech may be subsumed, in part, under language disorders. The cerebral-palsied child, for example, may be dysarthric; he also may suffer from grave temporal and spatial perceptual problems that will affect his ability to comprehend and use verbal symbols. The child with a repaired cleft palate often has nasal and poorly articulated speech. He has a speech disorder, but may he not also have a language disorder? We have taught numbers of children with repaired clefts who have very inadequate proprioceptive sensitivity and feedback, a neurological deficit that results in a *language,* not a *speech disorder.* Recently the delayed talker and the child with so-called infantile perseveration (it is atypical, not infantile) have come under the purview of the language specialists. They have taken a long look, and now they believe that the articulatory patterns of many of these children are the result of *poor perception* of the morpheme and/or the linguistic *form* of the sentence. Their problem is not the production of isolated sounds but of sound sequences, the continuum of speech. At some point neurological or psychological blocks have disturbed the integrative processes mediating language.

The Brain-Injured. There are groups of children whose language deficits are clearly recognized but the etiology of these deficits remains obscure. Some of them are called brain-injured, a diagnosis based upon the presumption of lesions of the CNS produced pre-, peri-, or post-natally. The Rh-infant who has suffered from foetal anoxia has, without doubt, an injured central nervous system. The injury possibly may be discrete, ablating neuronal assemblies and circuits of one modality, but its effects spread far afield. It is said, for example, that the child is handicapped by a central auditory disorder. The description is far too limited to accord with paradigms of neural activity. Lesions of the CNS may be caused, in other cases, by trauma attending birth. Most commonly cerebral-palsied children are thought to have suffered this misfortune. In one chapter we have discussed the profile of Sandy who is aphasic, the result of a skull fracture at 9 years. Encephalitis and other diseases which invade the CNS can produce equally dire effects upon the child's comprehension and use of language. Some of these children may have language deficits *and* speech defects. The severely handicapped, cerebral-palsied child has grave neuromuscular problems that cripple him in larynx and tongue.

The Brain-Different. Research in our own field has been limited largely to the intensive study of the input and output channels of oral language. Only scant attention has been paid to the continuous coding operations of the central nervous system which are required in the comprehension-expression of oral language. As a result, we have failed to recognize that a sizable group of children has an atypical neural organization, often genetically determined, which results in language disturbances. These children have no history-producing lesions. They are not brain-injured; they are brain-different. Presumably their *capacity* for learning is normal but their mode of learning is atypical. Such terms as *idiopathic language retardation* and *neurophrenic disturbance* have been applied to this group. Perhaps the most accurate description of their problem is contained in the term *neurogenic learning disability.*

Psychoneurological Language Disorders. The development of oral language can be disturbed by a combination of psychoneurological factors. The blind and the deaf have suffered impairment of the central nervous system but they also generally experience grave psychological blocks in learning oral language. The psychoneurological disabilities of autistic or schizophrenic children are reflected in profound disturbances in the integrative processes of coding oral symbols.

The Mentally Retarded. A group of children will be handicapped in oral language because they are mentally retarded. Their profiles are quite unlike those of brain-different children. The mental retardate shows an even depression of the profile. All dimensions of coding language—sensory-motor input, integration, retention, formulation, and expression—are uniformly affected. Because he suffers from a general *learning incapacity,* of which language retardation is one manifestation, he is not a major concern in this text.

I

Tracking Language in the Nervous System

1

Neural Substrates of Language Development

Complexity of the Central Nervous System

The nervous system no longer remains "a riddle wrapped in an enigma and cradled in a mystery" although it cannot yet be described with irrefutable clarity. The anatomist and the neurologist have gone far beyond the seventeenth century identification of hills and hollows, of gray islands and white channels in the brain; they must go farther yet before they reach a cogent and completely reliable explanation of the operation of the nervous system. The discovery of hardening and staining fluids gave to the biologist with his microscope an opportunity to trace cells and fibers. Then scholars in several fields—biology, physics, chemistry, embryology—combined their efforts in effecting a gigantic wiring system connecting ten billion cells. The results were intriguing but they raised more questions than they answered. In the late nineteenth century the chemical morphologist gave great assistance in understanding of the molecular constituents and action of neurones and tracts. And more recently, in this century, physicists have given to neurophysiologists expert electronic tools, notably the oscilloscope and the electroencephalograph by which the action circuits of the nervous system can be observed and recorded. With the advent of these electronic techniques it became apparent that any mechanical wiring system of input and output was not an acceptable or workable model of the central nervous system. The brain cannot be reduced to a mechanism. Because it is a dynamic organ, it is vastly more complex and variable. One must abandon, therefore, certain neurological concepts that have sidetracked those investigating the integrative action of the central nervous system, particularly at its most complex levels. Certainly no greater neural complex could be envisioned than that mediating language, involving as it does, the precursors or coexistence of the processes of motivation, attention, and perception.

At this point the student of language disorders may ask why he should be concerned with possible neural correlates of perception and use of verbal symbols. Of what value is it for him to understand brain-mind theories? There are two major gains in such a study. First, we cannot build a scheme of the comprehension and use of language upon a flimsy neural structure evolved by our imagination. To the extent that neural correlates of comprehension and use of language have been found, it is incumbent upon us to know them. We do not question the value of knowledge of the phonological, psychological, or phonetic bases of speech, much of which knowledge is hypothetical. Why then should we question the need to know the neurophysiological basis of language? There is a second return on our investment in such knowledge. If we understand neural patterning, for example, of perception of sound, movement, size, design, and color, we are in a better position to develop scientifically sound procedures of evaluation and training of the child handicapped by a linguistic disorder.[1]

No simple explanation of the function of the nervous system can be offered because its structure is not simple. If one regards the histological structure of the cortex and brainstem, he is impressed by the enormous wealth of detailed and patterned linkage and the masses of afferent and efferent fibers between which lie a vast assemblage of interneurones. "There are some ten thousand million neurones in the human cerebral cortex and each is a node in the network whose strands are woven from the numerous processes (dendrites and axons) that provide the multiple synaptic contacts."[2] On the basis of statistical computation, Eccles calculates that "the discharge of an impulse by any one neurone will have contributed directly and indirectly to the excitation of hundreds of thousands of other neurones within the very brief time of 20 msec."[3]

In the functioning of this system, moreover, the possibilities for connection seem infinite. Neurone X is a member of several networks so one cannot say that X is a part of one particular, closed, self-reexciting chain of stable character. In the advancing wave front A (many neurones in parallel), neurone X can be activated not only by A but also by other wave fronts. Through synaptic distribution of neurones activated in parallel with neurone X, it may activate neurones in distant wave fronts. In

[1] R. W. Sperry, Neurology and the mind-brain problem. In R. L. Isaacson, Ed., *Basic readings in neuropsychology*. New York: Harper & Row, 1964. Pp. 403–429.
[2] J. C. Eccles, *The neurophysiological basis of mind*. London: Oxford, 1953. P. 268.
[3] *Ibid.*, pp. 275–276.

the same way, other neurones, Y and Z, may influence X at one time; at another time neuronal assemblies or fronts, B and C, may influence neurone X.[4]

But why does an incoming sensory pattern modify or excite a specific neuronal network? Eccles believes that synaptic knobs in certain neuronal networks have developed a structural specificity for a particular sensory pattern and "respond" only to that pattern. He summarizes his concept in these words: "We are envisaging the pattern of activity in the cortex at any instant as being determined by two factors: (1) the immediate (and very recent) afferent input; (2) the developed structural specificity (inherited and acquired) of the neuronal networks." [5] In other words, the child's ability to comprehend and use language is conditional upon two things: (1) the integrity and operational unity, at a particular moment, of input modalities—audition, taction, vision, kinesthesis, and (2) the presence of neuronal networks or assemblies which have the potentiality, either genetic or acquired, to receive these sensory bits of information and to integrate them with previously coded information, present in the form of electronic patterns in neuronal networks. These networks, then, are not only acoustic, tactile, visual, and kinesthetic "processors," *per se;* they also contain the electronic codes of previously laid-down patterns. So meaning is determined by specific spatio-temporal patterns of activity occurring in the neuronal assemblies.

Genetic Potentiality for Language

In his description of the integration of neuronal networks, Eccles does not assume that language is an inherited function but he does predicate one's capacity to learn language upon patterns of structural specificity of neuronal networks, some of which are innate. Perhaps this is also what Ajuriaguerra [6] means when he says that there are no pre-formed centers of language but rather *preformed mechanisms which take shape as general maturation of the CNS proceeds.* Certainly the anatomical, biochemical, and electrophysiologic changes that are characteristic of maturation follow a genetic timetable. The infant's brain, for example, more than triples its weight in the first two years. The growth of dendritic plexuses results in dense arborization of neuronal networks so that by the baby's second birthday the nervous system normally has achieved sufficient anatomic maturation for the onset of speech. By 12 years, the central nervous system has reached maturity. The rapid increase in lipids, phosphatides, and ribonucleic acid in the

[4] *Ibid.*, pp. 240-244.

[5] *Ibid.*, pp. 269–270.

[6] J. de Ajuriaguerra, Speech disorders in childhood. In E. C. Carterette, Ed., *Brain function.* Berkeley: University of California Press, 1966. Pp. 118f.

same period, 2 years to 12 years, attests to the accompanying biochemical maturation. Physiological maturation has been assessed by the steady development of patterns of electrical activity in the nervous system. In the cortex certain brain waves are known as alpha patterns. In the year-old child, the alpha wave may be low in energy and will have a frequency of 3–5 cycles per second. At 12 years the alpha wave is stabilized at 10–12 cps. (A fuller discussion of the alpha and other wave patterns of electrical activity in the nervous system follows in a succeeding section of this chapter.)

Lateralization of function is further evidence of physiological maturation of the nervous system. Between 3 and 7 years a child normally develops preference in sidedness and by 9 years is strongly unimanual in most activities. By 12 years cerebral lateralization probably is irreversible. Failure to establish laterality even at this age is common among language-retarded children. We should remember, however, that manual preference is not an unfailing index of lateralization in the CNS. There are right handers who also do not demonstrate strong cerebral lateralization at 12 years. The acquisition of language seems to be dependent, in part, on these anatomical, biochemical, and physiological changes dictated by genetic factors.

Basic Neural Structures

The Neurone

The neurone is the basic unit of structure of the CNS.[7] The nerve cell has a central part or soma, and in its simplest form consists of this unipolar cell body with a single axone extending from the cell body. Actually the afferent and efferent limbs of this neurone have become fused together as they approach the cell body so it is, in fact, a bipolar unit. This type of neurone is of particular interest to us because it is located in sensory ganglia outside the CNS and in the mesencephalic nucleus of the fifth cranial nerve. The mesencephalic fifth, presumably, is concerned only with proprioception from the muscles of mastication. Bipolar cells possessing an axon and one dendrite are found characteristically in the auditory, visual, and olfactory systems. All other neurones may be classed as multipolar. They have a single axone but branching from the cell body are long dendrites that terminate in an intricate web or arborization. Multipolar cells also are of various types: stellate, fusi-

---

[7] The reflex arc, *per se,* is not discussed because it is no longer considered the unit of function of the nervous system. Probably such a description should not have been given for, as Sherrington pointed out, the functional unit of the CNS is the entire system and not a diagram of two or three neurones with synaptic connections.—C. S. Sherrington, Quantitative management of contraction in lowest level coordination. *Brain* (1931), 54 (Part 1): 1–28. See also J. M. Hunt, How children develop intellectually. *Children* (May–June 1964), 11: 86.

form, and pyramidal. Pyramidal cells are most familiar to us because they are found in the frontal cortex. Their axones have no myelin sheath for 100 or more microns, but before they enter the white matter of the cord, the sheath appears. The fibers that carry the impulse in the CNS are myelinated and possess a nodal structure. Around the neurone may be found glial or supporting cells. As the name suggests, they "glue" or form the embedding for neurones.

Although the number of individual neurones probably does not increase in early infancy, the neurones themselves grow considerably during early infancy. The growth in volume of the pyramidal cells of the middle frontal gyrus, for example, is rapid during the first two years, then slows down and presumably comes to a stop during puberty. In the period from infancy to 4 years a very significant proliferation in the interconnections of cells also occurs. Axones and dendrites grow from the cell body and form a dense net of interconnecting branches so that cell bodies are pushed apart by the increasing number of arborizations. Dendritic growth is notable first in the visual, then in the auditory and sensory-motor Rolandic and pre-Rolandic fields of the cortex. The schedule of development, it should be noted, parallels stages in the development of oral language.

Cerebellum

The cerebellum (Figures 1-1 and 1-2) is not part of the brain stem but is closely connected with it by three bridges: brachium conjunctivum, brachium pontis, and restiform body (superior, middle, and inferior peduncles respectively) (Figures 1-3 and 1-6). Lying beneath the occipital lobes of the cerebrum and above the pons-medulla section, the cerebellum is divided into two lobes: the corpus cerebelli, or cerebellar hemispheres, and the flocculus (Figure 1-4). The cerebellar hemispheres are divided into anterior and posterior lobes. A part of the posterior lobe, now called the middle lobe, has developed in conjunction with the cerebral cortex and suggests a close functional relationship both with the brain stem and the cortex. The fourth ventricle, as seen in the sagittal plane, forms a tent-like cavity (Figures 1-2 and 1-4).

Myriads of neural tracts enter and leave the cerebellum by way of the three bridges. Fibers from the vestibule (internal labyrinth of the ear), spinal cord, cranial nerve nuclei in the brain stem, nuclei of the reticular system, and the cortex make functional connections with cerebellar nuclei either on the same or opposite side. Heavy traffic apparently goes on with the reticular system. Every part of the reticular system, from the thalamus to the medulla, presumably receives projections from cerebellar nuclei which then may be directed either to the cortex or to the brain stem. So direct and rich are these connections that

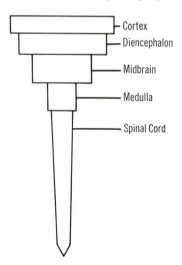

Figure 1-1. Diagram of anatomic divisions of CNS.

SOURCE: W. K. Livingston, F. P. Haugen, and J. M. Brookhart, Functional organization of the CNS. *Neurol* (Minneap) (1954) 4:488. Used by permission.

some neurologists include the cerebellum in the reticular system. The contribution of the cerebellum to speech must be considerable, for nuclear masses in both lobes provide feedback loops mediating motokinesthesis, touch, hearing, and sight.[8] One concludes that the cerebellum plays a significant role in the activation and inhibition of sensory-motor patterns through its intimate connections with reticular nuclei at every level of the brain stem and with nuclei in the thalamus, striate bodies, and cortex.

The Brain Stem: Medulla, Pons, Midbrain

Medulla. Although the medulla (Figure 1-5) represents a more complex arrangement, it is an extension of nuclear masses and their associated fiber tracts found in the spinal cord. Its importance in sensory-motor systems subserving speech is suggested by the location of the great nuclear masses subserving cranial nerves VII–XII. The medulla, in conjunction with the pons, is concerned with the regulation of respiration and cardiovascular mechanisms. Through the vestibular division of the VIIIth cranial nerve it assists in the mediation of equilibrium. Long ascending and descending tract systems also are present in the medulla. One great bundle, the pyramidal tract, containing both ascending and descending fibers, is named for its shape, the pyramids (Figure 1-6). The majority of the fibers of the pyramidal system will decussate

[8] R. Snider, The cerebellum. *Sci Amer* (August 1958), 199: 84–90.

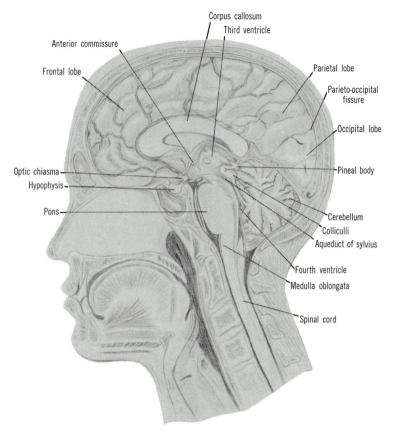

Corpus callosum
Third ventricle
Anterior commissure
Frontal lobe
Parietal lobe
Parieto-occipital fissure
Occipital lobe
Optic chiasma
Hypophysis
Pons
Pineal body
Cerebellum
Colliculi
Aqueduct of sylvius
Fourth ventricle
Medulla oblongata
Spinal cord

Figure 1-2. Median sagittal section of head and neck showing brain and upper cervical spinal cord in situ.

SOURCE: Adapted from O. Larsell, *Anatomy of the nervous system.* (2nd ed.) New York: Appleton-Century-Crofts, 1951. Used by permission.

(cross the midline) in the medulla. Other ascending bundles that project information concerned with position of body parts and muscle tonus will make synaptic connections in the cerebellum. Yet another large sensory bundle, the medial lemniscus, arising from cells at the caudal dorsal aspect of the medulla, is said to be concerned with discriminative processes of sensation. The medulla contains other highly specialized nuclei, the dorsal and ventral cochlear nuclei, which play a prominent role in primary levels of auditory discrimination. In addition to the great tracts entering and leaving the medulla, fibers emerge from auditory nuclei of the inferior olive, the medial lemniscus (somesthetic), lateral lemniscus, and the lateral reticulate nuclei to contribute to the reticular system at this level (Figure 1-7).

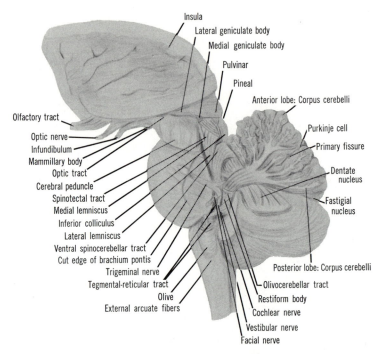

Insula
Lateral geniculate body
Medial geniculate body
Pulvinar
Pineal
Anterior lobe: Corpus cerebelli
Olfactory tract
Purkinje cell
Optic nerve
Primary fissure
Infundibulum
Mammillary body
Optic tract
Dentate nucleus
Cerebral peduncle
Spinotectal tract
Medial lemniscus
Fastigial nucleus
Inferior colliculus
Lateral lemniscus
Ventral spinocerebellar tract
Cut edge of brachium pontis
Posterior lobe: Corpus cerebelli
Trigeminal nerve
Tegmental-reticular tract
Olivocerebellar tract
Olive
Restiform body
External arcuate fibers
Cochlear nerve
Vestibular nerve
Facial nerve

Figure 1-3. Lateral view of internal structure of brainstem.

SOURCE: From *The neuroanatomic basis for clinical neurology*, by T. L. Peele. Copyright, 1961. Used by permission of McGraw-Hill Book Company.

Pons. A recent phyletic development, the pons (Figures 1-3 and 1-8), is truly a bridge uniting cerebral and cerebellar hemispheres. It is interposed between the medulla and the cerebral peduncles (midbrain) and lies ventral to the cerebellum. Externally it is identifiable by the middle cerebellar peduncle (*brachium pontis*) in its basilar portion and by the great roots of the trigeminal nerve. On the ventral surface of the pons are many scattered nuclear groups and great pyramidal tract systems from the basis pedunculi (midbrain). The nuclei undoubtedly unite both afferent and efferent tracts of the pyramidal trunk with the cerebellum via the *brachium pontis*. Tracts from reticular nuclear masses in the dorsal portion of the pons undoubtedly make functional connections with nuclei of origin for cranial nerves V, VI, VII, and part of VIII, situated in the pons-medulla sector (Figure 1-9). Reticular nuclei also send fibers to the cerebellum via the *brachium pontis.* The pons, like the medulla, makes substantial contribution to such basic language processes as respiration, auditory and tactile-kinesthetic discrimination, and to the sensory-motor synergies concerned with speech.

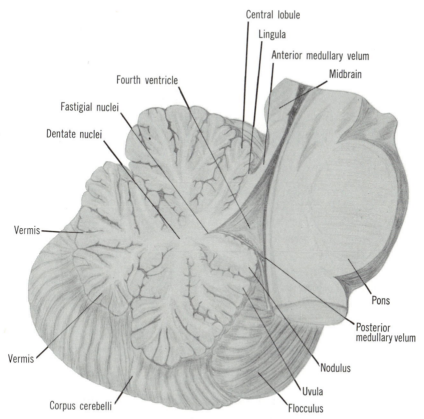

Figure 1-4. Median view of brain through cerebellum and pons.

SOURCE: Adapted from O. Larsell, *Anatomy of the nervous system.* (2nd ed.) New York: Appleton-Century-Crofts, 1951. Used by permission.

Midbrain. The midbrain, or mesencephalon, connects the pons and cerebellum with the cerebrum. Its well-defined, external landmarks are the superior and inferior colliculi in the dorsal section and the great cerebral peduncles in the ventrolateral portion. The ventral section of the cerebral peduncles marks the formation of the pyramidal tracts. Among the nuclear masses embedded in the reticular formation of the peduncles are the cells of origin of cranial nerves III (oculomotor) and IV (trochlear). The variety of activities to which the midbrain contributes is more readily apparent when one views it in transection (Figure 1-10). Auditory fibers from the lateral lemniscus make connection with nuclei of the inferior colliculus; optic fibers go to the superior colliculus. Other fibers from afferent-efferent trunk lines of the brain stem and cerebellum send fibers to reticular nuclei of the midbrain and thence to the geniculate bodies and the thalamus proper. The largest of these

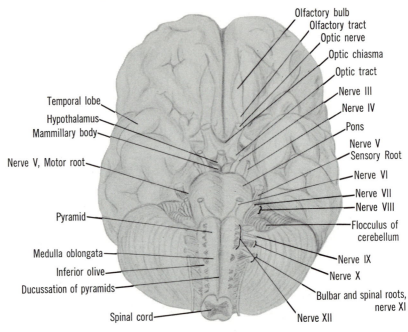

Olfactory bulb
Olfactory tract
Optic nerve
Optic chiasma
Optic tract
Nerve III
Nerve IV
Pons
Nerve V
Sensory Root
Nerve VI
Nerve VII
Nerve VIII
Flocculus of cerebellum
Nerve IX
Nerve X
Bulbar and spinal roots, nerve XI
Nerve XII

Temporal lobe
Hypothalamus
Mammillary body
Nerve V, Motor root
Pyramid
Medulla oblongata
Inferior olive
Ducussation of pyramids
Spinal cord

Figure 1-5. Base of brain.

SOURCE: From *The neuroanatomic basis for clinical neurology*, by T. L. Peele. Copyright, 1961. Used by permission of McGraw-Hill Book Company.

reticular masses, the red nuclei (nuclei Ruber), seem to be important agents in reticular organization. They send fibers not only into the spinal cord but also into the thalamus and parietal and temporal cortices; into the tegmental reticular nuclei of the midbrain, pons, and medulla; and into the cerebellum. The *substantia nigra,* embedded in the dorsal surface of the cerebral peduncles, is a thick layer of pigmented cells. It is also a part of the reticular system, having direct connections by its fiber tracts with the reticular nuclei in the tegmentum of the midbrain, nuclei of the thalamus, and basal nuclei (striate bodies) in the subcortex.

Thalamus

Above the midbrain and overlapping it in some areas are great clusters of nuclear masses and fibers known as the diencephalon or thalamus. It is usually divided into five regions: dorsal thalamus, hypothalamus, subthalamus, metathalamus, and epithalamus.

The external landmarks of the thalamus are distinguishable in the hypothalamus by the mammillary bodies, pituitary stock (infundibulum), and the optic chiasma (Figure 1-11), and in the epithalamus by the pineal body and posterior commissure.

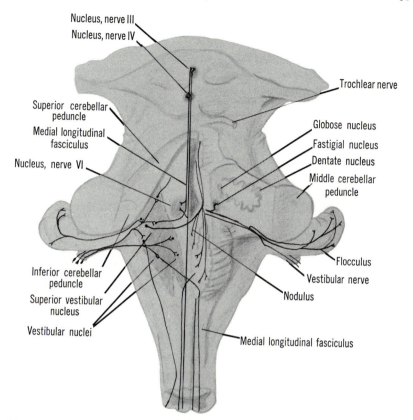

Nucleus, nerve III
Nucleus, nerve IV
Trochlear nerve
Superior cerebellar peduncle
Medial longitudinal fasciculus
Nucleus, nerve VI
Globose nucleus
Fastigial nucleus
Dentate nucleus
Middle cerebellar peduncle
Inferior cerebellar peduncle
Superior vestibular nucleus
Vestibular nuclei
Flocculus
Vestibular nerve
Nodulus
Medial longitudinal fasciculus

Figure 1-6. Basal portion of brain: medulla, cerebellum, and cerebellar peduncles.

SOURCE: Adapted from O. Larsell, *Anatomy of the nervous system.* (2nd ed.) New York: Appleton-Century-Crofts, 1951. Used by permission.

The thalamus proper, i.e., the dorsal thalamus, is formed of two large wing-like masses whose medial surfaces form the walls of the third ventricle (Figure 1-12). The nuclear composition of the thalamus proper is so complex that it is commonly divided into anterior, medial, lateral, and posterior nuclei. In a more useful classification based on function, they are grouped into I, nuclei with projections to localized cortical areas; II, nuclei belonging to the reticular system and possessing manifold connections with the cortex, subcortex, and brain stem; and III, interrelated nuclei without endbrain connections.[9]

Group I nuclei have demonstrated connections with somatic, visual, and auditory integrations of the cortex, brain stem, and cerebellum.

[9] T. L. Peele, *The neuroanatomic basis for clinical neurology.* New York: McGraw-Hill, 1961. Pp. 304–310.

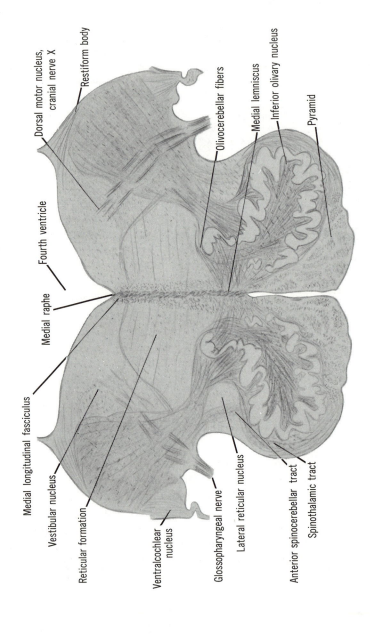

Figure 1-7. Transverse section of medulla at level of inferior olivary nucleus.

SOURCE:: Adapted from O. Larsell, *Anatomy of the nervous system.* (2nd ed.) New York: Appleton-Century-Crofts, 1951. Used by permission.

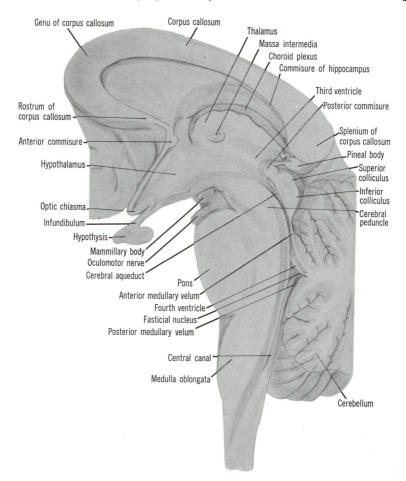

Figure 1-8. Median section through brainstem and cerebellum.

SOURCE: Adapted from O. Larsell, *Anatomy of the nervous system.* (2nd ed.) New York: Appleton-Century-Crofts, 1951. Used by permission.

Nuclei in the reticular complex, Group II, are instrumental in furthering the organization and integration (coding) of information, including that from the striatum and limbic system. Direct connections with motor and discriminative areas of the frontal cortex have been traced. Apparently this nuclear complex also affects the elaboration of information arriving in the cortex by direct, classical sensory routes. In other words, it plays a very definite role in perceptual processes. Finally it is believed that Group II nuclei are directly responsible for the replacement of the alpha rhythm of the cortex by the current rhythmic patterns of the thalamus. It should be remembered that tracts associated with nuclear

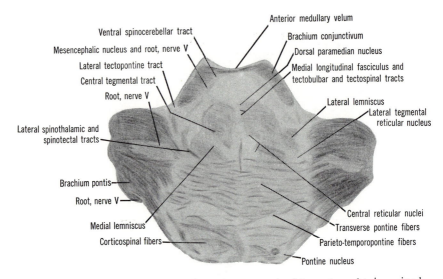

Figure 1-9. Transverse section of pons rostral to entry of trigeminal routes (cranial nerve V).

SOURCE: From *The neuroanatomic basis for clinical neurology*, by T. L. Peele. Copyright, 1961. Used by permission of McGraw-Hill Book Company.

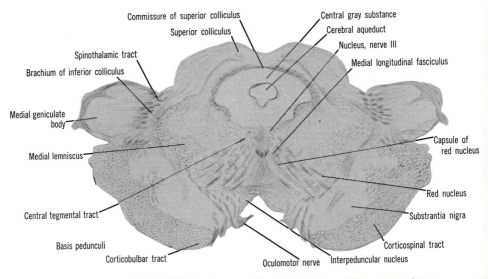

Figure 1-10. Transverse section through midbrain and hypothalamus.

SOURCE: Adapted from O. Larsell, *Anatomy of the nervous system.* (2nd ed.) New York: Appleton-Century-Crofts, 1951. Used by permission.

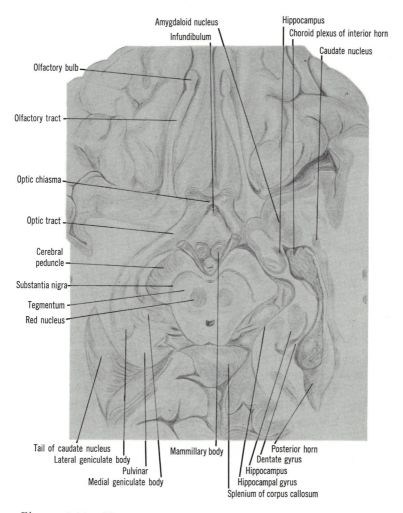

Figure 1-11. Transverse section (asymmetrical cut) showing thalamus on left and cerebral hemisphere on right.

SOURCE: Adapted from *Morris' Human Anatomy*, 11th ed. Edited by J. P. Schaeffer. Copyright, 1953. Used by permission of McGraw-Hill Book Company.

groups I and II are actually bidirectional, going to and coming from the cortex and brain stem, and hence are intimately concerned with the final stages of input-output information. Group III nuclei, as has been suggested, act to coordinate interthalamic activity. Many nuclei in this group are not modality specific. It would seem that the dorsal thalamus might be either a coeval or secondary cortical field. There are several investigators who consider it the primary field.

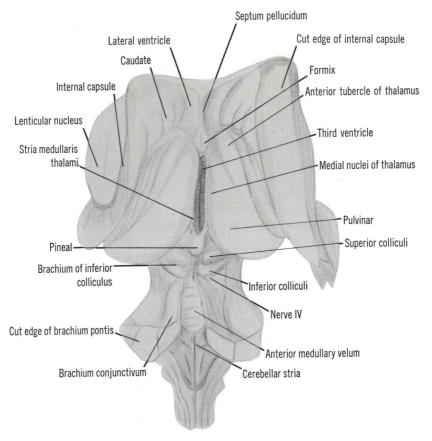

Figure 1-12.   Dorsal view of brainstem.

SOURCE: From *The neuroanatomic basis for clinical neurology*, by T. L. Peele. Copyright, 1961. Used by permission of McGraw-Hill Book Company.

The medial and lateral geniculate bodies making up the metathalamus are of special importance because they are concerned with discrimination of auditory and visual information, respectively. Other tracts in the thalamus proper and the subthalamus make connections with the hypothalamus and the epithalamus, thus presumably connecting the thalamus proper with some anatomical components of the limbic system. The limbic system, it is believed, provides the emotional and motivational matrices of behavior.

Cerebral Hemispheres

The cerebral hemispheres are incompletely separated from each other by the longitudinal cerebral fissure (Figure 1-13). In the middle

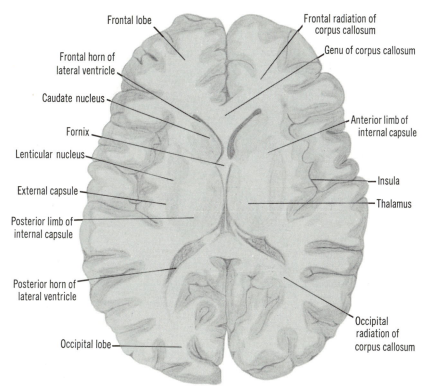

Frontal lobe

Frontal radiation of
corpus callosum

Genu of corpus callosum

Frontal horn of
lateral ventricle

Caudate nucleus

Anterior limb of
internal capsule

Fornix

Lenticular nucleus

External capsule

Insula

Thalamus

Posterior limb of
internal capsule

Posterior horn of
lateral ventricle

Occipital
radiation of
corpus callosum

Occipital lobe

Figure 1-13. Horizontal section of brain through corpus callosum.

SOURCE: From *The neuroanatomic basis for clinical neurology*, by T. L. Peele. Copyright, 1961. Used by permission of McGraw-Hill Book Company.

region of the hemispheres, a large band of nerve fibers, the *corpus callosum,* crosses in the midplane (Figure 1-14). Although there are two other small commissures, anterior and hippocampal, the great bridge between the cerebral hemispheres is the corpus callosum.

The surface of the hemispheres is thrown into folds, *gyri* or *convolutions,* and between these folds are *fissures* or *sulci* (Figure 1-15). The principal fissures are two: the *lateral fissure* or *fissure of Sylvius* that begins on the basal surface, and the *central fissure* or *fissure of Rolando* that starts on the upper medial surface of the hemisphere and runs downward and forward on the lateral surface. (See Figure 1-15 for the location of principal gyri.)

Basal Nuclei. Embedded in the base of each cerebral hemisphere are several masses of gray substance surrounded by the white substance of the hemisphere. They are called the caudate, lenticular, and amygdaloid nuclei (Figure 1-14). The caudate and lenticular nuclei are separated by the internal capsule; the amygdaloid is located in the rostral

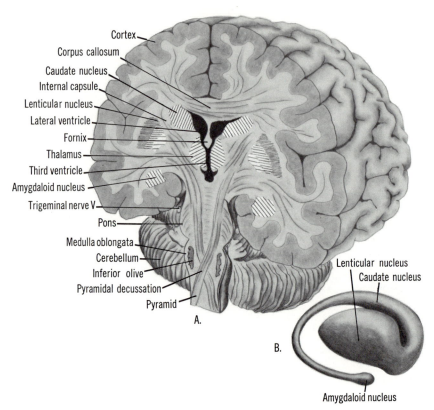

Cortex
Corpus callosum
Caudate nucleus
Internal capsule
Lenticular nucleus
Lateral ventricle
Fornix
Thalamus
Third ventricle
Amygdaloid nucleus
Trigeminal nerve V
Pons
Medulla oblongata
Cerebellum
Inferior olive
Pyramidal decussation
Pyramid
A.

Lenticular nucleus
Caudate nucleus
B.
Amygdaloid nucleus

Figure 1-14. Diagrammatic sketch of horizontal section of brain showing striate bodies (basal nuclei).

SOURCE: M. F. Berry and J. Eisenson, *Speech disorders.* New York: Appleton-Century-Crofts, 1956. P. 51.

tip of the temporal lobe and may bear little functional relation to the other two basal nuclei. The amygdaloid may well be a part of the limbic system. Since the lenticular nucleus no longer is considered an integer in terms of either histological structure or function, it becomes two separate nuclear masses: putamen and globus pallidus (or pallidum). The caudate and putamen have rich fiber connections with the frontal, temporal, and parietal cortices. All three nuclear masses—caudate, putamen, and pallidum—also project to and receive fibers from other sectors of the reticular system. These multiple connections have led to the inclusion of the nuclei in the reticular system, either as belonging to it absolutely or as being closely associated with it.[10] Although these nuclei have been associated primarily with fine motor synergies, current research

[10] *Ibid.,* pp. 401–407.

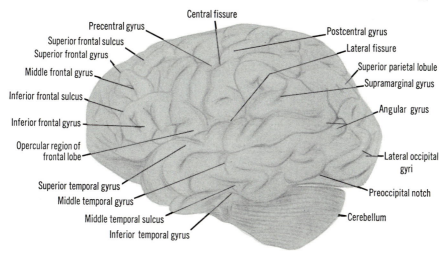

Figure 1-15. Lateral view of cerebral hemisphere and cerebellum.

SOURCE: From *The neuroanatomic basis for clinical neurology*, by T. L. Peele. Copyright, 1961. Used by permission of McGraw-Hill Book Company.

is being focused also on their joint influence with the cortex on other aspects of linguistic coding. They must be vitally concerned with the final stages of coding. Myriads of bidirectional pathways connect the cortex and the brain stem with the basal nuclei.

Cerebral Cortex. Immediately beneath the surface of gyri in the cerebral hemispheres are layers of neurones composing the *cerebral cortex*. These cells may number fourteen to sixteen billion. The cerebral white matter beneath the cell layers is a reticule of fibers, some of which connect various gyri; others are from the brain stem or from the cortical cell layers projecting into the brain stem. The majority of tracts to and from the cortex will go through the internal capsule.

Traditionally the cerebral cortex has been divided into frontal, parietal, occipital, and temporal regions corresponding to the cerebral lobes. More recently a fifth division, the limbic cortex, has been described; it includes parts of the frontal, parietal, and temporal lobes. It is a C-curved structure extending completely around the thalamus and includes the cingulate and hippocampal gyri, hypothalamic nuclei, and the amygdaloid, one of the basal nuclei.

Changing Concepts of Neural Structures and Functions

"Time makes ancient good uncouth" is a truism that can be applied to much neurological theory even up to the first quarter of this century.

Behavioral studies combined with electronic means of research have modified some venerable concepts of neural structure and function. These new ideas, evoked by current studies, undoubtedly will undergo change, but for the present they mark an advance in the synthesis of theory and observation of behavior. Certainly they provide a sounder foundation upon which to construct a language model.

Stimulation-Integration-Response (S-I-R Arc). Sherrington was the first to point out that the S-I-R, or the reflex arc, is a convenient abstraction, but like all abstractions, it often fails to check with the facts. The S-I-R arc, said Sherringon, is not truly the "unit of function" of the central nervous system; rather it is the entire system and not a diagram of two or three neurones with synapses which makes up the functional unit of the CNS. It is true that this arc may operate mechanically in spinal reflexes. In the brain stem and cortex, however, there is no proof of a functional one-to-one, automatic relation between stimulus and response. The nervous system cannot be operated as a vending machine. The sensation may go in but the desired response may not come out. Sensory input and motor output cannot be equated so neatly, perhaps because of the enigmatic I, Integration, about which little is known. The intrinsic (or integrative) systems, Pribram concludes, cannot be considered as "association centers upon which pathways from the extrinsic sensory sectors converge to bring together neural events anticipatory to spewing them out via the motor pathways." [11] There is, moreover, little proof of a topographical point-to-point relationship between the incoming battery of sensations and the response. Incoming sensation A may follow an entirely different route and reach quite a different terminus from sensation B, although both belong to the same modality. Integration is a continuous process beginning in the receptors and ending only as the response is made. It comprehends the total nervous system.

Livingston and colleagues have summed up some aspects of the integrative mechanism in their description of the "internuncial pool":

There is, interposed between the sensory and motor components of the simple reflex arc, a pool of neurons in which both spatial and temporal dispersion of the input can take place. It can be shown that the motor output resulting from a given stimulus applied to a posterior root is not only conditioned by preexistent activity in the internuncial pool, but is subject to modification from moment to moment by influences from the striatum and the brainstem reticular formation. They create a background activity in the internuncial pool which determines how the muscles can respond to stimulation of points on the sensory-motor cortex and in either reflex or voluntary movement. The study of the functions of the internuncial pool had two immediate effects on neuro-

[11] K. Pribram, Neocortical function in behavior. In H. F. Harlow and C. N. Woolsey, Eds., *Biological and biochemical bases of behavior.* Madison: The University of Wisconsin Press, 1958. P. 158.

logic interpretation: (1) it emphasized the factor of time as well as space in the patterning of neural activity; and (2) it suggested one way in which unity of action within the total organism might be achieved.[12]

These authors have suggested an essential operant in coding information, e.g., constant feedback and homeostatic control over input and output. The S-I-R arc, as a functional unit of neural activity, has been supplanted by the concept of a continuous monitor, feedback (p. 91).

Afferent and Efferent Systems. Traditionally, all great tracts were represented as being exclusively afferent (sensory) and carrying impulses toward the cerebral cortex, or as efferent (motor) and mediating impulses from the cerebral cortex toward the periphery. The third category, association fibers, remained ill-defined. In the last three decades neuroanatomists who have traced great trunk lines in the nervous system found that "afferent" tracts were not composed solely of sensory fibers and corresponding motor tracts were not exclusively effector or "efferent" pathways. As early as 1939 Adrian and Moruzzi found impulses traveling in the pyramidal tract which did not produce motor responses.[13] More recent work of Brodal and others demonstrates that sensory fibers, both tactile and proprioceptive, are found in the pyramidal tracts. Brodal has traced proprioceptive fibers from the tongue to the pons and finally to the cerebellum. He finds that they do not follow the usual course of the medial lemniscus to the upper brain stem, but course with motor fibers in the pyramidal pathway. "These fibers take origin from all levels of the cord and ascend among the *descending* fibers in the lateral and ventral corticospinal tracts, the pyramids, pons, and *capsula interna* and finally reach the cerebral cortex." [14]

Brodal's studies have been confirmed by others who find that even small efferent fibers in the ventral "motor" routes of mammals, when selectively stimulated, do not set up contractions but produce an *afferent* firing from muscle sense organs.[15] This important muscle sense organ, the muscle spindle, can be controlled either by activating or depressing the small motor horn cells or by stimulating the facilitatory or inhibitory mechanisms of the brain stem.[16] This control has been attributed to

[12] W. K. Livingston, F. P. Haugen, and J. M. Brookhart, Functional organization of the central nervous system. *Neurology* (Minneap), July 1954, 4: 491–492.

[13] E. D. Adrian and G. Moruzzi, Impulses in the pyramidal tract. *J Physiol* (London) (December 1939), 97: 153–99.

[14] A. Brodal and B. R. Kaada, Cutaneous and proprioceptive impulses in the pyramidal tract in cats. *Acta Physiol Scand* (August 1953), 29: 131. A. Brodal and F. Walberg, Ascending fibers in the pyramidal tract of the cat. *Arch Neurol* (Chicago) (December 1952), 68: 755–775.

[15] R. Granit, *Receptors and sensory perception.* New Haven: Yale, 1962. P. 191. R. Brain, *Recent advances in neurology and psychiatry.* Boston: Little, Brown, 1962. P. 12.

[16] R. Granit and B. R. Kaada, Influence of stimulation of central nervous structures on muscle spindles in the cat. *Acta Physiol Scand* (January 1952), 27: 130.

the Gamma fibers of the muscle spindle. Afferent fibers apparently may be found in all major tracts traditionally called "motor" or efferent.

Similarly in those tracts called *special sensory,* to the eye and the ear, efferent fibers have been traced. Galambos and others have demonstrated the presence of efferent tracts in the cochlear nerve, fibers which may be stimulated to action before they leave the inner ear or at several points in the brain stem, notably in the reticular system.[17] In the retinal relays of the eye, the same efferent innervation apparently exists. By stimulation of the tegmentum of the midbrain (a part of the reticular system), retinal relays may be enhanced or inhibited.

It is fairly clear that all these tracts facilitating or inhibiting responses are part of a feedback system that organizes and controls behavior. The neural response to oral symbols (language) may occur in the same millisecond of time as the aural sensation. Proprioceptive feedback coexists with the movement of the articulators in oral expression. In a succeeding section we shall discuss in greater detail the behavioral implications of this monitoring and adaptive mechanism, feedback, in the central nervous system. Suffice it to say now that we cannot describe sensory and motor tracts as separate entities. They run together and they act together. Ascending fibers, after a very short run in the pyramidal trunk, may synapse directly in reticular pools controlling motor units, and descending systems may project directly to reticular pools of "pure sensory" nuclei. Motor function without concomitant sensory phenomena is fiction.

Pyramidal and Extrapyramidal Areas. In the race to subdivide the CNS into increasingly small and particular parcels, the neuroanatomists in this century demarcated the section anterior to the traditional primary motor field as the extrapyramidal area and ascribed to it special functions. Electronic investigation in the last decade, however, has failed to separate pyramidal from extrapyramidal sectors. From a series of studies Brodal concludes that neither the origins nor the functions of pyramidal and extrapyramidal pathways can be differentiated.[18] Brodal points out that substantial contributions are made to the "primary motor" system by nuclei in the so-called extrapyramidal area (Brodmann's area 6), and by areas in the parietal and temporal lobes. Pribram goes so far as to include in the origin of the pyramidal tract the entire precentral cortex and much of the postcentral cortex.[19] Whereas it was

R. B. Livingston, Central control of afferent activity, Chapter 7. In H. H. Jasper, *et al.,* eds., *Reticular formation of the brain.* Boston: Little, Brown, 1958. P. 178.

[17] R. Galambos, Suppression of auditory nerve activity by stimulation of efferent fibers to the cochlea. *J Neurophysiol* (September 1956), 19: 424–437.

[18] A. Brodal, Some data and perspectives on the anatomy of the so-called "extrapyramidal system." *Acta Neurol Scand* (Copenhagen) (1963), Supplementum 4, 39: 2–60.

[19] K. Pribram, Neocortical function in behavior. In H. F. Harlow and C. N. Woolsey, Eds., *Biological and biochemical bases of behavior.* Madison: The University of Wisconsin Press, 1958. P. 157.

once thought that "primary motor" tracts (corticobulbar and cortico-spinal) originated only in the Betz cells of the primary motor area (Brod-mann's cortical area 4), now only 2–3 percent of the one million fibers comprising these tracts can be traced to this area. Pribram concludes, "The distinction between motor and pre-motor cortex fades . . . and makes unnecessary the classical distinction between the locus of origin of the pyramidal and extra-pyramidal systems which has already been called into question by anatomical data." [20]

If we accept these neurological data, we shall have to revise our concept of motor syndromes in cerebral palsy. Athetosis no longer can be assigned to lesions of extrapyramidal areas, spasticity to pyramidal areas.[21] Shifts from year to year in the description of motor syndromes of children enrolled for long-term pediatric care cast further doubt on the validity of pyramidal and extrapyramidal divisions. Many of these children originally diagnosed as spastic are described later as athetoid or tension-athetoid. The neat behavioral distinctions of motor systems to which we have held no longer seem to be valid.

Cortical Localization of Higher Functions. Students may be puzzled by the absence of the classical cytoarchitectural map of the cortex. Such a map no longer seems to accord with behavioral responses to experi-mental stimulation, ablation, or impairment restricted to discrete neural areas. Penfield and Rasmussen, among others, demonstrated that strict topographical mapping of the cerebral cortex no longer is valid.[22] Motor fields, previously limited to the frontal lobe, apparently can be demonstrated in the temporal and parietal areas.[23] The extrapyramidal zone seems to be only an extension of the classical pyramidal area 4.[24] Broca's area, traditionally located in the left hemisphere, undoubtedly is *one* field where many organizing tracts for final coding of "motor speech" are clustered. It is not the only field. As Lenneberg says, "there seems to be no more than a statistical relationship between Broca's area and the resultant deficit of aphasia. . . . There is no clear-cut evidence that Broca's area is more specifically related to speech than areas adjacent to it." [25] The margins of auditory fields have become equally indefinite. Auditory discrimination at the cortical level no longer can be restricted

[20] *Ibid.*
[21] T. L. Peele, *The neuroanatomic basis for clinical neurology.* New York: McGraw-Hill, 1961. Pp. 295–430. H. M. Kaplan, *Anatomy and physiology of speech.* New York: McGraw-Hill, 1960. P. 44. N. M. Levin, *Voice and speech disorders: Medical aspects.* Springfield, Ill.: Charles C Thomas, 1962. Pp. 672–673. Russell Brain, *Speech disorders.* London: Butterworth, 1961. P. 108.
[22] W. Penfield and T. Rasmussen, *The cerebral cortex of man: A clinical study of localization of function.* New York: Macmillan, 1950.
[23] W. Penfield and L. Roberts, *Speech and brain mechanisms.* Princeton, N. J.: Princeton, 1959.
[24] Brodal, *op. cit.*
[25] E. H. Lenneberg, *Biological foundations of language.* New York: Wiley, 1967. Pp. 59–61.

to Wernicke's area in the temporal lobe, for adjoining zones in the temporal and parietal lobes have demonstrated potentials in the acoustic analysis of speech. Memory circuits may emanate, in part, from the temporal cortex or from the limbic system. Sperry goes so far as to claim that activation of the same cortical areas may produce "sensations as diverse as those of red, black, green, and white, or of touch, cold, warmth, movement, pain, posture and pressure. . . ." [26] One may produce a response from the traditional "primary areas" but the same response has been produced by stimulation of other areas, not only in the cortex but also in the subcortex.

No "language repositories" can be found in the cortex. No engrams for words or syntactic rules have been tapped in cortical cell assemblies. Cortical areas traditionally assigned to language function possess no common cytoarchitectural features. Sensory aspects of language cannot be separated from motor gesture projection systems and neither sensory nor motor components of the cortex act independently of subcortical and brain-stem nuclear assemblies. In the comprehension of oral language, for example, interdependent structures and interlocking directorates of neuronal networks are involved. An injury to one set of analyzers or coders perforce must adversely affect other analyzers in the circuit. Analyzers are located all along the line to the periphery. A cortical lesion among auditory nuclear aggregations, for example, could affect the analyzer in the cochlea or in the cochlear nuclei of the medulla; they, in turn, would involve other analyzers intimately associated in the language function. Similarly a disturbance of a cortical wave front in the left parietal and in rostral aspects of the temporal lobes could disturb all other sectors of the auditory-analyzer system.[27] The result is that one cannot determine the effect of a specific lesion on a specific area because the effect may be one of hypersynchrony in distant neuronal assemblies. When hypersynchrony is not great, it would allow some assemblies to function, particularly those that are long established, but would tend to interfere with recent memory, decrease responsiveness, and interfere with complex intellectual activities.[28] Tactile-kinesthetic analyzers must be associated with visual parietal and motor cortical fields, although the exact role of the frontal cortex in motor patterns of speech is not clearly defined.

Clinical research also has demonstrated the control of sensory-motor cortical fields for speech by subcortical systems. Dysarthria, for example, is not prominent in cortical lesions but is notable and dramatic in diencephalic (thalamic), mesencephalic (midbrain), and pontine

[26] R. W. Sperry, Neurology and the mind-brain problem. In R. L. Isaacson, Ed., *Basic Readings in Neuropsychology.* New York: Harper & Row, 1964. P. 406.
[27] A. R. Luria, *Restoration of function after brain injury.* New York: Macmillan, 1963, pp. 49–54. A. R. Luria, Traumatic aphasia, *Izv Akad Med Nauk USSR*, 1947.
[28] D. O. Hebb, *The organization of behavior.* New York: Wiley, 1949. P. 283.

lesions, surgical interference, and stimulation.[29] Specifically, these sub-cortical systems must include nuclear organizations of the reticular net-work, including those in the basal nuclei (corpus striatum), thalamus (geniculate bodies, thalamus proper), midbrain, and pons. Purpura says in this connection, "Recent studies from several laboratories have now shown that stimulation of these ventrolateral nuclear groups of the thalamus as well as some related basal nuclei structures may severely disturb the ordering and motivational factors of speech." [30] If the frontal and parietal fields of the cortex play a part in motor gesture patterns of speech, it must be in the activation of this common projection system arising in the ponto-mesencephalic-thalamic-strial reticular system. The cortical "localization" fields of motor speech, specifically Broca's area, precentral gyrus, postcentral gyrus, and adjacent gyri in the frontal and parietal lobes of the major hemisphere are parts of a single system sub-serving sensory-motor circuits mediating oral expression.[31]

Localization of processes of attention, long-term memory and emo-tional motivation involved in language learning, likewise, cannot be pinpointed in the cortex. Temporal-parietal and hippocampal-fornix areas have been connected with these functions. If they are associated more closely with these mechanisms than other parts of the cortex, they can act only as convergent fields *in conjunction with* the entire nervous system.

So for the classical doctrine of static, invariable, specific localization we would substitute the concept of dynamic cortical fields, sensitive to classes of information, controlling and controlled by feedback processes of peripheral and brainstem analyzers. Thus the cortex takes part in a continuous coding process in which it is potentially bound with all sub-cortical and brain-stem neuronal assemblies mediating language.[32]

Characteristics of Neural Function

The Nerve Impulse

Action Potential. It is more than 175 years since Galvani of Bologna demonstrated that the muscles of a frog could produce an

[29] E. H. Lenneberg, Discussion of paper: Language following surgical discon-nection of the hemispheres, by R. W. Sperry and M. S. Gazzaniga. In F. L. Darley, Ed., *Brain Mechanisms Underlying Speech and Language.* New York: Grune & Stratton, 1967. P. 121.

[30] D. P. Purpura, Discussion of paper: The output side of information processing, by E. V. Evarts. In F. L. Darley, Ed., *Brain Mechanisms Underlying Speech and Language.* New York: Grune & Stratton, 1967. P. 49.

[31] R. E. Myers, Cerebral connectionism and brain function. In F. L. Darley, Ed., *Brain mechanisms underlying speech and language.* New York: Grune & Stratton, 1967. Pp. 61–72.

[32] W. R. Ashby, *Design for a brain.* New York: Norton, 1952. D. B. Lindsley, Higher functions of the central nervous system. *Ann Rev Physiol.* (July 1955), 17: 311–338.

electric current. From Galvani's historical, accidental experiment came two fundamental conclusions of use to us in considering the neurophysiology of language, (1) that a current of stimulation will produce activity in nerve and muscle, and (2) that both tissues during activity develop their own current or action potential. The initiation of activity probably does not begin in the soma of the nerve cell, as Du Bois-Reymond first surmised, but in a small section of the emerging axon. It enjoys a lower threshold of excitability than the cell body, and this is true both of myelinated and unmyelinated fibers. As a result, the initial segment of the axon will fire more quickly and easily than the cell body. But when the segment has fired, its depolarization works backward over the same membrane to produce a wave of hyperpolarization, thus inducing inhibition.

The resultant wave of negativity that sweeps down the nerve fiber depends for its conduction upon the inherent electrical properties of the fiber, not upon the intensity of the stimulus. The action potential, the electrical sign of excitation, in other words, is induced from a series of ionic changes which derive their energy from the metabolism of the fiber itself. The fiber, then, is no passive conductor but an important determinant of the strength of the action current.

Speed and Composition. Speed of conduction depends upon the state and size of the fiber. In the large motor fibers in the adult, for example, the impulse may fire at the rate of 100 meters per second. Here again the strength of the stimulus does not seem to be a factor. The activity at any point on a nerve is very short lived, lasting no more than a few thousandths of a second. Trains of diphasic waves of activity follow, one upon another, and thus the impulse is swept along to its first synaptic junction. The frequency or temporal pattern of the impulse presumably is determined by the number of fibers responding to the stimulus. A single fiber in the auditory nerve, it has been found, does not respond at rates as high as 6,000 or even 1,000 per second for long periods. The high frequency of a *composite wave* most probably is the result of the response of many fibers, "each responding at a submultiple of the stimulus frequency and arranged so that each wave of the stimulus finds some fibers ready to respond to it." [33]

The *kind of sensation* resulting from the stimulus probably cannot be ascertained by the form or composition of the wave pattern. We cannot differentiate, for example, among auditory, proprioceptive, tactile, or optic impulses upon the basis of appearance. "Nerve impulses are essentially homogeneous in quality and are transmitted as 'common currency' throughout the nervous system." [34] We do not perceive sensations, in

---

[33] E. D. Adrian, *The mechanism of nervous action.* Philadelphia: University of Pennsylvania Press, 1959. P. 39.

[34] R. W. Sperry, Neurology and the mind-brain problem. In R. L. Isaacson, Ed., *Basic readings in neuropsychology.* New York: Harper & Row, 1964. P. 405.

other words, by the kind or quality of the impulses but by variance in timing and distribution of nervous excitation. Thus impulses that are similar in temporal-spatial patterning and in synaptic potential will be linked with their counterparts in other neural assemblies.

The All-or-None Principle. Formerly it was held that neurones responded to the maximum of their capacity or not at all. The neural impulse was a yes-no proposition. We now know that only one section of the neurone, the axone, follows this rule. The all-or-none principle applies, however, only to the discharge into the axon, not to the activity of other parts of the neurone. It does not apply to the receptor and effector endings, to the dendrites, or to the cell body itself. Neither does it apply to the neural events taking place at synaptic junctions or in peripheral or central analyzers of the nervous system.[35] The new concept, in short, suggests that grading and modification of neuronal activity takes place in all sectors of the nervous system. Output cannot be matched against input because the character of the activity may vary from second to second.

Coding of verbal symbols may be affected by a multiplicity of factors. Coding can be influenced by shifting response potentials in dendritic transmission, in synaptic junctions, in any or all neural analyzers mediating comprehension and expression of oral language. The shifts may be genetically determined or they may be dependent upon nutritional states, i.e., upon the amount and availability of ribonucleic acid and other metabolic constituents provided by the glia. On this point, neuroscientists have postulated a nucleic acid base for encoding and read-out in the nervous system. Learning and memory, in their view, depend upon a specified and replicated neuronal RNA which provides the template for elaboration of enzyme-like, neuronal transmitter substances, responsible for consequent patterns of neural firing, and serving interneuronal transmission of excitation and expressive behavior. Magoun goes so far as to hypothesize that

rehabilitative therapy might be considered a kind of applied combination of sensory neurophysiology and neurochemistry which seeks, by manipulating input signals, to specify the nucleic-acid and protein metabolism of residual cortical neural aggregates in a way to improve or restore functions that are impaired or missing following disease.[36]

Sometimes shifts in neural potentials may be caused by purely temporal factors, the result of emotional or motivational states. In children with neurological disturbances, a complex of sensory informa-

[35] M. A. B. Brazier, The biologist and the communication sciences. In R. W. Gerard and J. W. Duyff, Eds., *Information processing in the nervous system.* Internat'l. congress series, no. 49. Amsterdam: Excerpta Medica Fdtn, 1964. Pp. 88–89.
[36] H. W. Magoun, Lacunae and research approaches to them. II. In F. L. Darley, Ed., *Brain mechanisms underlying speech and language.* New York: Grune & Stratton, 1967. P. 217.

tional bits presumably may enter the CNS but their transmission and synthesis may be blocked by delays of grading in the neuronal network. In this split second of time, in this hour of this day, in this required speech, and in this state of metabolic, emotional, and motivational stability, X's nervous system is not able to process the information.

Synaptic Junctions and Neural Activity

Intellectually we are as old or as young as our synapses. The problem of "retrieval" of language that plagues both the aphasic and, less frequently, the nonaphasic is directly related to the vitality and malleability of the synapse. New synaptic connections in the aging no longer are easily established nor are old ones easily maintained. The ability to learn and to recall ideas has declined with the decline in synaptic potential.

Synaptic Potential in Facilitation and Inhibition. The ability of a nerve impulse to make "functional" contact with other neurones at a synapse depends largely upon the number and chemical state of synaptic knobs—the small, bulbous endings of fine fibers which impinge on the surface of the cell. They are, in fact, the terminal branches of axones from other nerve cells. Within the knob, which is enclosed in a membrane, are numerous, small vesicular structures, containing specific chemical substances essential for synaptic transmission.[37] What these substances are remains *sub judice*. Both acetylcholine and ribonucleic acid (RNA) are supported by considerable research. The RNA advocates find that when primary motor neurones in the cortex are subjected to transsynaptic bombardment, ribonucleic acid increases in amount. Since RNA molecules pass into the cytoplasm of the cell, it provides a potential medium for memory coding just as DNA (deoxy-ribonucleic acid) forms a basis for genetic coding.[38] In learning, RNA may be one of the chemical substances that alter the ionic balance of the receptor membranes at the synapse, thus lowering the threshold and effecting the discharge of an electrical (code-carrying) signal. If it heightens the "imprint" of the information, then it must be an active force in insuring recall.

Coding is dependent upon the ability of synaptic junctions, not only to accelerate information processing, but also to inhibit information not useful to the code at the moment. Just as RNA may be the exciting agent so acetylcholine may act as the effective inhibiting agent in the process. Such inhibitory action by acetylcholine was demonstrated in a study of the electronic activity of the hair cells of the cochlea. In this study it acted to suppress both the cochlear microphonic and the

[37] J. C. Eccles, Ionic mechanism of postsynaptic inhibition, *Science* (September 11, 1964), 145: 1140.

[38] H. W. Magoun, *The Waking Brain.* Springfield, Ill.: Charles C Thomas, 1958. Pp. 148–153.

neural responses.[39] The *mode* of transmission of RNA and acetylcholine probably is similar. Acetylcholine, for example, presumably diffuses across the narrow synaptic gap and combines with the receptor sites on the pre-synaptic or postsynaptic membrane to prevent depolarization and so "hold" the threshold against excitation.[40] If the hold is maintained, the impulse does not enter into the temporal-spatial pattern. In other words, the neurone is not a part of the cell assembly network of that code. Eccles maintains that all presynaptic action is depressing or inhibitory and has its purpose the erasure of specific inputs.[41]

The organization and priority of excitatory and inhibitory potentials in coding sensory information has been explored from many angles. We do not know the priority of one sensory modality over another in preempting multimodal neurones, but if we may judge from studies of animal behavior, sensory priority in the CNS exists. Hernandez-Peon and coworkers have found that inhibitory synapses operate in the cat when auditory impulses to which the cat has previously responded are blocked by powerful visual stimuli (the presentation of a mouse in a glass box). The inhibition apparently is effected through the action of the reticular system upon the cochlear nerve before the impulse reaches the ventral and dorsal cochlear nuclei in the medulla. No electrical "response" could be detected in the subcortical auditory assemblies in the ventral and dorsal cochlear nuclei, the medial geniculate body, or in the temporal areas of the cortex.[42] Galambos also found that the impulses from the cochlear nerve could be inhibited by the stimulation of the olivocochlear efferent auditory pathway at its decussation point near the midline on the floor of the medulla. Apparently inhibition of auditory impulses may occur at any point from medulla to cortex.[43]

Whether synaptic inhibitory or facilitatory potentials win out de-termines the final character of the code. It will be determined by the algebraic sum of their potentials. Much information being transmitted in coded pattern along a line undoubtedly is lost at synaptic relays, or certain segments of the pattern may fade and others persist.[44] This

[39] T. H. Bullock, Neurophysiology: U. S. and Japan joint symposium. *Science* (June 12, 1964), 144: 1361–1364.

[40] G. C. Salmoiraghi and F. E. Floom, Pharmacology of individual neurons. *Science* (May 1, 1964), 144: 493–498.

[41] J. C. Eccles, Inhibitory controls on the flow of sensory information in the nervous system. In R. W. Gerard and J. W. Duyff, Eds., *Information processing in the nervous system.* Internat'l congress series, no. 49. Amsterdam: Excerpta Medica Foundation, 1964. Pp. 24–40.

[42] P. Hernandez-Peon, H. Scherrer, and M. Jouvet, Modification of electric activity in the cochlear nucleus during "attention" in unanesthetized cats. *Science* (February 24, 1956), 123: 331–332.

[43] R. Galambos, Suppression of auditory nerve activity by stimulation of efferent fibers to cochlea. *J Neurophysiol* (September 1956), 19: 424–437.

[44] J. C. Eccles, Discussion, in *Information processing in the nervous system.* Internat'l congress series, no. 49. Amsterdam: Excerpta Medica Foundation, 1964. Pp. 141–144.

is a normal operation of the synaptic junction. Serious problems arise when the nervous system attempts to process both essential and non-essential information. Many language-handicapped children must have low inhibitory potentials for all stimuli. They attend to auditory verbal symbols until other stimuli—visual, tactile, kinesthetic—enter the environment. Without apparent priority these nonserviceable, extraneous stimuli compete for attention. Gating at synaptic junctions in the reticular and other systems mediating feedback breaks down with a resulting welter of "noise" in the nervous system. The pattern—if there was a pattern—is erased. Perhaps one day we will find a way to establish sensory priority and heightened synaptic inhibition of "alien stimuli" in the child suffering from deficits or injury to the nervous system.

Spontaneous Neural Rhythm

Fiber Tracts. Many ganglion cells and their tracts exhibit a spontaneous rhythm, the result of constant, active metabolism.[45] A spontaneous discharge by ganglion cells, even in the absence of excitation, has been recorded and amplified both for vision and audition. Galambos, reporting on the spontaneous activity in auditory nerve fibers, concludes that the spontaneous rhythm is the background against which effects of stimulation are displayed. By a comparison of the effects against the background, the individual is able to discriminate sound.[46] Is it possible that responses also rely on a spontaneous rhythm of the nervous system, an underlying pulse on which motor speech patterns are built? Perhaps we perceive and execute articulate speech against this background of a basic neural rhythm, an innate temporal pattern. Stetson,[47] McDonald,[48] and Lenneberg [49] lend their support to this belief in a carrier pulse for motor gestures of speech.

Another purpose of spontaneous rhythms is the maintenance of an "activity quotient" in the cortex and brain stem.[50] Audition, a primal modality, has a tonic influence upon the level of spontaneous activity in the entire brain. The spontaneous pattern goes on independently of the stimulation by sound. Loss of hearing, hence, is something more

    [45] R. W. Gerard, in J. F. Delafresnaye, Ed., *Brain mechanisms and learning: A symposium.* Oxford: Blackwell, 1961. P. 650.
    [46] R. Galambos, Inhibition of activity in single auditory nerve fibers by acoustic stimulation. *J Neurophysiol* (September 1944), 7: 287–303.
    [47] R. H. Stetson, *Motor phonetics.* Amsterdam: North Holland Publishing Company, 1951.
    [48] E. T. McDonald, *Articulation testing and treatment: A sensory-motor approach.* Pittsburgh: Stanwix House, 1964.
    [49] E. H. Lenneberg, *Biological foundations of language.* New York: Wiley, 1967. Pp. 108–116.
    [50] W. A. Rosenblith, *Sensory communication,* W. A. Rosenblith, Ed. Cambridge, Mass.: M. I. T., 1961. Pp. 818–819.

than the absence of stimulation—deafness. It means the loss of the spontaneous rhythm, a most important contributor to the "activity quotient" and stability of the central nervous system. If the spontaneous rhythm in the auditory circuit is impaired, it could upset the stability of allied modalities. An illustration comes to mind. While riding with friends through a sundrenched countryside, a suggestion was made to the driver that he put on his dark glasses. "No," he protested, "I can't hear as well when I wear them." Did the driver, an audiologist, mean that muting one basic sensory modality had an adverse effect upon the readiness of other sensory modalities to respond?

Cortical and Subcortical Rhythms. Other sectors of the nervous system possess their own innate rhythms. The cortex, thalamus, and perhaps parts of the brainstem exhibit spontaneous rhythms of electrical activity that Eccles believes are the result of "closed self-reexciting chains of cortical neurones." [51]

Alpha Rhythm. This rhythm is the best known of the autonomous potentials. In the development of the cortex in the infant of 3 months, the pattern exhibits a frequency of three per second waves; at 1 year, the frequency has risen to five or six; by 12 years the wave pattern has reached adult frequency of ten to twelve per second.[52] The potential of these waves varies from zero to 100 microvolts and must be determined, in large part, by metabolic factors. Such waves are most often recorded from the parietotemporal regions but similar waves have also been recorded from the frontal regions. Alpha waves are in phase in normal physiological states, and their frequency usually is the same in the two hemispheres. The rhythm of 10–12 Hz is maintained in the waking state but apparently only in conditions of mental relaxation, low cortical activity, and inattention. During sleep the alpha waves disappear and large, slow, irregular waves appear.[53]

Beta Rhythm. Other rhythms have been ascribed to the cortex but their significance is not clear. The *Beta rhythm* is reported by Penfield to have a frequency higher than 14 Hz, with an average frequency of 25 Hz. These waves are sometimes superimposed on the alpha rhythm, and are frequently recorded in the absence of the alpha rhythm. They are predominant in the precentral areas of the cortex. Attention to certain tactile and kinesthetic stimuli and to voluntary movements interrupts or completely blocks this rhythm. Penfield, reporting on his study of the Beta rhythm by means of electrodes placed on the precentral gyrus, claims to have established the presence of the Beta rhythm in inattentive states

[51] J. C. Eccles, *The neurophysiological basis of mind.* London: Oxford, 1953. P. 253.

[52] D. B. Lindsley, Higher functions of the central nervous system. *Ann Rev Physiol* (July 1955), 17: 318.

[53] J. C. Eccles, *The neurophysiological basis of mind.* London: Oxford, 1953. Pp. 254–255.

and its interruption by movement. Movement of the fingers, for example, blocked the rhythmic activity in the hand area of the pre- and postcentral gyri. Penfield found, however, that this response could occur only in the sensory-motor area without affecting the alpha rhythm simultaneously recorded from the parietal zone, posterior to the postcentral gyrus.[54]

Delta Rhythm. A third projected cortical pattern is the *Delta rhythm,* 1–4 Hz, which is said to occur with deep sleep in infants and in organic brain disease in adults. In infancy, this rhythm is a characteristic phenomenon but when it is found in children, 10 to 12 years of age, it is thought to be indicative of mental immaturity or of personality disorders.[55]

Although cortical dysrhythmia has been an excellent diagnostic tool in epilepsy, dysrhythmia in the population of the United States certainly is not limited to epileptics. Peele estimates that at least 10 percent of the people have abnormal wave patterns. The incidence of cortical dysrhythmia is 25 times greater than the clinical incidence of epilepsy.[56]

Alteration of the Alpha Rhythm. The basic resting alpha pattern of 10–12 Hz may be interrupted by states of tension, fear, or by active attention, the result of internal stimuli or of external stimuli initiating sensory impulses. The reticular system presumably acts as the major interruptive agent although thalamocortical and limbic circuits may assist.[57] The way in which this alerting mechanism works is (1) to desynchronize the wave pattern in specific cortical fields destined, let us say, to analyze sensory information, and (2) to inhibit adjoining areas by decreasing their potential.[58] In a sense the arrest of the alpha rhythm may be regarded as an inhibitory process involving several areas of the cortex so that the focus of attention can be directed to a specific area or field. Freed of the alpha wave, the cortical field possesses a heightened responsiveness.[59] The central processing of sensory information, however, cannot be measured by peripheral input. Information not useful

[54] H. Jasper, Reticular-cortical systems and theories of the integrative action of the brain. In H. F. Harlow and C. N. Woolsey, Eds., *Biological and biochemical bases of behavior.* Madison: The University of Wisconsin Press, 1958. Pp. 43–44.

[55] T. L. Peele, *The neuroanatomic basis for clinical neurology.* New York: McGraw-Hill, 1961. P. 360.

[56] *Ibid.,* pp. 360–361.

[57] D. B. Lindsley, The reticular system and perceptual discrimination. In H. H. Jasper, *et al.,* Eds., *Reticular formation of the brain.* Boston: Little, Brown, 1958. Pp. 517–518.

[58] O. S. Adrianov and M. Ya. Rabinovich, *Nekotorye teoreticheskiye voprosy stroyeniya i deyatel'nosti mozga (Theoretical questions on brain structure and activity).* Moscow: U.S.S.R. Press, 1960). Pp. 152–178. H. Jasper, Reticular-cortical systems and theories of the integrative action of the brain. In H. F. Harlow and C. N. Woolsey, Eds., *Biological and biochemical bases of behavior.* Madison: The University of Wisconsin Press, 1958. P. 42f.

[59] Hans Berger, Über das elektroenkephalogramm des menschen, I. mitteilung. *Arch Psychiat Nervenkr* (April 1929), 87: 527–570.

to the organism at the moment will be inhibited by the alerting mechanism so that only sensory patterns having significance for the subject will be admitted to cortical analysis. Cortical discrimination or perception seems tied to facilitatory and inhibitory activity of brainstem systems.[60]

The belief that attention always produces a simple blocking of the alpha rhythm is not entirely accurate. Electrical activity of the cortex, in the first place, will depend on the excitatory state of the cortex when the sensory pattern arrives. Fatigue, drugs, emotional disturbances, undue tension, and the significance of the sensation to the individual, result in markedly different patterns of electrical activity in the cortex.

This account of the relation of the alpha rhythm to perception obviously is incomplete. The prevailing view seems to be that the cortex is alerted by reticular and correlative brainstem circuits; the basic resting pattern of the cortex is interrupted; low amplitude, fast waves take the place of the alpha rhythm. The alerting mechanism not only blocks the alpha waves on certain neuronal fronts; it also resets the rhythmic beats and excitability cycles of these fronts so that incoming rhythmic patterns coincide in their temporal and spatial aspects with activated neuronal assemblies in the cortex. So connections are made, differentiated, and elaborated; perception is the result.

Some linguistically retarded children, we believe, do not possess this kind of normal rhythmic activity in the nervous system. The incoming impulses may arrive in the cortex without definite temporal-spatial patterning, and hence cannot be synthesized with the activated neuronal assemblies of the cortex. The cortical neuronal assemblies themselves may reflect a basic dysrhythmia and so preclude the synthesis and elaboration of incoming neural patterns. In either event, perception is distorted or blocked.

Cerebral Dominance

Does Man need two brains? This question of the dispensability of one cerebral hemisphere has been raised persistently for more than two centuries. The answer remains an enigma. After reading current literature on the question, we agree with Sperry that we are faced with "almost intellectually paralyzing complexities and contradictions." [61] From our survey of contradictions and complexities of research, some questions emerge that highlight the issues in this debate. They are as follows: (1) Does the child begin life with a potential in both hemispheres for the development of oral language? (2) Assuming that speech functions

[60] E. C. Adrian, *The physical background of perception* Oxford: Clarendon Press, 1947. Pp. 76–78.
[61] R. W. Sperry and M. S. Gazzaniga, Language following surgical disconnection of the hemispheres. In F. L. Darley, Ed., *Brain mechanisms underlying speech and language.* New York: Grune & Stratton, 1967. P. 109.

are lateralized in the course of development in the left or major hemisphere, at what age is lateralization or cerebral dominance achieved? (3) Does each hemisphere possess discriminatory processes (even in older children and adults), and do they contribute equally to the sensory-motor patterns of speech? (4) In the event of injury to the major hemisphere does the minor hemisphere have a potential for motor speech so that it may be trained to take over speech functions normally located in older children and adults in the major (left) hemisphere?

Development of Dominance. On the basis of the evidence that we have reviewed, the first question should be answered affirmatively. In the average child, progressive lateralization of language in the left hemisphere (even in left-handed individuals) normally occurs *as language develops.* The process usually begins about the age of 2 years. Elementary stages of lateralization may be completed when the child is 5 to 6 years of age, but the higher nervous integration of the human brain probably has not been set completely by that time because some functional plasticity is still evident up to the twelfth or thirteen year.[62] Prepotency for speech in the dominant hemisphere, however, is marked after the fifth year.[63] After that time one's ability to employ the minor hemisphere in speech functions probably declines.

We could settle the second question more easily if all authorities agreed that 5 years was the cut-off point for the establishment of cerebral dominance for speech, but they do not agree. Some scholars claim that the removal for medical reasons of one hemisphere, either right or left, in children below the age of 10–12 years has not produced irreparable impairment of language.[64] Basser, on the other side, concluded from exhaustive studies of cortical lesions in very young children (3 to 5 years) that "when brain damage was sustained *before* the acquisition of speech, speech was developed and maintained in the intact hemisphere alone. . . ."[65] In the writer's experience, children below the age range of 10–12 years, who have incurred serious and presumably permanent lesions in one hemisphere, are still impaired in all facets of language despite years of reeducation in speech and language (p. 328). The improvement often has been quite remarkable, but the potential of the minor hemisphere for language learning is far below the pretraumatic potential of the major hemisphere. Perhaps disturbed and enfeebled potentials in

[62] S. Obrador, Nervous integration after hemispherectomy in man. In G. Schaltenbrand and C. Woolsey, Eds., *Cerebral Localization and Organization.* Madison: The University of Wisconsin Press, 1964. P. 141.

[63] D. Kimura, Functional asymmetry of the brain in dichotic listening. *Cortex* (June 1967), 3: 167–169.

[64] E. H. Lenneberg, Speech development: Its anatomical and physical concomitants. In E. C. Carterette, Ed., *Brain function III: Speech, language and communication.* Berkeley: University of California Press, 1966. Pp. 46–47.

[65] L. S. Basser, Hemiplegia of early onset and the faculty of speech with special reference to the effects of hemispherectomy. *Brain* (September 1962), 85: 427–459.

the ailing major hemisphere interfere with the potentials of the minor hemisphere and thus retard learning, a disturbance which would not occur in children after total hemispherectomy. The recent case report of an adult who was able to comprehend and use oral language following hemispherectomy of the major hemisphere supports this argument that the minor hemisphere may assume linguistic functions more adequately if there is no interference from the damaged hemisphere.

The following are extracts from a report of dominant hemispherectomy of a 47-year-old male who was "right-handed and right-eyed":

Improving comprehension of spoken words was reflected in E. C.'s increasing scores in the Peabody Picture Vocabulary Test (PPVT). On 3 June (six months following hemispherectomy) he correctly selected 85 of 112 items. The marked improvement in PPVT scores shows an increasing attention span and capacity for prolonged testing, as well as increasing verbal comprehension which was evident in conversation and in performances on other psychological tests. . . . In the fifth postoperative month, E. C. showed sudden recall of whole familiar songs, and he now sings with little hesitation and with few errors in articulation. . . . (He) can now tell time, keeps appointments on other floors without being reminded. . . . Most important, perhaps, he demonstrates a capacity to enjoy and participate in human relationships despite his marked disabilities. . . . The ability to discriminate color, solve abstract and concrete mathematical problems, engage in purposeful movements with the left hand, and to perform at a nearly normal level in nonlanguage tests of "higher" mental functions indicates either that these functions are not exclusively or predominantly "localized" in the adult dominant hemisphere, or that, following removal of this hemisphere, the right hemisphere has the capacity to amplify previously smaller contributions to these functions.[66]

One must also reckon with the factor of individual differences in the development of dominance. Children vary greatly in the rate and extent of maturation of the nervous system, and cerebral lateralization, a maturation process, varies in the same way. In some individuals lateralization is never realized with the result that even as adults they possess a type of cerebral organization particularly vulnerable to all types of stress.[67] Their neural organization is not ambilateral; on the contrary, it reflects a lack of laterality or dominance in both hemispheres. When the issue is finally settled, we probably shall find that the development of dominance depends on many factors, both genetic and acquired: intel-

[66] A. Smith and C. W. Burklund, Dominant hemispherectomy: Preliminary report on neuropsychological sequelae. *Science,* (September 9, 1966), 153: 1281–1282.

[67] M. Critchley, Speech and speech-loss in relation to duality of the brain. In V. Mountcastle, Ed., *Interhemispheric relations and cerebral dominance.* Baltimore: Johns Hopkins, 1962. Pp. 208–213. L. Roberts, Central brain mechanisms in speech. In E. C. Carterette, Ed., *Brain function III: Speech, language and communication.* Berkeley: University of California Press, 1966. Pp. 18–19. O. L. Zangwill, *Cerebral dominance and its relation to psychological function.* Edinburgh: Oliver and Boyd, 1960. Pp. 26–27.

ligence, neural potential and organization, and in the event of injury, the age at the time of insult and the level of premorbid mental maturity

Equipotentiality and Discrimination. Whereas there seems to be a developing dominance in the major or left hemisphere in motor speech, we have less clear evidence of the respective roles of the hemispheres in the discriminatory processes mediating language. Some authorities hold that in older children both hemispheres contribute to sensory-motor patterning but certain modalities of discrimination may not be equally represented in the same hemisphere. Auditory and tactile-kinesthetic discriminations, in particular, seem to be more diffusely represented in the right than in the major left hemisphere.[68] Although each cochlea, for example, has fiber connections with both hemispheres, apparently the *quality* of projection to the two sides is different.[69] In the minor hemisphere it seems to result in diffuse, less distinctive patterns. Similarly a parietal lesion in the minor hemisphere produces deficits in spatial summation, an important requisite for proprioception. The resulting pattern may not be "lost," but it is not sufficiently intense to produce discrimination.[70] Lesions in the parietal-temporal areas in either hemisphere, it is believed, more frequently interfere with the perception of meaning than with the motoric processes of language.[71] Apparently each hemisphere normally makes some contribution to discrimination.

A recent report probably increases the complexity of the question but it also throws new light on the role of the two hemispheres in discrimination. Gazzaniga, in collaboration with Sperry, investigated brain mechanisms mediating behavior in a group of adult patients in whom the corpus callosum and other commissural structures had been sectioned.[72] They found that the major or dominant hemisphere may

[68] B. Milner, Laterality effects in audition. In V. Mountcastle, Ed., *Interhemispheric relations and cerebral dominance.* Baltimore: Johns Hopkins, 1962. P. 188. S. Weinstein, Differential effects on certain intellectual and complex perceptual functions. In V. Mountcastle, Ed., *Interhemispheric relations and cerebral dominance.* Baltimore: Johns Hopkins, 1962. P. 176.

[69] W. D. Neff, Differences in the function of the two cerebral hemispheres. In V. Mountcastle, Ed., *Interhemispheric relations and cerebral dominance.* Baltimore: Johns Hopkins, 1962. P. 198.

[70] D. Denny-Brown, Discussion. In V. Mountcastle, Ed., *Interhemispheric relations and cerebral dominance.* Baltimore: Johns Hopkins, 1962. P. 245.

[71] R. W. Sperry and M. S. Gazzaniga, Language following surgical disconnection of the hemispheres. In F. L. Darley, Ed., *Brain mechanisms underlying speech and language.* New York: Grune & Stratton, 1967. Pp. 108–145. C. Branch, B. Milner and T. Rasmussen, Intra-carotid sodium amytal for the lateralization of cerebral speech dominance. Observations in 123 patients. *J Neurosurg* (May 1964), 21: 399–405. R. L. Masland, Lacunae and research approaches to them. In F. L. Darley, Ed., *Brain mechanisms underlying speech and language.* New York: Grune & Stratton, 1967. Pp. 232–236. H-L. Teuber, Effects of brain wounds implicating right or left hemisphere in man: Hemisphere differences and hemisphere interaction in vision, audition, and somesthesis. In V. Mountcastle, Ed., *Interhemispheric relations and cerebral dominance.* Baltimore: Johns Hopkins, 1962. Pp. 156–157.

[72] M. S. Gazzaniga, The split brain in man. *Sci Amer* (August 1967), 217: 24–29.

act independently of the minor hemisphere in discrimination, but the minor hemisphere also had a remarkable power to discriminate meaningful stimuli and to make *nonverbal* responses. When an object was presented visually to the right or minor hemisphere, for example, the "split brain" patient was able to select the object from a group of objects placed out of his view by tactile exploration with the left hand. When the same information was presented to the dominant left hemisphere the patient was able to deal with and describe it quite normally both orally and in writing. Could these adults with split brains also make the proper nonverbal response to auditory stimulation? Gazzaniga found that they could select the object (screened from their sight) even when it was not named directly but was described. ("Retrieve the fruit monkeys like best.") The minor hemisphere could make high-level discriminatory responses on the nonverbal plane; it also could make fairly complex emotional responses to stimuli; but its power of oral response was feeble.

Equipotentiality and Oral Expression.   The final question pertains to the assumption of speech function by the minor hemisphere in the event of injury to the major hemisphere. We pointed out earlier that very young children probably employ diffuse areas in both hemispheres in learning to comprehend and use speech. As the child learns, cortical fields of influence are more clearly defined and motor speech particularly tends to develop high potentials in one hemisphere. We know that in the majority of individuals Broca's area in the left hemisphere has a higher potentiation of circuits mediating vocal and articulatory patterns than its counterpart in the right hemisphere. We would expect, then, that lesions in the major hemisphere, particularly in children over 5 years of age, affect more frequently and more seriously the use of oral language. It is difficult, however, to distinguish *use* in a circuit of which proprioceptive, auditory, visual, and somatic patterns also are integral parts. The *act* of expression cannot be divorced from the sensory arm of the sensory-motor components that go to make up the final effector pattern. It also is difficult to distinguish the upper limit of linguistic ability for each hemisphere because it seems to vary greatly from subject to subject. The patient in Smith and Burklund's study (p. 43), who underwent hemispherectomy of the major hemisphere, made a rather remarkable recovery in comprehension and use of oral language. In Gazzaniga's study (above), the patient could respond to a concrete noun such as *pencil* when the stimulus was presented only to the minor hemisphere, but he found it very difficult to employ predication in any response. Grammar, Gazzaniga thought, was poorly developed in the minor hemisphere. The ability of the minor hemisphere to take over the sensory-motor functions of speech when the major hemisphere no longer is operative depends, as does the development of cerebral dominance, on intelligence, genetic capacity of the minor hemisphere for neural potential and organization, the age of the individual at the time of insult, and the level of premorbid mental maturity. Adult man may get along fairly well with one hemisphere, but he operates better on the two-hemisphere plan in which division of labor occurs. The division of labor is not equal, for the participation of the two hemispheres may be qualitatively different in handling the same sensory-motor event. Oral expression, we are fairly sure, has its higher potential in the left hemisphere, even in left-handed individuals. We are less sure of the superiority of the left hemisphere in the representation of discriminatory patterns in the sensory-motor processing of oral language.

2

Operational Systems

Primary Sensory Systems

Many sensory modalities—vision, olfaction, taction, audition, and proprioception—enter directly or indirectly into the comprehension-use of oral language. Vision is important in the visuomotor perception of speech and its gestural accompaniment. Taction is so closely allied with proprioception in modes of stimulation, end organs, and function that we shall frequently link them in the term, tactile-kinesthesis. Touch, strictly speaking, should be delimited as the kind of light pressure that may be discriminated in two-point discrimination. When the pressure or tension becomes slightly heavier, it stimulates proprioceptor end organs in muscles, tendons, joints, and the vestibular apparatus of the ear. The end organs of taction and proprioception, in other words, both require a stimulus of mechanical deformation. The difference in stimulation is largely one of degree, and in many aspects of fine movement and postural shifts taction seems to operate as an integral part of kinesthesis. Both are instrumental in perception of vibration because both respond to repetitive mechanical stimuli. Impulses arising in end organs of taction and in proprioceptors in muscles, tendons, and joints may follow a common route in the brainstem. Integration of tactile and proprioceptive impulses underlies gnosis or appreciation of form, and extent, and sequence of motor activity in the performance of such complex movements as speech. In this chapter we shall discuss only two modalities in detail, proprioception and auditory perception, but in succeeding chapters shall refer frequently to visuomotor and tactile-motor function in oral language.

Variable Factors of Speech Discrimination. A complex of factors must go into the hopper of discrimination. If it were not so, we could not account for the unlimited variability in perception among individuals. The way in which an organism's nervous system will process these neural signals depends not only upon the stimulus pattern but upon other events in the organism's environment and the organism's needs, as well as the response behavior that it expects to emit.[1] Success in coding will depend also upon neural organization and operation. The variables may be genetic or adventitious in origin.

Neural Plasticity. A basic differential in a nervous system is its plasticity. Plasticity will determine its stimulability, the strength and viability of synaptic potentials, the rate of fusion frequency, the competence of feedback loops to effect facilitation and inhibition, and the regularity of spontaneous wave patterns in the cortex. When certain neural highways are closed to the tactile-kinesthetic and auditory signals of speech, for example, the possibility of alternate routes will be determined largely by neural plasticity. A dramatic case in point is the report of Landau and colleagues at the Central Institute for the Deaf. They reported on the terminal history of a 10-year-old congenitally aphasic boy who, during his residence at the institute, developed an oral vocabulary and the ability to carry on simple conversations. After his death (from causes unrelated to the cerebral disorder), autopsy disclosed that there were extensive bilateral lesions of the temperoparietal regions and complete bilateral degeneration of the medial geniculate bodies. Despite a complete destruction of "critical" auditory routes this child dealt reasonably well with the verbal world about him. Apparently he was able to use indirect pathways that provided a measure of auditory perception.[2]

Developmental Variances. Sometimes the variables of speech discrimination must be accounted for on a developmental basis. The most elementary speech signals meaningful to a baby probably are intonational patterns, yet this perceptual ability often is not well developed in children of school age. Lieberman presents an interesting account of the emergence of intonational contours from primitive breath-group patterns or archetypes appearing in the baby's early cries. The intonational signal, Lieberman finds, is perceived in terms of these archetypal patterns because they represent the most basic way in which intonational signals can be produced using the human vocal tract.[3] In this early stage of oral comprehension the baby will not perceive such components of an intonational pattern as fundamental frequency, amplitude, and duration.

[1] W. A. Rosenblith, Editor's comment. In W. A. Rosenblith, Ed., *Sensory communication.* Cambridge, Mass.: M. I. T., 1961. P. 818.

[2] W. M. Landau, R. Goldstein, and F. R. Kleffner, Congenital aphasia; a clinicopathologic study. *Neurology* (Minneap) (October 1960), 10: 915–921.

[3] P. Lieberman, *Intonation, perception, and language.* Cambridge, Mass.: M. I. T. 1967. Pp. 61–103.

He certainly will not interpret the words encompassed in the intonation contour.[4] He responds in the beginning to the melodic, rhythmic pattern as a whole. Later he will comprehend the significance of stressed syllables and words making up the phrase. Phonetic signals, once considered the key to the perception of speech, are not significant at this stage. The child of 4 years normally will incorporate the phoneme *by hypothesis* into syntactic and semantic interpretation. He will construct mentally those phonemic signals that hypothetically fit into a reasonable syntactic and semantic interpretation of the message. Ask a child of 4 to repeat a series of nonsense syllables and one readily discovers his inability to discriminate phonemes out of context. Only when one speaks with great articulatory precision and slow rate can the child hypothesize about the character or order of phonemic signals in nonsense syllables. Another phonological variable is the articulatory competence of the speaker in connected speech and the mimetic competence of the listener in forming motor-proprioceptive patterns of the sequence.

The perception [5] of syntactic and semantic cues hinges primarily upon the earlier perception of intonational patterns, for they furnish natural guides to these linguistic features. Later other cues will assist the comprehension of syntactic and semantic units. Before speech can become intelligible they must be consistent with each other and with the more basic intonational patterns emerging from archetypal breath-groups. Note that the question, a syntactic unit, generally is perceived by its rising intonational curve. Note, too, that one who must speak a foreign tongue after a short period of training relies first upon intonational patterns. He knows that if he can produce the basic melody of a foreign speech, meaning is greatly facilitated. The writer once suggested to her phonetician-colleague occupying an adjoining deck chair on a Norwegian ship that she would like tea but she did not know how to ask for it. The colleague spoke to the steward. "What did you say?" the writer asked. "I just grafted a bit of English on a Norsk intonation curve," she said. Tea came promptly.

As comprehension of verbal sequences develops, semantic markers more precise than intonational contours are employed. Among these markers are contextual cues resulting from constraints on phoneme and word sequences.[6] From a ground of noise the individual perceives those sequences that must go together because they complete meaning. If the message is not intelligible, he interjects sequences, supplying by hypothesis missing parts. The acoustic and kinesthetic signals are none-

[4] M. M. Lewis, *Language, thought, and personality.* London: Harrap, 1963. Pp. 27–30.
[5] The terms *discrimination* and *perception* are synonymous in this book.
[6] P. Denes, Understanding and creating sentences. In E. C. Carterette, Ed., *Brain function III: Speech, language, and communication.* Berkeley: University of California Press, 1966. Pp. 224–225.

theless real, albeit he has constructed them by "internal computation." Sometimes he ignores these signals altogether, using his knowledge of semantic and syntactic constraints of language and the social context of the message to comprehend acoustic signals. Tests of verbal closure assess one's ability to hypothecate missing semantic segments on the basis of a core of cues.[7] Results indicate a wide range of ability among children in the school population in perception of syntactic and semantic cues.

Other variables of perception center in motor speech—in speech rate, vocal quality, facial and bodily gestures, in the total neuromuscular pattern of speech production. Internal and external environmental factors of noise levels, dialectal surrounds, and emotional instability may adversely affect verbal comprehension. Genetic factors responsible for perceptual immaturity and atypical neural organization undoubtedly enter into coding. And finally perception of speech may be facilitated or deterred by psychological determinants of attention, motivation, reinforcement, and memory.

Proprioception (Kinesthesis) of Speech

Primacy of Proprioception in Language Learning. Proprioceptive impulses originate in stretch or tension receptors in muscles, tendons, joints, and in the vestibular apparatus of the ear. The resulting appreciation of position, movement, balance, and changes in equilibrium on the part of the muscular system is called proprioception or kinesthesis. Proprioception employs bidirectional tracts in the nervous system so its pathways might more properly be called sensory-motor loops. Comparatively little attention has been paid to kinesthesis in the comprehension and use of verbal symbols, yet this modality is as important as auditory perception. Research in widely separated academic areas attests to its significance in every aspect of language learning. Psychologists find that a child's first ideas are related primarily to movement, not to sound. Vernon, among others, believes that the tendency to perceive the simplest type of movement may be unlearned, innate.[8] Brain, a neurologist and speech pathologist, argues that since motor patterns are the earliest events in the comprehension of speech, neurological processes of kinesthetic feedback must mediate between the acoustic stimulus and its perception.[9] Gelhorn, a physiologist, does not call basic movements innate but he finds that they are organized in neural patterns very early in a child's life. It is a patterned response and not the response of a single neurone because a proprioceptive impulse originating in a

[7] R. L. Schiefelbusch, Language studies of mentally retarded children. *J Speech Hearing Dis [Monogr]* Supplement (January 1963), 10: 3–7.
[8] M. D. Vernon, *The psychology of perception.* Baltimore: Penguin, 1962. Pp. 153–156.
[9] R. Brain, *Speech disorders.* Washington: Butterworth, 1961. Pp. 80–83.

certain muscle will modify not only its own responsiveness to cortical stimulation but also that of other muscles associated with it in the response.[10] In the synergic action involved in articulating the word *baby,* for example, signals from the gamma spindles in the orbicularis oris muscle will trip off the sequence of muscle activation and inhibition which may include phasic sequences in the lingualis, styloglossus, palatoglossus, and hyoglossus muscles. There is a built-in mechanism that requires stimulation only of one neuronal assembly in order to initiate a sequence of action. There is, in short, a kind of built-in proprioceptive-motor mechanism for sequential action that may be triggered by a single neuronal assembly.

Even more important, perhaps, is the research concerned specifically with the function of proprioception in language learning. When Novikova found that there was a noticeable increase in tongue muscle potentials of deaf children engaged in learning speech he was able to accelerate their learning by the stimulation of proprioceptive feedback through "verbal movements." [11] As a result of their extensive research of perceptual processes in language learning, Liberman and colleagues conclude that the appreciation of kinesthesis (proprioception) is even more important than auditory perception. The articulatory movements that the listener makes in reproducing the acoustic patterns, they believe, determine the fine cues to perception of words. They may be only short-circuited neural equivalents of these movements but they are essential to his understanding and use of speech. The phonemic cues to key words, /p/ and /k/ for example, may be entirely identical acoustically yet they will be clearly differentiated in proprioceptive terms. Even more important in teaching methods is their finding that the kinesthetic cue to perception arises *primarily* "from the articulatory movement . . . made in going from consonant to the next phoneme." [12] In terms of movement patterns it is the shift in muscular action (accompanied by proprioceptive feedback) from one series of articulatory sequences to the next which governs our ability to perceive language and to repeat what we have comprehended. Man's superiority over other higher animals in acquiring language presumably resides in this singular ability to organize and master sequences of combinative information.[13] He can hold in memory the sequences of articulatory movement, the pattern not only of a word

[10] E. Gellhorn, Proprioception and the motor cortex. *Brain* (March 1949), 72: 35–62.

[11] L. A. Novikova, Electrophysiological investigation of speech. In N. O'Connor, Ed., *Recent soviet psychology.* New York: Liveright, 1961. P. 225.

[12] A. M. Liberman, F. S. Cooper, K. S. Harris, and P. F. MacNeilage, A motor theory of speech perception. In *Proceedings of the Speech Communications Seminar.* Stockholm: Royal Inst. Tech., 1963. L. Lisker, F. Cooper, and A. M. Liberman, The uses of experiment in language description. *Word* (April–August 1962), 18: 103.

[13] Hans G. Furth, Sequence learning in aphasic and deaf children. *J Speech Hearing Dis* (May 1964), 29: 171–177.

but of phrases and sentences. As Broadbent says, "Speech is the most obvious case of stimuli being dealt with in sequences. . . . It is normal for the whole sequence to be delivered before any response is required." [14] If this is true, a child's perception of oral language must be predicated on *sound sequences,* not on sound in isolation.

The case for proprioception as a prime modality in language learning gains support from the experimental synthesis of speech. Computer-generated speech, it has been found, would be more accurate if more attention were paid to the articulatory shapes that fit the audiowave form. Cooper says in this connection, "The significant aspect of speech is not so much the shape of the articulatory tract as the sequence of muscle contractions which produce that shape, even earlier, the neural motor commands that activate the muscles of the articulatory apparatus." [15]

Some workers in the field hold that tactile-kinesthetic feedback becomes relatively more important than the auditory in language comprehension-use as one reaches adulthood, but we find little scientific support for this view. The majority who hold that proprioception, first and last, is as important as audition in mediating language argue in this vein: 1. Since motor patterns are the earliest events in the comprehension of speech, proprioceptive feedback must mediate between the acoustic stimulus and its perception. 2. Proprioceptive feedback signals from articulatory movements apparently are more distinctive than acoustic signals. 3. Phonemic sequences are truly motor command patterns, i.e., they are temporal-spatial, neural patterns that activate entire muscle groups responsible for articulation of syllables, words, or phrases. These concepts, strongly fortified by research, suggest that our clinical practice of teaching the sound in isolation is completely unsound.

Proprioceptive Feedback. The function of proprioceptive feedback in speech should be recognized, not only in articulation but in all aspects of speech production: postural set, gesture, respiration, and phonation. Speech production is a neuromuscular synergy involving the entire body. The baby learning to speak must learn sensory-motor patterns *tout d'une pièce.* Upon basic bodily postures he builds fundamental movement patterns and they, in turn, provoke the development of a sequence of differentiated phasic motor movements: postural shifts, directional signals, the rhythmic breath pulse associated with phonation, bodily and facial gestures, and articulatory patterns.[16] Even in the last step—articulatory patterning—the child must learn a synergy of movements, not a single movement or even a pattern of stationary concepts about a single sound.

[14] D. E. Broadbent, *Perception and communication.* New York: Macmillan, 1958. Pp. 44, 47.

[15] F. S. Cooper, Speech from stored data. In *IEEE international convention record, part 7.* New York: Inst. Elec. Electron. Eng., 1963. P. 143.

[16] M. M. Shirley, The motor sequence. In W. Dennis, Ed., *Readings in child psychology.* New York: Prentice-Hall, 1963. P. 81.

An articulatory synergy embraces more than a syllable or foot or word; it is a complex, singly directed, integrated pattern that may include the whole phrase.

No part of the sequence of motor learning apparently can be slighted. If basic postures are not established, the child's appreciation of his body image—the balance and position of body parts—will be deficient. Upon this inadequate perceptual base he cannot build the series of motor learnings leading finally to the variable, adaptive purposeful movements of speech. Early deficits in perceptual-motor awareness must be offset, if possible, before more complex motor patterns are attempted.[17]

Neural Track in Proprioception (Kinesthesis). Neurone networks enter into the transaction mediating proprioception much as they do in the visual or auditory systems. There is not one track but several tracks by which proprioceptive impulses enter and influence the final pattern of the code. Many proprioceptive impulses will course with efferent impulses in the pyramidal tracts. Those that have joined tactile fiber tracts may synapse in cuneate nuclei at the dorsal end of the brainstem. After decussation (crossing), a portion of these fibers may ascend via the medial lemniscus to the upper brainstem, thalamus, basal nuclei, and cortex. Others will join with proprioceptive fibers from the pyramidal tract and enter synaptic areas in the reticular formation, from which feedback loops will be projected to cerebellar, pontine, and midbrain nuclei. Still others possibly may travel the entire distance without synapse to subcortical and cortical areas [18] and circle back to thalamic and brainstem nuclei. By countless synapses with cell aggregates in reticular, subcortical, and cortical areas, activation and inhibition operate to refine and elaborate the proprioceptive patterns and to integrate them with patterns of other modalities (visual, auditory) mediating discrimination of the verbal sequences.[19] Some patterns may not match basic time-space relations and will be excluded. Critical synaptic junctions, essen-

[17] J. R. Kershner, and D. H. Bauer, *Neuropsychological and perceptual motor theories of treatment of children with educational inadequacies.* Philadelphia: Bureau of Research, Dept. Public Instruc., 1966.

[18] In tracing proprioceptive fibers from the front tongue to the cortex, Brodal observed that they send collaterals to the reticular formation at the pontine and midbrain level.—A. Brodal and B. Kaada, Cutaneous and proprioceptive impulses in the pyramidal tract of the cat. *Acta Physiol Scand.* Copenhagen: Munksgaard Press, (1953), 29 (1): 131–132. Cooper has described stretch receptors in the intrinsic muscles of the tongue.—S. Cooper, Muscle spindles in the intrinsic muscles of the human tongue. *J Physiol* (London) (October 1953), 122: 193–202.

[19] "Responses to different modalities of stimulation could be recorded at a single reticular site and, when two stimuli of differing modality were presented in rapid succession, attenuation of the second response indicated convergence from different afferent sources upon common neural elements, with consequent lack of modality segregation."—H. W. Magoun, *The waking brain.* Springfield, Ill.: Charles C Thomas, 1963. P. 83.

tial to coding, may be temporarily or permanently weakened in power. Temporal-parietal areas may not have been alerted and sensitized to incoming impulses by the reticular activating system. Success of the operation depends upon the several neurological variables of coding (p. 102).

Proprioception (Kinesthesis) and Language Learning. Proprioception is difficult to trace and to measure both in linguistic and non-linguistic functions because muscle memory patterns are largely un-analyzable. Let the driver of a car attempt to describe exactly what he does in avoiding a collision with another car. He rarely is able to verbalize his action, but he can show you how he acted, and accurately too. One cannot be taught to dance by verbal analysis of the steps involved. He is aided in learning by visual, auditory, and tactile perception, but he must rely fundamentally upon the proprioceptive patterns to ensure his success. Another example of the use of unanalyzed proprioceptive feedback is the check we make when we are in doubt about the spelling of a word. We write it quickly, wishing to rely completely upon muscle memory without interference from the enfeebled auditory or visual patterns of spelling. We brook no intrusion of analysis based on memory of cues from other sensory modalities. For muscle memory we rely on uninterrupted motor sequences. Some children with perceptual deficits depend so heavily on muscle memory in copying a drawing, for example, that they exclude visual or oral stimuli during the *act* of copying.

We often observe spontaneous, overt proprioceptive reinforcement in language learning of very young children. Watch an alert 2-year-old child follow the story being told by an adult and one probably will note articulatory mimesis by the child. These movements which wax and wane with interest are not a replication of sounds but of sequences of sounds—of phrases or sentences. And the mimetic pattern includes not only the articulators but all coeval activities: postural adaptation, breathing synergy, facial expression and gesture. Any kind of serial learning that employs perceptual-motor tracts must lean heavily upon proprioception. The young child who successfully produces a difficult series of syllables in a sentence often reports that he knows it is right because "it feels right." Awareness of synergic relation and progression results from effective proprioceptive feedback.

Experimental Studies of Proprioceptive Feedback. We may recognize the importance of proprioception in oral language but experimental studies are meager in providing scientific support of its importance in speech training. There is reason for it. Auditory stimuli can be initiated by external means; the child himself must initiate proprioceptive movements of specific muscle synergies. Auditory impulses can be measured electronically in the cochlea; no reliable measure of proprioceptive response has been found. Gastaut, Mochava, and their colleagues have supported mimetic practice of facial expression, hand gesture, tongue and lip movements in speech. In their respective laboratories they found that the basic rhythm of the motor area of the cortex was not altered by a clicking sound (unconditioned stimulus), but when the sound was combined with an active or passive movement of the head, conditioning of the sound was effected. Whereas the sound originally had no effect on the "Rolandic rhythm," by the simultaneous repetition of the two stimuli, the sound alone finally produced a Rolandic block (indication of a response of the stimulus of sound).[20] Perhaps this laboratory experiment explains why a renowned actor when he falters over a line increases the vigor of the established gestural pattern and so recovers the line.

Hefferline used an electronic method by which the individual could monitor the proprioceptive feedback of his own jaw muscle (masseter). Two recording electrodes were placed over the muscle which picked up the action potentials; they were amplified and recorded on two meters, one of which was visible to the subject. The subject was told that signals of light and sound would be given for him to begin work.

What you are to do is to close your mouth by the smallest amount you can. This will make the needle rise on the scale. It will take only the tiniest bit of movement from you to make the needle go to the top of the scale. . . . We want you to try to make the needle go to midscale . . . try to keep it there. After you have done this for 10 seconds you will hear another "beep." The middle light will come on and your meter will go dead. The needle will drop down to zero and stay there. But what you are doing with your jaw will now show up on a meter just like yours that we have out here. What we want you to do during this 10 seconds is to keep your meter at midscale . . . even though you can't see it.[21]

We have reported the experiment in some detail because it might be adapted to the teaching of proprioceptive control of muscular activity to individuals with slight neuromotor disabilities.

Experimental studies of proprioceptive feedback by speech scientists are promising but inconclusive. Work at present has been limited to the establishment of the value of tactile-kinesthetic cues in speech.[22] Undoubtedly tests of stereognosis employing tactile-kinesthetic cues will become one reliable index of sensory-motor integrity of the articulatory mechanisms (p. 118).

[20] H. Gastaut, *et al.*, Etude topographique des réactions électroencéphalographiques conditionnées chez l'homme. *Electroenceph Clin Neurophysiol* (February 1957), 9: 1–34.

[21] R. F. Hefferline, The role of proprioception in the control of behavior. *New York Acad Sci: Series II* (June 1958), 20: 739–764.

[22] R. McCroskey, The relative contributions of auditory and tactile cues to certain aspects of speech. *Southern Speech J* (1958), 24: 84–90. R. L. Ringel and M. D. Steer, Some effects of tactile and auditory alteration on speech output. *J Speech Hearing Dis* (December 1963), 6: 369–378.

Clinical Reports of Disordered Proprioception. These reports, although fragmentary, present clearer evidence than experimental studies of the role of proprioception in language learning. In his study of perceptual-motor deficits in children with developmental language disorders, Professor A. R. Plum (Chief, Pediatrics Division, Riks-hospital, Copenhagen, Denmark) found that more than 60 percent of the preschool group (4–6 years) were unable to skip, hop, or pantomime very simple action sequences of nursery rhymes, even after several months of instruction. In another report, ability in lip reading is positively correlated with "conceptualization abilities." [23] Since lip reading manifestly is a skill based on visual and tactile-kinesthetic perception, deaf children who are able lip readers must be superior in these modes of perception. In a study of differential diagnosis of aphasia, the author concludes that the inability of aphasic children to learn to lip-read must be associated with deficient visual motor-proprioceptive feedback.[24]

Although Parkinson's Syndrome does not appear in children, research on this syndrome has disclosed another effect of proprioceptive disturbance on language. Chesni found that proprioceptive deterioration in Parkinsonian rigidity not only affects articulatory patterning but also *la formulation verbale intérieure* (implicit speech). As rigidity increased in phonatory muscles, implicit speech, measured by electromyographic means, diminished. In his words there was "an abatement of internal speech in correlation with the abatement of phonatory movements." [25]

We have been accustomed to think of the speech of cleft palate children as a problem resulting solely from the structural anomaly. Stark provides evidence to support our position that proprioceptive deficiencies also are a contributing cause of the poor language and speech of this group of children.[26] Stark established a lack in *volume* of facial muscles in complete palatal clefts; nerves follow the muscle anlage; hence the nerve supply to the muscle also was found to be meager. The resulting deficiency, particularly in motor-proprioceptive circuits, reduces the cleft palate child's ability in patterning articulatory movement and facial gesture. From clinical observation of more than four hundred young children with repaired facial clefts, we have gathered corroborative evidence of impaired tactile-kinesthetic perception. Such

[23] R. Tiffany and S. Kates, Concept attainment and lip reading ability among deaf adolescents. *J Speech Hearing Dis* (August 1962), 27: 265–274.

[24] J. L. Olson, *A comparison of sensory aphasic, expressive aphasic and deaf children in the Illinois test of language ability.* Ann Arbor: University Microfilms, 61–81, 1964. Pp. 52–56.

[25] Y. Chesni, Sur le rôle des propriocepteurs dans le contrôle de la parole. *Rev Laryng* (Bordeaux) (July–August 1963), 84: 451–457.

[26] R. B. Stark, Pathogenesis of harelip and cleft palate. *J Plast Reconstru Surg* (January 1954), 13: 20–39.

an impairment affects the total dimension of language, its comprehension-use.

In the cerebral-palsied individual, proprioceptive facilitation and inhibition work at cross purposes in motor patterning. When agonists in the pattern are contracting, their antagonists are not inhibited, with the result that all muscle groups, agonist and antagonist, exhibit hypertension. Obviously the motor synergy of speech will be completely disrupted by such a breakdown in proprioceptive feedback. The effect on other centrally directed pathways important in language learning, although less apparent, also is significant. Uninhibited, spasmodic movements of the head and neck can produce distortions in auditory feedback with serious effects on auditory discrimination. Held and Freedman also conclude that the coordination of visual and auditory responses suffers a marked deterioration when disorder is introduced in the proprioceptive-motor loops of basic postural and movement patterns.[27] If auditory discrimination and basic postural and movement patterns are related, we assume that auditory perception of language should improve as general sensory-motor loops controlling the head and neck of the cerebral palsied are conditioned by training.

Tactile-kinesthetic cues are also important to the child handicapped by developmental perceptual deficits affecting language. They are important not only in word and phrase discrimination; they are invaluable aids in the comprehension and use of syntactical sequences.[28] Just as sounds are influenced by those which precede and follow, so words and phrases are modified by their arrangement in the sentence or complex of sentences. Children handicapped by perceptual deficits are wont to comprehend tactile-kinesthetic cues *seriatim,* and hence they have no gestalt of the phrase or sentence. As de Hirsch has said, "Movement . . . has to be experienced (perceived) as an entity. A summation of small units will never result in smooth fluid performance. . . . The most careful execution of single movements will not produce a flowing hand. A succession of correct sounds will not result in speech." [29]

Reinforcement of Proprioception (Kinesthesis) by Training. Bobath and colleagues have recognized the need of basic motor patterning in habilitating cerebral-palsied children. Their method is predicated on the development of reflex-inhibiting postures by tactile-kinesthetic training. Only as normal basic postures are established can controlled, organized, sequential movements develop. When postural movements

[27] R. Held and S. J. Freedman, Plasticity in human sensorimotor control. *Science* (October 25, 1963), 142: 455–462.

[28] K. de Hirsch, J. Jansky, and W. Langford, The oral language performance of premature children and controls. *J Speech Hearing Dis* (February 1964), 29: 64. E. K. Monsees, Aphasia in children. *J Speech Hearing Dis* (February 1961), 26: 83–86.

[29] K. de Hirsch, Gestalt psychology as applied to language disturbances. *J Nerv Ment Dis* (September–October 1954), 120: 260.

of the chest, shoulders, and neck are normal, training of precise vocal and articulatory muscle synergies is greatly facilitated.[30] The problems of Per (see ch. 10), a 16-year-old athetoid, illustrate this failure in basic perceptual-motor patterning. His postural control is very poor; tonic neck reflexes are intensified as soon as he attempts to communicate. With the aid of a mirror, he is able to produce single sounds and syllables, but he cannot join these syllables in order to produce a phrase. Proprioceptive cues to motor events *between* syllables apparently are absent. Per's proprioceptive feedback, both in postural patterning and in motor patterning for speech is seriously impaired.

The importance of tactile-kinesthesis in speech training has gained impetus from the work of Stetson, McDonald, and others. The title of McDonald's recent book, *Articulation and Treatment: A Sensory-Motor Approach,* denotes his position that articulation must be studied as "an organized system of skilled movements" which are part of a "larger pattern of speech producing movements." [31] Building upon a foundation laid by Stetson,[32] McDonald discards the isolated sound unit and develops the concept of patterns of movement and contexts. We would go beyond McDonald's concern for articulation. Speech is a total bodily response, and hence we believe that the child must be taught sequential bodily and facial gestural patterns just as he is taught sequences of articulatory gestures. He must be taught to mimic, as the well-taught deaf child does when he learns to "speech-read." When we asked a child why he made a spontaneous correction in syntax, he said, "It didn't *feel* right the other way." Perceptual-motor deficits affect both the phonological and syntactic perception of language.

Auditory Perception of Speech

At the outset we must define our view of the boundaries of this discussion. With some exceptions gross auditory acuity for sound is beyond the limits inasmuch as auditory perception generally presupposes an energy level of conduction above the threshold of hearing. Occasionally a child may have suffered both a physiologically impaired auditory structure and a central loss in hearing for speech. Sometimes threshold variances, produced by internal or external disturbances, may alter perception. In these unusual circumstances the peripheral hearing mecha-

[30] K. Bobath and B. Bobath, A treatment of cerebral palsy based on the analysis of the patient's motor behavior. *Brit J Phys Med* (May 1952), 5: 107–117. M. Crickmay, *Description and orientation of the Bobath method with reference to speech rehabilitation in cerebral palsy.* Chicago: Natl. Soc. Crippled Children and Adults, 1955.

[31] E. T. McDonald, *Articulation testing and treatment: A sensory-motor approach.* Pittsburgh: Stanwix House, 1964. Pp. 1–5.

[32] R. H. Stetson, *Motor phonetics.* Amsterdam: North Holland Publishing Company, 1961.

nism may be a consideration in perception. In other words, a general factor, common to both acuity for pure tones and hearing for speech may be hypothesized, but each function also has its own constellation of distinct features. In the perceptual failure of audition, we are dealing mainly with short-circuits in speech analyzers, not in the conductors of sound, and speech analyzers extend from the cochlea to the cortex. Our primary concern, then, is not with auditory acuity as it is assessed by pure-tone audiometry, but with a child's ability in hearing for speech. This process sometimes is referred to as *auding;* we call it the auditory comprehension-use of language.[33]

Although the perception of pure tones is not our province, the attributes of tone—fundamental frequency, amplitude, and duration— are embedded in the discrimination of cues to phonemic sequences of speech. We do not know precisely how these tonal attributes are perceived but we know they are not perceived independently. These temporal aspects of physical sound, *per se,* are secondary to the *sequences of information* contained in acoustic wave patterns. They cannot be considered primary acoustic correlates of linguistic information. The perception of attributes of tone and the perception of speech are not significantly correlated.[34] Discrimination of the isolated phone and/or phoneme also is not focal to speech perception in children although the adult occasionally may employ phonemic cues. The distinctive auditory cue to speech is rarely correlated with the phoneme segment which purportedly includes it. Tests of discrimination of sounds or even of consonant-vowel syllables tell us relatively little about the discrimination of speech (p. 131). The perceptual elements of the speech continuum transcend phonic data.[35] They transcend audiometric tests employing single words. They transcend even Myerson's test[36] since it, too, is posited on a single word as the perceptual cue in a three-word carrier phrase.

Auditory perception of speech *per se* deals mainly with the temporal management of information from the input. It is a process by which one explains how a child's nervous system learns to comprehend and make use of auditory information. We do not know all the processes operative in auditory circuits, but presumably the following should be included: (1) analysis at the initial stage of rapidly successive bits of information;

[33] W. G. Hardy, *Dyslexia in relation to diagnostic methodology in hearing and speech disorders.* In J. Money, Ed., *Reading disability.* Baltimore: Johns Hopkins, 1962. Pp. 171–178.

[34] I. J. Hirsh, Audition in relation to perception of speech. In E. C. Carterette, Ed., *Brain function III: Speech, language, and communication.* Berkeley: University of California Press, 1966. Pp. 93–116. L. Meyerson, Hearing for speech in children: A verbal audiometric test. *Acta Otolaryng* (Stockholm) (1956), Suppl. 128: 126.

[35] I. J. Hirsh, Auditory perception of speech. In E. C. Carterette, *op. cit.*, pp. 106–107.

[36] Myerson, *op. cit.*, pp. 54–69.

(2) primary patterning through activating and inhibitory feedback processes until new patterns are joined with wave patterns from other modalities; (3) further modification of wave patterns effected, in part, by earlier patterns activated in cortical and subcortical areas. That these three phases are not discrete divisions is immediately apparent. We do not perceive the elements of speech in a stepwise function of time.[37] If perception is a continuous process, all phases probably are represented throughout coding. The close integration of modalities (2 above) was suggested in the preceding discussion of proprioception. The motor theory of speech perception presupposes that auditory discrimination of speech rests upon kinesthetic discrimination. Words assume sharp profiles, "faces," in auditory comprehension because motor speech and its motor feedback help to provide them. It is a process of analysis by synthesis in which the child makes use of his knowledge of the articulatory gestures that are involved in the production of speech.[38] As Bastian puts it, "The effective perception of linguistic events is based on much more than well-developed auditory discriminations. . . . The necessary extra ingredients for the perceptual processes arise from the fact that any really competent listener is also a competent speaker." [39] Stockwell calls it "a simultaneous encoding and matching process." [40] Auditory perception of speech also hinges upon memory, the retention of auditory patterns that have previously been laid down in the nervous system (3 above). Presumably the matching of current auditory patterns with past patterns is a major function of the continuous process of analysis by synthesis. Myerson discusses other variables operative in the auditory perception of speech (auding):

Hearing for speech is not a constant. It is not an inevitably fixed function resting completely upon simple physiological and sensory factors; it is a complex skill. Like other skills it is subject to learning and to improvement. It is certain that at various points the auditory apparatus sets physiological limits which cannot be exceeded or compensated for, just as the visual apparatus sets limits upon reading print and the musculature sets limits upon the speed of typewriting. There is no reason to believe, however, that the average individual approaches any closer to his physiological limits in hearing for speech than he does in other complex tasks such as reading or typing. Moreover, the possession of sensory capacities does not determine how these capacities may function in meaningful tasks or how effectively they may be used. . . . It is unlikely, therefore, that it will ever be possible to demonstrate an identity

[37] W. H. Fay, *Temporal sequence in the perception of speech*. The Hague: Mouton, 1966. P. 19.

[38] P. Lieberman, *Intonation, perception, and language*. Cambridge, Mass.: M. I. T., 1967. Pp. 162–170.

[39] J. Bastian, The biological background of man's languages. In C. Stuart, Ed., *Languages and linguistics: Monograph series 17*. Washington: Georgetown University Press, 1964. P. 144.

[40] R. Stockwell, Discussion. In E. C. Carterette, *op. cit.*, p. 203.

between a relatively simple sensory function such as hearing pure tones and the vastly more complex function of hearing speech.[41]

Auditory Perceptual System. In auditory perception we are concerned with every part of the auditory analyzing system from the cochlea to the cortex. Dysacusis (deficit in auditory recognition and discrimination) may stem from deficits or disturbances in the cochlea, in the acoustic nerve before it joins the CNS, or in other sectors of the brain stem and cortex. The chief sectors to which we shall pay attention are the cochlea, the direct classical lemniscal route, indirect reticular route, and cortical-subcortical bidirectional pathways.

Cochlea. Although the Organ of Corti in the cochlea may not be the most effective analyzer, it marks the beginning of analysis, particularly in the higher-frequency ranges of speech perception.[42] Preliminary organization of auditory information must begin in the cochlea (Figure 2-1) but the processing track will have many switches, radial tangents, and nuclear stations—and in defective states—dead-end spurs on its "run" to brainstem and cortical stations of perception. We assume that the peripheral auditory mechanism is intact and in good working order. Air pressure cycles will be picked up by the tympanum and the ossicular chain of the middle ear. They, in turn, will transmit the air pressure cycles intact via the basilar membrane to the hair cells, the sensitive receptive endings of the Organ of Corti. From the spiral ganglion encased in the modiolus emerges the axonal fiber bundle, the acoustic branch of the eighth cranial nerve. This branch contains both afferent (centrally directed) and efferent (peripherally directed) fibers, thus providing for immediate feedback control. In the cochlea a secondary acoustic correlate, frequency, probably undergoes initial analysis. The cochlea acts as a mechanical acoustic analyzer of some tonal characteristics of speech, particularly those of high frequency. It is mechanical in the sense that the position of maximum activity along the basilar membrane changes as a function of frequency. Pitch fluctuations, in common with variations in amplitude and duration, provide acoustic cues to the perception of stressed syllables and phrase boundaries.[43]

Direct Lemniscal Route. The great fiber bundle of the acoustic nerve will course through the internal auditory meatus and make its first synapses in the ventral and dorsal cochlear nuclei as it enters the medulla (Figure 2-1). At the point at which the nerve passes through the internal auditory meatus, impulses separated in a given fiber by time

[41] L. Myerson, *op. cit.*, p. 144.

[42] H. Davis, Peripheral coding of auditory information. In W. A. Rosenblith, Ed., *Sensory communication.* Cambridge, Mass.: M. I. T., 1961. Pp. 119–121. R. Granit, *Receptors and sensory perception.* New Haven: Yale, 1962. Pp. 294–295.

[43] P. Lieberman, *op. cit.*, pp. 44–47.

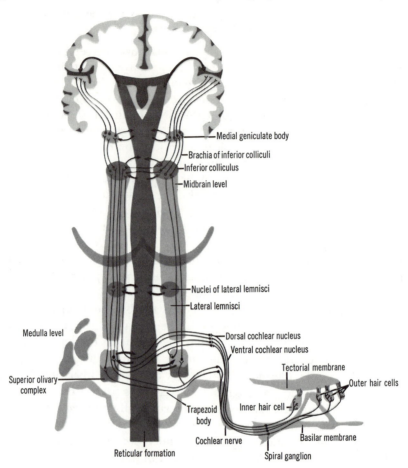

Figure 2-1.   Classical (lemniscal) and indirect routes of the cochlear
division of the VIIIth nerve.

SOURCE: Adapted from D. Myers, W. D. Schlosser, and R. A. Winchester, Otologic
diagnosis and treatment of deafness. *Clin Sympos,* 14: 39, 1962, published by CIBA
Pharmaceutical Company. Used by permission.

intervals of at least 1 msec. have been recorded.[44] The majority of the
fibers will cross the median line in the trapezoid body and course upward
in the lateral lemniscus, making collateral connections at every opportunity in the brainstem and the geniculate bodies of the thalamus.
Finally these impulses, organized into patterns and synchronized with
auditory patterns from the reticular route and with other sensory

[44] H. Davis, Peripheral coding of auditory information. In W. A. Rosenblith,
Ed., *Sensory communication.* Cambridge, Mass.: M. I. T., 1961. Pp. 119–121.

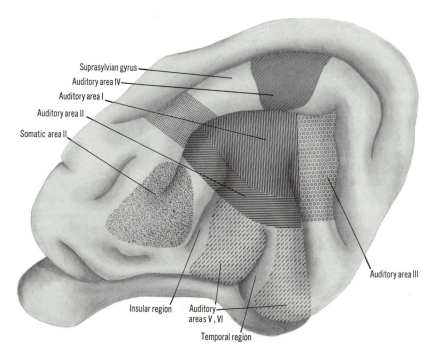

Suprasylvian gyrus
Auditory area IV
Auditory area I
Auditory area II
Somatic area II
Auditory area III
Insular region
Auditory areas V, VI
Temporal region

Figure 2-2. Diagrammatic sketch of some auditory perceptual fields of cerebral cortex.

SOURCE: Adapted from W. D. Neff, Discriminatory capacity of different divisions of the auditory system. In M. A. B. Brazier, Ed., *Brain and behavior*, Vol. I. Washington, D. C.: Amer. Inst. Biol. Sci. Used by permission.

patterns mediating speech perception, will synapse with nuclear assemblies in cortex and subcortex (Figure 2-2).

Indirect Reticular Route. As the afferent fibers of the cochlear tract course centralward, they send fibers into the reticular complex which synapse with nuclear areas in the brainstem (Figures 2-1; 2-3). All the nuclei making up the indirect auditory route are not known. Nuclei of the olivary tracts, inferior colliculi, reticular and thalamic nuclei, and possibly the medial geniculate bodies belong to the indirect, reticular route. Electrical responses to auditory stimuli in the reticular system indicate that many processes of facilitation, inhibition, and modification occur here. Selective tuning operates chiefly by suppressing the excitatory effects of certain acoustic patterns. When one considers the great amount of traffic which moves over this track, the reticular channeling of auditory impulses becomes a very important route.

Cortical and Subcortical Pathways. Bidirectional pathways from the cortex and subcortex have exerted constant influence over developing

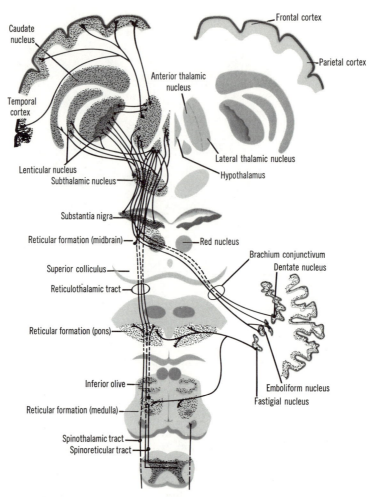

Figure 2-3.   Diagram of ascending pathways showing their
connections with reticular system.

SOURCE: A. Brodal, Some data and perspectives on the anatomy of the so-called "extra-pyramidal system." *Acta Neurol Scand*, 39 (4): 27, 1963. Copenhagen: Munksgaard Press. Used by permission.

auditory patterns through functional connections with both direct and indirect routes (Figure 2-4). We cannot say that final coding begins in the cortex. Much emphasis now is being placed on subcortical mechanisms of learning and it could well be that final coding has a subcortical rather than a cortical genesis.[45] Even after temporal-spatial patterns have been subjected to cortical activity, further modification in

[45] H. Magoun, *The waking brain.* Springfield, Ill.: Charles C Thomas, 1963. Pp. 116–126.

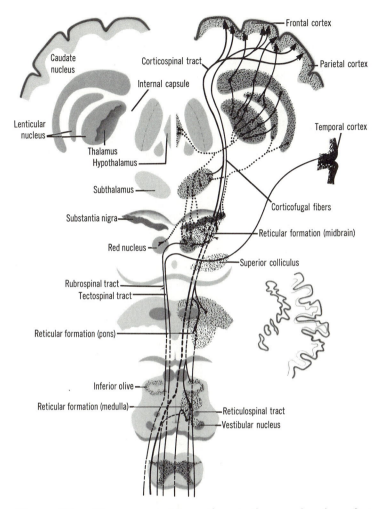

Figure 2-4. Diagram of descending pathways showing their connections with reticular system.

SOURCE: A. Brodal, Some data and perspectives on the anatomy of the so-called "extra-pyramidal system." *Acta Neurol Scand*, 39 (4): 23, 1963. Copenhagen: Munksgaard Press. Used by permission.

subcortical networks may take place.[46] The chief subcortical areas possessing rich auditory connections with cortical fields are the striate bodies, thalamus, and geniculate bodies of the metathalamus. Their bidirec-

[46] Penfield and Roberts suggest that sensory areas of the cerebral cortex are way stations in the current of afferent neuronal impulses. From the cortex they may pass inward again to the higher brainstem where final reorganization of sensory material takes place.—W. Penfield and L. Roberts, *Speech and brain mechanisms.* Princeton, N. J.: Princeton, 1959. P. 26f.

tional fiber bundles converge in several areas of the cortex, notably in temporal and parietal regions (Figure 2-2).

Phases of Auditory Coding of Speech. Auditory perception of speech, as we have said earlier, is not a stepwise phenomenon but a continuous modulation as a function of time. Time is the measure in such complex neural events as frequency variations, duration of input signals, periodicity of neural excitation, segmentation of the stream of speech into elements, identification and match of elements, and in the production of speech patterns.[47] The arbitrary division of coding into phases may be somewhat chimerical, a kind of convenient abstraction. It is useful in the sense that specific neural activity can be matched with the temporal phase.

Phase 1. Activation of neurones requires (1) a chemical mediator responsible for the specific sensitivity of the end organs, and (2) generator potentials to transform the change in end organs into a form of energy capable of discharging the nerve terminals. In the Organ of Corti mechanical pressure on its hair cells fires the chemical catalyst. It, in turn, incites a potential of sufficient magnitude to initiate impulses in a rhythmic flow in the acoustic nerve. The modification of these impulses by feedback probably begins immediately in the cochlea and continues throughout the brainstem and cortex. A few tracts conceivably could bypass the lower stages and carry as much temporal detail as the nervous system can retain all the way to the cerebral cortex. The usual pattern, however, is a cyclic process in which constant erosion occurs from the millisecond the stimulation is received in the cochlea until the response of perception is made.[48]

What is coded in the first phase is hypothetical. Possibly the stream of impulses is partially differentiated in terms of fundamental frequency, amplitude, and duration. Some impulses may diminish in strength or fade out in this phase either because the generator potential is insufficient to maintain a flow of impulses required for the formation of a rhythmic pattern or because feedback has inhibited them from entering central channels.

Phase 2. Modification and discrimination of the auditory pattern continues as the wave pattern makes connections with the ventral and dorsal cochlear nuclei, inferior colliculi, medial geniculate body, and other nuclear assemblies along the lemniscal or direct auditory route (Figure 2-1).

The indirect route via the reticular system may be even more important in organizing and focusing the perceptive field of audition since interconnections are rich and multisensory convergences abound in this

[47] Fay, *op. cit.*, pp. 13–24.
[48] W. K. Livingston, F. P. Haugen, and J. W. Brookhart, Functional organization of the CNS. *Neurology* (Minneap) (July 1954), 4: 485–496.

system.[49] Many circuits embracing nuclear masses in the brainstem and cortex send information to the reticular system. Within the reticular networks several events have been postulated. Waves similar in frequency, amplitude, and duration may be joined through facilitation at synaptic junctions. Inhibitory processes in the same millisecond may hold up or prevent other impulses from entering the channel. Waves mediating visual and tactile-kinesthetic patterns may converge upon the auditory pattern. One effect of intermodal organization in this phase may be the synthesis of pitch, amplitude, and duration so that intonational patterns now emerge and are recognizable. This critical stage in interpreting auditory information depends heavily upon the temporal resolving power of the nervous system, i.e., its ability to resolve time patterns, and in this phase to resolve them in terms of basic intonation patterns.[50] Since the perception of intonation contours is aided by the breath group employed in speech, motor patterns of speech also must enter the coding process.[51] Success in this phase will depend, in large part, on power at synaptic junctions and on interconnection patterns within the reticular system (p. 71).

Phase 3. Bearing in mind the continuous nature of coding, we suggest nonetheless certain neural events that may occur in the third phase in order to further perceptual processes of audition. The rostral reticular system, thalamus, and cortex probably combine forces over numerous bidirectional pathways. Gastaut believes that the thalamo-cortical pathways, which he calls the "rostral-reticular stem," are of particular importance in differentiating between two sets of neural events that differ only in temporal patterning.[52] In order to make such a differentiation between time patterns Neff postulates a short-term memory (between a fraction of a second and a few seconds) to be essential.[53] Specific cortical fields undoubtedly are alerted and sensitized by the reticular system (Figure 2-2), and emotional reinforcement via the limbic system is simultaneously activated.[54] As a result, wave fronts cours-

[49] Neurones making up the reticular network are multisensory or plurivalent, i.e., they are not specific for one modality. The same cell may fire in response to visual, auditory, or somatic stimuli.—A. Fessard, The role of neuronal networks in sensory communication within the brain. In W. A. Rosenblith, Ed., *Sensory communication.* Cambridge, Mass.: M. I. T., 1961. Pp. 588–599.

[50] P. Lieberman, *Intonation, perception, and language.* Cambridge, Mass.: M. I. T., 1967. Pp. 48–107. H-L. Teuber, Summation. In M. A. B. Brazier, Ed., *Brain and Behavior I.* Washington: Am. Inst. Biol. Sci., 1961. Pp. 393–417.

[51] Lieberman, *op. cit.,* pp. 41–47.

[52] H. Gastaut, The neurophysiological basis of conditioned reflexes and behavior. In G. Wolstenholme and C. O'Connor, Eds., *Neurological basis of behavior.* Boston: Little, Brown, 1958. P. 265.

[53] W. D. Neff, Neural mechanisms of auditory discrimination. In W. A. Rosenblith, Ed., *Sensory communication.* Cambridge, Mass.: M. I. T., 1961. P. 274.

[54] J. C. Eccles, *The neurophysiological basis of mind.* London: Oxford, 1953. P. 274f.

ing through dendritic-glial layers in the sensitized areas of cortex and sub-cortex are able to impose their temporal-spatial patterns upon patterns similar in form and derived from earlier inputs. In this phase of analysis by synthesis, the determinant is again the temporal resolving power to order and sequence syllables, words, phrases, and the sentence. Perception is approaching completion.

To what extent intercortical activity is necessary in coding verbal symbols we do not know (p. 41). From her study of audition, Milner hypothesizes that "auditory functions are more diffusely represented in the right than the left hemisphere." [55] A recent report throws additional doubt on man's need for "two brains." An adult patient was subjected to complete left hemispherectomy, his natively dominant hemisphere. Immediately upon his recovery from surgery it was noted by his physicians that he was able to follow simple oral commands, and "tests showed normal hearing in both ears at 250 to 2000 Hz in each ear." After completing further tests fourteen months later, they conclude:

> Since language functions are not destroyed, and since speaking, reading, writing, and understanding language show continuing improvement in E. C. after left hemispherectomy, the right hemisphere apparently contributes to all these functions, although in varying proportions. . . . Perhaps the right hemisphere has the capacity to amplify previously small contributions to these functions.[56]

As has been suggested in an earlier chapter (p. 45), children endowed with functional plasticity probably employ areas in both hemispheres in learning a language. As maturation proceeds the essential circuits are clustered in the left hemisphere even in left-handed persons. Presumably one can build up the neural patterning of language in the minor hemisphere in the event of injury or insult to the major hemisphere.

We have presented a molar view of the way in which auditory information may be handled in the nervous system. The view encompasses feedback loops extending from cochlea to the cortex and from cortex to cochlea, thus forming cyclic rings of activity.[57] It is predicated upon a multiplicity of modal and intermodal connections embracing sensory-motor, visual, and auditory circuits in brainstem and cortex. Finally it is dependent upon the activation of similar neural patterns derived from earlier input.

[55] B. Milner, Laterality effects in audition. In V. Mountcastle, Ed., *Inter-hemispheric relations and cerebral dominance.* Baltimore: Johns Hopkins, 1962. Pp. 187–188.

[56] A. Smith and C. W. Burklund, Dominant hemispherectomy: Preliminary report on neuropsychological sequelae. *Science* (September 9, 1966), 153: 1281–1282.

[57] For a more complete discussion of auditory feedback, see p. 94.

Auditory Imperception and Language Disorders

Deficits in Peripheral Coding. Coding may be interrupted initially in the cochlea, either by a defective analyzer within the Organ of Corti or by distorted feedback from the brainstem.[58] Children with language deficits frequently experience much greater fluctuation in tone reception than normal children, although reports of two studies of this problem are contradictory.[59] Neither study dealt specifically, however, with the perception of the speech continuum. In one study fluctuation of tone was used; in the other, W-22 word lists. The total *complex* of acoustic events determines "speech hearing," not tones or single words, and this they did not assess.

In an EEG study of audition an impaired set-to-attend mechanism was found to be a cause of threshold fluctuation in auditory perception. Spong and coworkers tried various experimental situations in which auditory (and visual) stimuli were presented. They found that the magnitude of the response, measured electronically, always varied "according to whether or not the subject is attending to stimuli in that or another modality." [60] The amplitude of the cortical-evoked responses varied with the attention set of the subject. When a "vigilance condition" was established, it was by far the most successful of the three experimental conditions. Probably when we have the proper means of measurement, and when we know what we should be measuring, we will find that in some groups of linguistically handicapped children interruptions and distortions of auditory perception of the speech continuum are caused mainly by impairment of the set-to-attend mechanism.

The peripheral analysis of sound may be defective in another way. If the cochlear mechanism receives and transmits distorted cues to the CNS, these cues will not be coded properly when they reach the main analyzing circuits. Perhaps the child may be taught to interpret these inadequate, imperfect cues. Certainly he will not be able to learn them without special training.

Deficits in Central Coding. Auditory impulses may start out well; they may reach the ventral and dorsal cochlear nuclei in the brainstem before they encounter synaptic junctions so weak in potential or neuronal assemblies so sparse in number that they can proceed no further in the organization of temporal-spatial patterns. The impulses may reach subcortical or even cortical fields. They are imperfect, stunted patterns. A

[58] T. T. S. Ingram, Developmental disorders of speech in childhood. *Brain* (September 1959), 82: 450–467.

[59] J. Reichstein and J. Rosenstein, Differential diagnosis of auditory deficits. *Exceptional Child* (October 1964), 31: 64–82. H. A. Grey, M. J. D'Asaro, and M. Sklar, Auditory perceptual thresholds in brain-injured children. *J Speech Hearing Res* (March 1965), 8: 49–57.

[60] H. Spong, R. Haider, and D. B. Lindsley, Selective attentiveness and cortical evoked responses to visual and auditory stimuli. *Science* (April 17, 1965), 48: 397.

failure at synaptic junctions may be caused by genetic defects, injury, or general retrogression associated with aging.

Another central deficit is associated with *timing.* The temporal factor is exceedingly important in auditory perception. Auditory symbols must be perceived within a time interval that varies slightly among children. A delay of milliseconds at this stage of perception can distort verbal meaning. A plausible cause is that the activator and organizer of the sequence, the reticular system, is defective. A slight alteration in the time sequences (rhythmic patterns) can place the auditory cycle out of phase with other auditory cycles and with neural circuits of other modalities that also are contributing in this split second to the perceptual pattern. The resultant pattern may be distorted or excluded from final coding. If the distorted auditory cycles are passed along, they cannot easily be imposed upon earlier temporal-spatial patterns already activated in cortical and subcortical circuits.

Ineffective gating also produces perceptual distortion in many children. Integrative systems have limited capacity, and if the traffic is excessive the mechanism of facilitation and inhibition (operated through feedback control) may break down. If it is an inherently weak mechanism it may break with only a modicum of sensory traffic. With the aid of a built-in monitor, both direct and indirect auditory systems in normal states are able to facilitate or inhibit impulses. They will shut out those auditory impulses that do not contribute to the specific percept, delay slightly, or speed the arrival of others in order to bring all impulses in proper phase relations. But if the integrative mechanism itself is weak, if certain wave patterns are late in arriving, or if gating is so ineffective in the peripheral receptors that the traffic load in the reticular complex is overwhelming, then we may expect a breakdown. Auditory perception is seriously disturbed. We have observed linguistically disturbed children who apparently are trying to cope with a welter of unprocessed sensations and ungoverned circuits. Their nervous systems receive "busy signals" at every turn. They have no lines open for reception of the relevant auditory signals. They cannot order their sensory world. They grasp at cues but they are often the wrong ones. The limbic system probably has its own organizing potential and may make some contribution to discrimination of sound sequences. We alluded earlier to inhibitor-selectors influencing receptor end organs of the cochlea. Ganglionic clusters outside the nervous system also may fail to eliminate impulses that are aberrant (i.e., they have varying temporal-spatial patterns) and hence disturb normal patterning.

Deficits in Terminal Coding. Deficit or injury of crucial cortical fields of audition may cause profound interference in auditory perception. Konorski believes that auditory memory of verbal symbols is a specific effect of lesions in the anterior and Sylvian gyri.[61] Since we cannot support the concept of areas for memory storage (see p. 107), we suggest that the more basic destruction involves auditory discrimination, of which memory is adjunct.[62]

One must be constantly reminded that a cortical lesion is rarely discrete in its effect upon such a dimension as auditory perception. A lesion in the superior temporal gyrus, for instance, will have its effect on many networks *functionally* connected with the site. Through the loss in feedback control, it can affect the cochlear analyzers, the reticular and limbic systems, the specialized corticofugal and thalamocortical pathways. Since cell assemblies in the posterior deep masses of temporal and parietal lobes also contribute significantly to final auditory discrimination, they too could be affected by a lesion in the superior temporal gyrus.

The Reticular Activating-Adapting System

Because relatively recent research has brought the reticular system out of limbo and put it in an orbit of great importance, it demands a consideration that long established systems do not require. The existence of a reticular core in the brainstem has been recognized for a century, but as its name implies, it was simply a kind of reticule to which was assigned nebulous properties of association or transfer. Now with the advent of electrophysiologic techniques, it has assumed an important role in both centrally and peripherally directed neural activity. Moruzzi and Magoun describe the system as a "cephalically directed brain-stem system, apparently consisting of reticular relays ascending to the basal diencephalon and further to the cortex where it was found to desynchronize the high-voltage slow waves and create a pattern of low voltage, high frequency activity, the so-called arousal reaction." [63]

The concept of this system has been extended far beyond the function of arousal, although this remains one of its primary roles. It might be designated more accurately as an energizing and organizing system. It must act both as an augmentor and inhibitor of impulses coursing via conventional tracts through the nervous system. Through its direct influence over brainstem and cortical function, it insures efficient opera-

[61] J. Konorski, The physiological approach to the problem of recent memory. In J. F. Delafresnaye, Ed., *Brain mechanisms and learning.* Oxford: Blackwell, 1961. P. 129.

[62] W. D. Neff, Discriminatory capacity of different divisions of the auditory system. In M. A. B. Brazier, Ed., *Brain and behavior I.* Washington: Amer. Inst. Biol. Sci., 1961. Pp. 222–223.

[63] G. Moruzzi and H. W. Magoun, Brain stem reticular formation and activation of the EEG. *Electroenceph Clin Neurophysiol* (November 1949), 1: 455–473.

tion. It possesses, in short, the potentialities which Coghill attributed to the fundamental dynamics of coordination [64] (Figures 2-3 and 2-4).

Reticular Structure. In 1932, a time when almost no attention had been paid to the reticular formation by óther scientists, W. F. Allen presented an excellent morphological description of the reticular formation and suggested its functions. Allen said, "It is known from embryology that most of the left-over cells of the brain stem and spinal cord which are not concerned in the formation of motor root nuclei and purely sensory relay nuclei are utilized in the production of the *formatio reticularis*. This is a very old structure phylogenetically. It is but little differentiated in the lower vertebrates, where it apparently serves as an effective mechanism which enables these animals to adapt themselves properly to their various inside and outside conditions. In the higher vertebrates there is but little reticular formation in the spinal cord, but considerable in both the medial and lateral portions of the medulla, pons, and midbrain, where for the most part it exists anatomically in its original undifferentiated state. The reticular formation surrounds or partially surrounds the sensory nuclei of the thalamus, and when considered phylogenetically the nucleus ruber, substantia nigra, and other differentiated hypothalamic and midbrain nuclei should probably be considered as specialized derivatives." [65]

The reticular system now is thought to be represented by all those neuronal structures from the basal nuclei (striate bodies) into the medulla which are not included in the classical afferent-efferent pathways.[66] Its nuclear masses and pathways are found throughout the entire central core of the neuraxis and have intimate connections with the cerebellum and the cerebral cortex (Figures 2-3, 2-4). They are characterized by diffuse aggregations of cells of different types and sizes, and separated by a reticule of fibers traveling in all directions.[67]

The fibers of this system pursue a course largely independent of the traditional sensory-motor pathways, passing over a different route even from the thalamus to the cortex.[68] Sectors of the reticular system that purvey sensory-motor information are sometimes called indirect routes. The indirect auditory pathway, for example, does not run with the classical auditory route via the lateral lemniscus. All major, centrally di-

[64] R. Granit, *Receptors and sensory perception.* New Haven: Yale, 1962. P. 91.
[65] W. F. Allen, *Formatio reticularis* and reticulospinal tracts, their visceral functions and possible relationships to tonicity and clonic contraction. *J Washington Acad Sci* (Seattle) (October 1932), 22: 490–495.
[66] H. Jasper, Reticular-cortical systems and theories. In H. F. Harlow and C. N. Woolsey, Eds., *Biological and Biochemical Bases of Behavior.* Madison: The University of Wisconsin Press, 1958. P. 39.
[67] A. Brodal, *The reticular formation of the brain stem.* Springfield, Ill.: Charles C Thomas, 1958. P. 2.
[68] D. F. Lindsley and W. R. Adey, Availability of peripheral input to the midbrain reticular formation. *Exp Neurol* (October 1961), 4: 358–376.

rected routes, however, send collaterals to the reticular system and hence have an intimate connection with it. The arousal properties of the system may be mediated by collateral connections from the direct primary sensory route (lemniscal paths) which turn into the ascending reticular system in the brainstem.[69]

The functional difference in the two systems has been described by Livingston: "The traditional sensory routes seem to represent the route by which highly specific information can reach the cortex in the shortest possible time," whereas "the second route through the reticular formation seems to represent a much more plastic and diffuse system in which the input from many different sources can be *integrated* and *modulated* before it reaches the cortex as a whole." [70] Lindsley presents some evidence to support this difference in sensory processing. He found that when the indirect system was put out of commission by barbiturates, cortical areas apparently still received information via the direct system, but the cortex could not discriminate or decode the messages.[71] Direct and indirect motor routes have been described in much the same way: "The influences which play on the motor horn cells can reach them by the direct, rapidly-conducting and relatively specific pyramidal route or by the slower-conducting, more diffuse pathway through the striatum and the reticular formation." [72]

Functions of the Reticular System. So numerous and diverse are the functions ascribed to the reticular system that several neurophysiologists have predicted the abdication of the cortex. Sir Geoffrey Jefferson entertained such dire possibilities in his remarks at an international symposium: The reticular formation has turned

into a system which, like a big flourishing and expanding business, has bought up all its competitors. . . . I have watched parts of the cerebellar function disappear into the reticular system—and there are some indications that the sympathetic nervous system, too, is in danger of a merger, perhaps only as a subsidiary.[73]

We do not anticipate such a gloomy future for the cortex. The nature of its traffic will be described in different terms—that is all. The reticular system is important; and cogent to our concern in language learning are its activities associated with arousal and drive-setting mechanisms,

[69] H. W. Magoun, Non-specific brain mechanisms. In H. Harlow and C. N. Woolsey, Eds., *Biological and biochemical bases of behavior*. Madison: The University of Wisconsin Press, 1958. P. 26.

[70] W. K. Livingston, F. P. Haugen, and J. M. Brookhart, Functional organization of the central nervous system. *Neurology* (Minneap) (July 1954), 4: 495.

[71] D. B. Lindsley, The reticular system and perceptual discrimination. In H. Jasper, *et al.*, Eds., *Reticular formation of the brain*. Boston: Little, Brown, 1958. P. 517.

[72] Livingston, *et al.*, *op. cit.*, p. 491.

[73] G. Jefferson, The reticular formation and clinical neurology. In H. H. Jasper, *et al.*, Eds., *Reticular formation of the brain*. Boston: Little, Brown, 1958. P. 729.

facilitation and inhibition, differentiated phasic movements, voluntary motor activity, and perception. We shall postulate its functions in language learning in some detail.

Alerting Function. In order to sensitize certain cortical fields to respond to stimuli significant to them, to prepare them, as it were, for the arrival of sensory-motor patterns, impulses from the reticular-cortical complex presumably desynchronize the high voltage, slow waves of the alpha pattern and impose a pattern of low voltage, high-frequency activity in cortical areas.[74] These "fields of influence" are surrounded by areas whose thresholds in the same millisecond have been raised. In other words, the reticular system has sensitized specific cortical areas to the reception of certain temporal-spatial wave patterns and at the same time, has prevented noncritical assemblies from exhibiting responses of attention.[75] The "alerter" also may exclude or interrupt certain impulses when others of greater importance to the individual enter the internuncial pool in the reticular formation. In this process the feedback mechanism that began its modification of the sensory impulses at input is of vital assistance (p. 91).

The alerting mechanism of the reticular system is a neurological correlate of attention. This mechanism, Hebb says, provides "the immediate facilitation from one phase sequence or assembly action (of neurones) to the ensuing one. . . . This is the way the reticular system bids the individual 'to attend.' " [76] How the reticular system establishes priority of attention among stimuli is a moot question. Galambos, *et al.*, have made interesting observations on priority with respect to auditory stimuli in animals. They state that "the neural processes responsible for attention play an important role in determining whether or not a given acoustic stimulus proves adequate." [77] Apparently auditory response to sound is secondary to visual-visceral stimuli in importance to some animals. Attention of a cat, for example, to a stimulus of prime importance (mice in a glass jar) resulted in complete inhibition of the auditory response to the sound. Competing stimuli were much stronger and hence commanded the cat's attention. According to Galambos attention may be so powerful that the reticular system will exclude the incoming signal at the peripheral or pickup point of sensory input, or at several points after it has entered the central nervous system. Unless conditioning is deeply set and motivation extraordinarily keen, sensations from the viscera will take precedence over such sensory modalities

[74] Moruzzi and Magoun, *op. cit.*, pp. 455–473.

[75] H. W. Magoun, *The waking brain.* Springfield, Ill.: Charles C Thomas, 1963. Pp. 103–105. H. H. Jasper, Ascending activities of the reticular system. In H. H. Jasper, *et al.*, Eds., *Reticular formation of the brain.* Boston: Little, Brown, 1958. Pp. 320–321.

[76] D. O. Hebb, *The organization of behavior.* New York: Wiley, 1949. P. 152f.

[77] R. Galambos, Suppression of auditory nerve activity by stimulation of efferent fibers to cochlea. *J Neurophysiol* (September 1956), 19: 424–437.

as vision, audition, proprioception, and taction. But if visceral stimuli are held in abeyance, then vision probably will take precedence over audition, proprioception, and taction, providing the intensity of the competing stimuli is equal, or nearly so. The auditory potential, for example, will be reduced or ablated in favor of the visual potential. Lindsley concludes that "the very essence of attention and consciousness now seems to reside in shifting processes and states within the central nervous system, some of which are detectable through changes in electrical potentials recorded . . . directly and focally in certain regions of the brain." [78]

Linguistically handicapped children quite regularly exhibit behavior that may be caused by disturbance of the reticular mechanism controlling attention. The inability of certain groups of children to attend and to make selective responses is the concern of all who teach in the field of special education. One is aware, for example, of the mental retardate's lack of set-to-attend. He cannot prepare to receive the information because he cannot habituate himself readily to insignificant, irrelevant stimuli. Intense and repeated stimulation may heighten synaptic power momentarily. In that short span he does attend. Gordon, an adult aphasic with whom we have worked, experiences diurnal shifts in attention. On Monday Gordon is very receptive to language retraining. He is alert and attends strictly to the problem at hand. He corrects his own mistakes in grammar, his errors in identification of phrases; he notes his failure to catch quickly the total significance of a passage and discusses it. Gordon returns for his second session on Wednesday, but on this day he learns little. He is listless, withdrawn. We resort to dictation. He asks us to repeat again and again. Finally he shakes his head and gives up. Why, you ask. We know that fatigue, stress, depression undoubtedly have a deleterious effect on the nervous system, and particularly on the synaptic potentials in the adapter-organizing sectors. Possibly he may surmount these diurnal changes through a process of habituation. One hopes that he can be taught not to respond to certain sounds but to be highly responsive to other combinations of sound. And having established these sound combinations by repeated exercise of the circuits, he may have learned another lesson in language.

Facilitation and Inhibition. Exactly *how* the reticular system effects a synchrony, an harmonious pattern, we can only postulate on the basis of current research. Much must be accomplished by facilitation and inhibition (gating, p. 36). The system certainly possesses all the capacities for selection, modification, and organization. One sensory modality has a potential connection either directly or indirectly with every other

[78] D. B. Lindsley, *Attention, consciousness, sleep and wakefulness.* In J. Field, *et al.,* Eds., *Handbook of physiology; 1: Neurophysiology,* vol. III. Washington: Amer. Physiol. Soc., 1960. Pp. 1554-1555.

sensory modality within the reticular system. Presumably it controls the elaboration or reduction of impulses from both routes, the direct route into the primary cortical receiving zones and the indirect reticular route. In order to bring the incoming impulses into proper spatial-temporal relationships, the reticular system must reset the excitability cycles of many neuronal assemblies so that they can be fitted into a matrix of sustained excitatory or inhibitory patterns held in the reticular formation and the dendritic meshwork of the cortex. The process of continuous modulation of the pattern will be carried on by intracortical and transcortical networks. Repeated activation of the reticulocortical networks increases synaptic efficiency throughout the neuronal assemblies.[79] The final form of the pattern begins to emerge as figure upon ground.

Whether facilitation or inhibition is the stronger agent in the reticular organizing process we do not know. Probably inhibition pulls the longer oar. The reticular system is a main thoroughfare to the cortex and consequently is loaded with sensory traffic. In producing coordination and interaction among impulses, the reticular monitor necessarily must be busy eliminating or restricting impulses that do not contribute effectively to the total pattern of perception. The suppression of these impulses apparently can take place at any point. Galambos has demonstrated by electrogenic means that stimulation of the olivocochlear efferent bundle on the floor of the medulla suppresses the activity of the auditory nerve.[80] The olivocochlear pathway probably belongs to the reticular complex and through a "special system of centrifugally conducting dorsal root fibers" (feedback circuit) it is capable of conditioning the auditory nerve endings. Others have reported a thalamocortical ring of inhibition within the reticular system. Stimulation can be incited in this ring by a loop of fibers from the rhinencephalon and caudate nucleus (basal nucleus) or by loops from the medulla and pons. Such stimulation incites low-frequency excitation that synchronizes the EEG pattern and so blocks higher sensory and motor action. The consequent total effect, the internal inhibition of higher nervous activity, is the opposite of the activating mechanism of the reticular system. It establishes "a learning not to respond," and this becomes a significant factor in discrimination.

Reticular facilitation and inhibition can best be described, perhaps, by observing their breakdown in children with deficits or injuries of the nervous system. Afferent patterns cannot be discriminated or organized. One hypothesizes that the major networks are battered by an army of disorganized impulses and excitability cycles which bear no spatial and, what is more important, no temporal relation to each other. The alpha

[79] Eccles, *op. cit.*, p. 227.
[80] R. Galambos, Suppression of auditory nerve activity by stimulation of efferent fibers to cochlea. *J. Neurophysiol* (September 1956), 19: 424–437.

rhythm runs on but superimposed on it are strange, nonrhythmic spikes of electrical activity. Disintegrating emotional states also pervade the CNS without inhibition.

In many children in this group the alerting mechanism operates, perhaps too well, but the reticular system is not selective. It cannot inhibit those sensory-motor patterns which are not useful to the present behavioral response. These children may try to shunt into the background sensations deleterious to perception and learning, but they rarely are successful. The sluice gates are open. They overreact to class bells; the light is too bright; the room too warm. On a higher level they experience even greater difficulty. "I try," one says, "but I cannot see what you see in that picture." Another complains, "I always seem to fall over the very thing I am trying to avoid." "I get that tune mixed up with other songs I know," yet another says. We presume that reticular networks, or the cortex in conjunction with the reticulum, cannot suppress aberrant impulses, step up necessary potentials, and modulate still others. The effect in speech perception may be likened to visual perception in a fog. Words, phrases have no faces; they do not emerge as clear figures upon a ground.[81]

Control of Phasic Movement. Closely allied to the sensory functions of the reticular system is the regulation of such motor aspects of behavior as phasic movement, muscle tone, and righting reactions. These impairments, sensory-motor in origin, can be observed in cerebral palsy. In severe cases, excitations flow in uninhibited fashion until tonic contraction has virtually paralyzed, for instance, the movement of the articulators in speech. The fine gradations of tension and relaxation which one sees normally in posture and movement are gone. The system responds nonselectively; all stimuli apparently share "equal time and force." A frequent accompaniment to these manifestations is a lack of control of the righting reflexes. As the cerebral-palsied child develops, his head and neck assume bizarre positions. Voluntary effort to control them only results in more extreme responses. Little wonder that the athetoid exclaims, "But the harder I try to relax, the more tense I become."

Injury to the motor cortex has been the classical etiological explanation of cerebral palsy. This explanation is being supplanted by etiologies that include other sectors of the nervous system. The reticular system is one sector. In some types of cerebral palsy, undoubtedly this system, not the motor cortex, has suffered primal insult. A. A. Ward states that the efferent functions of the reticular formation encompass the basic substrates of all motor activity. "In higher forms, it is thus directly responsible for postural reflexes and righting reactions, and plays a critical

[81] D. F. Lindsley and W. R. Adey, Availability of peripheral input to the midbrain reticular formation. *Exp Neurol* (October 1961), 4: 358–376.

role in phasic movement and in maintenance of muscle tone." Ward goes on to show that the reticular formation also mediates the general static reactions, which include the tonic neck reflexes and the tonic labyrinthine reflexes.[82]

Voluntary Motor Activity. The reticular system also must be concerned with the efficient projection of voluntary motor impulses. The gamma-spindle cells are generally considered to be self-regulators of muscle activity. We must recognize, however, the power of the reticular system to impose its regulation on the gamma-spindle in the interest of expert muscle coordination, and especially in complex muscle activities.[83] The articulation of speech is a complex activity. It demands a satisfactory range, level, and duration of tonic attack which must extend beyond the requisites of single sounds or syllables. In the rapid fire of the speech continuum, is the gamma-efferent, reticular control able to effect smooth coordination? Or is the whole synergy out of tune? Perhaps speech characterized by an "awkward tongue," "slightly spastic tongue," or cluttering is the result of a breakdown in reticular controls over voluntary motor activities.

The explicit nature of control of corticoreticular loops has been demonstrated in experimentally produced lesions of the reticular system. Impulses initiated by the primary motor neurones in the cortex travel as usual in the pyramidal tract *but* they do not result in contraction. Some neurologists believe that what has been lost is the ability to *initiate* motor movement. Since muscles do not respond singly but in patterned synergies, motor impulses probably cannot be started because they cannot be organized into synergies without the help of the reticular system. In this connection one remembers the muscular rigidity characteristic of the Parkinson syndrome. Rigidity, *per se,* however, is not the central problem in speech. The greater handicap is the inability to initiate organized movement patterns of the jaw and tongue. This disability could result from the deterioration of corticofugal circuits connecting cortex, basal nuclei, and the reticular formation.[84] The rigidity of Parkinsonism may be likened to that of the cerebral-palsied child or the stutterer who also is unable to initiate movement patterns of the speech organs.

The control of the reticular system over respiratory rhythms has been well established. These activities are additional proof of its contribution toward homeostasis, the establishment of an internal milieu which permits the motor functions of the body to operate smoothly and *tout d'une pièce.*

[82] A. A. Ward, Efferent functions of the reticular formation. In H. H. Jasper, *et al.,* Eds., *Reticular Formation of the Brain.* Boston: Little, Brown, 1958. Pp. 263–264.
[83] Granit, *op. cit.,* pp. 244, 268.
[84] A. Brodal and B. R. Kaada, Cutaneous and proprioceptive impulses in the pyramidal tract of the cat. *Acta Physiol Scand* (August, 1953), 29: 131–132.

Summary. We have presented current theories of structure and function of the reticular system and have related its function to the comprehension and use of language. Future research may modify aspects of its activity. Its place as a prime alerter and integrator of the nervous system, we believe, is well established.

In recapitulation, the reticular system assists discrimination (perception) and motor response in this way: It has alerted the cortex, sensitizing certain "fields of influence" and decreasing the potential of adjacent areas. By determining the rate (frequency code) and patterning of nerve impulses, it brings those of a kind into a space relation and shunts to particular areas certain "packets" of information. In order to effect this organization and direction, it must shut out extraneous impulses, increase the potential of faint but significant impulses, modulate slightly the form of some temporal patterns, and thus bring the whole complex of sensory-motor circuits into a meaningful whole. It assists, in short, in the coding of all varieties of integration, including perception, learning, and motor response. It is solely or largely responsible for the "development and maintenance of a dynamically ordered economy of behavioral response and adjustment." [85]

The Limbic System

In 1878 Broca named the large cerebral convolution surrounding the brainstem the limbic lobe, assigned olfaction to it, and thereby halted all investigation for more than a half-century (Figure 2-5). Until 1937 when Papez presented the results of his research on limbic structures in a paper entitled, "A proposed mechanism of emotion," [86] this cerebral lobe was still called the "olfactory brain." As an outgrowth of researches by Papez, Adey, and others, functions in addition to olfaction-gustation have been ascribed to the limbic system.

Structures and Connections. The limbic system is called a functionally integrated system; certainly it is not a structural unit. Presumably such substructures of the cortex as the hippocampal gyrus lying in the posterior horn of the lateral ventricle and the adjacent nuclear masses in the hypothalamus belong to the limbic system. Considerable support also has been found for the inclusion of thalamic nuclei and the basal section of the frontal-temporal cortex in the limbic complex. As the diagrammatic sketch indicates (Figure 2-5), all these nuclear structures are located in the basal portion of the cerebrum. Their axons are bidirec-

---

[85] D. B. Lindsley, Physiological psychology. In P. Farnsworth, Ed., *Ann Rev Psychol* (1956), 7: 324–348.

[86] J. W. Papez, A proposed mechanism of emotion. *Arch Neurol* (Chicago) (October 1937), 38: 725–744.

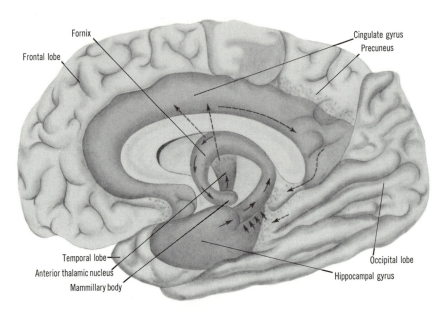

Figure 2-5. Diagrammatic sketch of limbic areas mediating effective behavior.

SOURCE: P. D. MacLean, Psychosomatic disease and the "visceral brain": Recent developments bearing on the Papez theory of emotion. *Psychosom Med*, 11:338–353, 1949.

tional and have synaptic junction with fibers of the cortex, basal nuclei, and thalamus (Figures 2-3 and 2-4). The wealth of fiber connections within the limbic system and with cortex and adjacent nuclear bodies suggests a general reinforcement of many aspects of learning.

Functions. The control of metabolism by the limbic system will not be considered, although the link between extreme emotional states and hunger or thirst, for example, is well known. Limiting our discussion to its role in higher learning we may say that the limbic system operates in three areas: (1) emotional reinforcement and motivation, (2) recent memory, and (3) mastery of purposive motor response (Figure 2-6). Memory and purposive motor patterning, however, might well be assisted by emotional dynamics and therefore be subject to indirect mediation by the limbic system.

The dominant effect of limbic activity on learning patterns is a general emotional coloration, a pervasive reinforcement. Excitation of the hippocampus either by electrical stimulation or by the presentation of haptic, auditory, and visual stimuli, for example, will elicit trains of rhythmically recurring potentials which persist well beyond the dura-

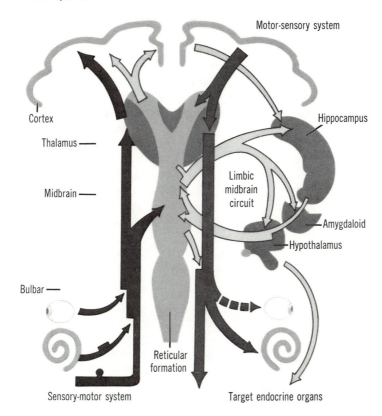

*Figure 2-6. Simplified anatomical plan of neural connections
involved in learning.*

SOURCE: R. Galambos and C. T. Morgan, The neural basis of learning. In J. Field,
Ed., *Handbook of physiology, sec. I: Neurophysiology*, Vol. III. Washington, D. C.:
Amer. Physiol. Soc., 1960. Used by permission.

tion of stimulation and will outlast the rapid activity of the neocortex.[87]
Protein metabolism during such a period is sometimes higher than that of
the cortex. Possibly this response is the biological counterpart of the
effects of emotional resurgence often experienced in learning situations.
At what point does emotional facilitation by the limbic system become
great enough to stimulate learning; at what point does it paralyze
thought? The level of emotional control may lie in the gating power of
the reticular system (p. 71). The two systems, midbrain reticular and
limbic, must be related for they exhibit the same spontaneous rhythms
and appear to function in a similar way. Adey suggests that the limbic

[87] P. D. MacLean, Psychosomatics. In J. Field, Ed., *Handbook of physiology,
sec. 1: Neurophysiology III*. Washington: Amer. Physiol. Soc., 1960). P. 1738.

impulses may act as a phase-comparator mechanism, altering the patterns in a phase relation in order to facilitate or inhibit elements of the code.[88]

Recent memory, it has been postulated, may be disturbed by interference specifically with limbic areas in the deep masses of the frontotemporal lobes.[89] Milner in her study of impaired recall of verbal material also assigns the impairment to these areas.[90] The question is whether these tracts contribute specifically to the retention of what has been learned or whether they are instrumental in sharpening the focus of the pattern by emotional reinforcement so that once the pattern is laid down, it will be retained. Similarly the third contribution of the limbic system, *viz.*, to planned motor expression would seem also to be one effect of a more basic function, the facilitation of learning by emotional reinforcement.[91] It is reasonable to assume that since its fibers join thalamocortical, midbrain reticular, and striocortical circuits, it shares their responsibility in integrating specific spatio-temporal patterns useful to the purposive behavior of the individual at the moment. Emotional reinforcement often is the crucial catalyst in establishing learning.

Cortical and Subcortical Adapting-Projecting Systems

Review of Neural Concepts. Again we are making an arbitrary division when we attempt to separate brainstem adapting-projecting systems from cortical and subcortical systems (Figures 2-3, 2-4). If coding is a continuous process they are a single system. No sector of the coding process can be autonomous or independent (Figure 2-6). At this juncture we turn to bidirectional cortical and subcortical circuits engaged in the final stages of coding motor speech. Their function may best be understood by reviewing some cornerstones supporting our concept of the neural processing of oral language.

1. Traditional pathways called motor (pyramidal) and sensory (auditory, visual, haptic) are comprised both of afferent and efferent fibers (p. 29). The efferent sections of the motor-sensory or pyramidal pathway originate not only in precentral gyri of the frontal lobe but also in adjacent areas of the frontal and parietal cortices (Figure 3-1).[92]

[88] W. R. Adey, Brain mechanisms and the learning process. *Fed Proc* (July 1961), 20(2; part 1): 617–627.

[89] Adey, *ibid.*, p. 625.

[90] B. Milner, Laterality effects in audition. In V. Mountcastle, Ed., *Interhemispheric relations and cerebral dominance.* Baltimore: Johns Hopkins, 1962. P. 179.

[91] W. R. Adey, Studies of hippocampal electrical activity during approach learning. In J. F. Delafresnaye, Ed., *Brain mechanisms and learning.* Oxford: Blackwell, 1961. P. 585.

[92] A. Brodal, Some data and perspectives on the anatomy of the so-called "extrapyramidal system." *Acta Neurol Scand* (Copenhagen) (1963), Supplementum 4, 39: 2–49. C. N. Woolsey, Organization of sensory and motor areas. In H. F. Harlow and

The axones of the giant pyramidal cells in the precentral gyrus actually contribute only three percent of the fibers of the pyramidal tract.[93] Incorporated into sensory-motor fields are the old "extrapyramidal" area and other motor areas in the parietal and temporal lobes. They have been designated as primary sensory-motor areas.[94]

2. The classical sensory fields of the cortex must be extended to include other fields particularly in the posterior temporal and parietal sections of the cortex (Figure 2-3).

3. Cortical areas are functionally efficient only in connection with other structures. The functional *unit,* of which Broca's area is one component, is made up of other cortical structures (connected by transcortical fibers) and also of subcortical structures.[95] The interruption of linguistic comprehension-expression may be caused by the impairment of sensory-motor and transcortical systems whose final synaptic junctions lie in cortical and subcortical structures.

4. No cortical association areas have been established upon which pathways from sensory sectors converge, and from which neural events will be spewed out via motor pathways (Figures 2-3 and 2-4).[96] Since all sensory-motor pathways are subject to uninterrupted feedback control, integration (association) is presumed to be continuous throughout coding. The high point of cortical integration does not seem to center in the traditional association areas of the frontal lobe but in temporal-parietal fields where countless sensory-motor patterns converge. Lesions in these fields produce greater intellectual deficits than lesions in the traditional frontal areas.[97]

5. Both cerebral hemispheres undoubtedly contribute to sensory-motor discrimination of oral language, but circuits mediating certain aspects of verbal discrimination may not be equally represented in the same hemisphere. In older children and adults areas of maximal activity in discrimination and expression generally will be found in one hemisphere. Presumably in the first years of life the higher nervous integration of the human brain has not been fixed by use, and the so-called functional

C. N. Woolsey, Eds., *Biological and chemical foundations of behavior.* Madison: The University of Wisconsin Press, 1958. Pp. 69–74.

[93] J. Paillard, The patterning of skilled movements. In J. Field, Ed., *Handbook of physiology; sec. 1: Neurophysiology III.* Washington: Amer. Physiol. Soc., 1960. P. 1687.

[94] C. N. Woolsey, Cortical localization as defined by evoked potential and electrical stimulation studies. In G. Schaltenbrand and C. N. Woolsey, Eds., *Cerebral localization and organization.* Madison: The University of Wisconsin Press, 1964. Pp. 18–32.

[95] P. Bucy, Discussion, In G. Schaltenbrand and C. N. Woolsey, Eds., *Cerebral localization and organization.* Madison: The University of Wisconsin Press, 1964. P. 13.

[96] K. Pribram, Neocortical function in behavior. In H. F. Harlow and C. N. Woolsey, Eds., *Biological and biochemical foundations of behavior.* Madison: The University of Wisconsin Press, 1958. P. 158.

[97] M. Piercy, The effects of cerebral lesions on intellectual function: A review of current research trends. *Brit J Psychiat* (May 1964), 110: 310–352.

plasticity is still very marked. Laterality, as demonstrated by handedness, may not be regularly associated with the dominance of either hemisphere. Although cerebral ambilaterality may assist those who have had a cerebral injury to recover speech, it probably is a hindrance to children in such learning activities as speech and reading.

6. The very complex motor performance of oral expression is not the result of "more and more detailed patterns of neuronal pathways to individual muscles" but of an increasing complexity of many sectors of the coding mechanism coordinating groups of muscles into great synergic patterns.[98] Visual, haptic, auditory, and somatic patterns contribute to the *act* of oral expression. Indeed, if we are to understand the *act* of oral expression we shall have to follow Paillard's direction: "In our ascending search for the origins of patterning of motor commands, we are thus led to leave the fields of motor integration and to draw progressively nearer the field of sensory integration." [99] Feedback from cortical circuits subserving these modalities may extend only to the thalamus, to the reticulum, or they may go all the way to visual, auditory, and gamma fibers in the muscle spindle.[100] The cerebellum also receives many kinds of information from cortical circuits pertaining to movement patterns and also returns information by way of the reticular system to assist the cortex in motor patterning (Figures 2-3, 2-4). It has been demonstrated that thalamocortical bidirectional pathways enter actively into motor expression. Broca's area has clear and manifold connections with sensory-motor fields in frontal, temporal, and parietal regions. But Broca's area does not comprise the "speech area." It contains no patterns of language "but only patterns of how to make vocal organs utter words," and it probably is but one of several areas concerned with this function. It cannot be called an independent area in the projection of propositional speech.[101]

7. Although we are considering at this point the *act* of oral expression we must emphasize that this is but one type of response. The *act* of perception is a response just as is the response of inner language (p. 125). And even in the act of oral expression we have found nothing to suggest where perception might end and motor processes begin.[102]

Adaptation-Projection in Motor Speech. If these concepts are valid,

[98] D. Denny-Brown, *The basal ganglia.* London: Oxford, 1963. P. 129.

[99] J. Paillard, The patterning of skilled movements. In J. Field, Ed., *Handbook of physiology, sec. 1: Neurophysiology III.* Washington: Amer. Physiol. Soc., 1960. P. 1692.

[100] M. A. B. Brazier, The electrical activity of the nervous system. *Science* (December 11, 1964), 146: 1427.

[101] E. A. V. Busch, Discussion. In G. Schaltenbrand and C. N. Woolsey, Eds., *Cerebral localization and organization.* Madison: The University of Wisconsin Press, 1964. P. 56.

[102] R. W. Sperry, Neurology and the mind-brain problem. In R. Isaacson, Ed., *Basic readings in neuropsychology.* New York: Harper & Row, 1964. P. 415.

motor expression is a circular phenomenon. Adaptive and projectional tracts are not unidirectional because feedback proceeds in both directions. The CNS does not project up or down, or for that matter, horizontally or vertically. In our view there is no single point at which an impulse ceases to travel *toward* the cortex or is projected *from* the cortex. Patterned impulses are contained in circle networks, providing interchanges for ingress and egress but at no point on the circle can we say, "Here motor expression begins." In this circle, the sensory-motor cortical fields, from which primary effectors join the circle, may be thought of as "funnels of convergence" for the stream of impulses that have gone into the making of the motor pattern.

In Penfield's view, this volitional stream of impulses impinging on the precentral gyrus does not arise cortically since neither removal of the area anterior to the precentral gyrus nor ablation of the postcentral gyrus can entirely abolish skilled movements. Penfield looks to the centre encephalic system of the brain stem as initiating a stream of willed impulses capable of producing the action that is appropriate to all previously received information. . . . Walshe has also directed attention to the possible subcortical origin of these streams of controlling impulses, stating that "the human pyramidal system of itself initiates nothing," and to speak of it as responsible for this or that category of movements is to ignore the source and motive power of its activities.[103]

The patterned activity represented finally in the act of oral expression is that of groups of muscles organized in a synergy of sequential activity. In a sense the sequences may not rightly be differentiated from the postural changes from which they emerged.[104]

Language Impairment and Adapting-Projecting Systems. We have presented evidence to show that the response in speech is an integral part of the entire coding process, and hence intake cannot be separated from output. In the preceding sections in this chapter we have described specific language disturbances that might be caused by an initial deficit or malfunction of the peripheral receptive system subserving language, or of the reticular or limbic systems. It goes almost without saying that the malfunction, wherever it begins, will be experienced in the entire circuit. Since the "higher" adaptive-projection systems belong to the circuit, they too will be affected adversely. In this sense, all the examples of language disorders we have given may be thought of as the result of impairment of several circuits of the nervous system subserving function. We are particularly aware of neural disorganization when the

[103] C. Terzuolo and W. R. Adey, Sensorimotor cortical activities. In J. Field, Ed., *Handbook of physiology, sec. 1: Neurophysiology II.* Washington: Amer. Physiol. Soc., 1959. P. 825.

[104] Postural reactions are a part of a motor act inasmuch as all movement is a modification of basic postural response.—D. Denny-Brown, The general principles of motor integration. In J. Field, Ed., *Handbook of physiology, section 1: Neurophysiology II.* Washington: Amer. Physiol. Soc., 1959. Pp. 781–795.

cortical and subcortical networks are not functioning properly in the comprehension-expression of language. As was true in other systems we have considered, the failure may be occasioned either by a functional interruption at synaptic junctions or by a damage to one or several nuclear assemblies in the circuit.[105] In either case, the electrochemical upset at synaptic junctions affects the entire potential of all circuits sub-serving language. A patent example of proprioceptive distortion occurs in cerebral-palsied speech. Interrupted or impaired feedback loops of sensory-motor fields of the cortex and subcortex may distort the response of perception of language and the motor patterning of the speech organs. The distortions sometimes produce a veritable explosion of muscular adjustments in tongue, lips, and jaw in the cerebral-palsied. Failures in muscle gradation and sequence shifts of movement produce grotesque gyrations instead of skilled patterned movement. Although an adult aphasic may have a "discrete" cortical lesion, it undoubtedly affects the potential of a wide field of neural circuits. The lack of synaptic potential is apparent in the failure to synthesize patterns in discrimination. Paul, the victim of such a "discrete" lesion at 45 years of age, describes the living room furniture as individual, unrelated items. He goes from chair to sofa to lamp to a second lamp and to a third lamp. When the clinician bids him speak of all the lamps in the room, he says, "Well you see one lamp and two lamp and three lamp." He can make no generalization be-cause he cannot fuse these "flicker patterns" of visual discrimination. We have tried to help him to focus and stabilize the discrimination pattern by fusing it with other patterns. So far we have had only a modicum of success.

[105] A. Brodal, Some data and perspectives on the anatomy of the so-called "extrapyramidal system." *Acta Neurol Scand* (1963), Supplementum 4, 39: 31.

3

Operational Mechanisms

In this chapter we shall describe certain operational mechanisms of the nervous system which are basic to language learning. Undoubtedly other mechanisms will be added as the study of neural patterning of language continues. The operational mechanisms included in this discussion are homeostasis, the set-to-attend, feedback, coding, and fixation.

Homeostasis (Controlled Lability)

In notes of a class lecture by W. B. Cannon, homeostasis is defined as the regulated balancing of nervous and endocrine factors in the organism in order to preserve an internal steady state.[1] Cannon developed and modified the concept of inner stability which Claude Bernard earlier had called, *la fixité du milieu intérieur.*[2] In Cannon's view, however, stability is not fixed; it is labile. A homeostat is stable only so long as it maintains an adaptively modifiable equilibrium. The central nervous and endocrine systems act as master homeostats exercising control over minor homeostats—respiratory, thermal, vascular, and lymphatic—which assist in the maintenance of physiological equilibrium. All homeostats, master and subordinate, will make self-adjustments by means of error-detecting and error-correcting devices of feedback.

Homeostatic Control in Speech. Learning a language demands much of a plastic nervous system so its homeostatic overseers must be

[1] Notes taken by the writer at Harvard University, 1934.
[2] W. B. Cannon, *The wisdom of the body.* New York: Norton, 1939.

on constant alert. They must be sensitive to such factors as traffic load, potential strength of neural circuits, efficacy of feedback, and the diverse components to be patterned. In every case homeostatic controls will be governed by the relation of the neural events to the total behavior of the individual.[3] Normally the *milieu intérieur* will not be disturbed by unexpected events of a certain magnitude. In motor speech, for example, a considerable margin of safety may be exercised before homeostatic controls are taxed. Note the adaptations that one must make in respiration, phonation, resonation, and articulation for speech, yet equilibrium normally is maintained. Study of a single aspect, respiration, reveals that it is markedly different from the patterns of quiet breathing. The number of breaths per minute is sharply reduced. Inspiration is shorter and more shallow than expiration. The normal CO_2/O_2 balance regulating quiet respiration is upset. Electrical activities of inspiratory muscles may continue through part of the expiratory phase. Despite all these modifications of breathing for speech the individual normally is able to tolerate them without adverse effect. Homeostasis operates. A cerebral-palsied child whose homeostasis is impaired, on the other hand, complains frequently of dizziness during speech production.

The agent or agents that act to effect a stable neural lability have not been fully substantiated. Pribram believes that the reticular system is the "bias wheel," the major homeostatic control (p. 71).[4] Undoubtedly the limbic system (p. 79) and other neural-endocrine mechanisms contribute to the operative principle of controlled lability.

Defective Homeostasis and Language Learning. In the normal process of learning a language we presume that the systems of neural-endocrine control are in a state of stable lability. The central regulators, reticular and limbic systems, are set at an optimum, at the level of equilibrium. The child is set-to-attend, to learn. Homeostatic controls, however, vary greatly both because of genetic and adventitious factors. Some children from birth are not able to achieve an operative biological equilibrium. The physical organism succumbs to every ill wind; the constitution is a frail reed, indeed. The higher functions of the nervous system show a similar failure in adaptation. In the actuation of synergies of excitation and inhibition, of attention and motivation, the neural and hormonal machinery seems weak, ineffective, out of gear. It cannot produce a state of stable lability.

[3] P. Hernandez-Peon, H. Scherrer, and M. Jouvet, Modification of electrical activity in cochlear nucleus during "attention" in unanesthetized cats. *Science* (February 24, 1956), 123: 331–332. R. Galambos, Suppression of auditory activity by stimulation of efferent fibers to cochlea. *J Neurophysiol* (September 1956), 19: 424–437. R. Galambos, G. Sheatz, and V. G. Vernier, Electro-physiological correlates of a conditioned response in cats. *Science* (March 2, 1956), 123: 376–377.

[4] K. Pribram, Control systems and behavior. In M. A. B. Brazier, Ed., *Brain and behavior*. Washington: Amer. Inst. Biol. Sci., 1963, 11: 376.

In another group of children physicochemical events have conspired to upset homeostasis. Disease or trauma has left its effect, sometimes only a subtle effect, upon learning. Feedback triggering the neurocouple of the reticular system may have broken down either partially or completely. It is no longer sensitive to the changing milieu and hence does not contribute effectively to stability. The limbic system may attempt to stabilize the emotional matrix and if the events are of short duration, occasionally it may be successful. In such an unstable and uncontrolled state of "free energy," auditory, visual, and tactile-kinesthetic streams of impulses course through the nervous system but it is unable to organize them into temporospatial patterns of perception. Sometimes such an individual attempts to block certain impulses from entering the CNS. A child of 10 years who had suffered serious cortical injury in an accident found that he was more successful in the first stages of relearning language when all stimuli except auditory impulses were eliminated. As he proceeded, however, he discovered that language was imprinted more effectively in terms of recall when tactile-kinesthetic and visual modalities were linked with auditory impulses.

Set-to-Attend Mechanism

Neurological Bases. In discussing alpha wave activity of the cortex (p. 40), we alluded to its interruption as a signal of arousal of the cortex. Attention develops in the child as alpha wave frequency increases. In a 4-month-old baby, the wave has a frequency of 3–4 Hz; at 1 year the rhythm has increased to 5–6 Hz; by the age of 12 years, it has reached the adult frequency of 10–12 Hz.[5] The neurological events producing an excitatory focus (attention) in specific cortical and subcortical fields probably follow this sequence: (1) interruption of electronic waves of many sectors of the CNS, resulting in increased potential in these sectors, (2) inhibition or blockade of certain sensory receptors (visceral and somatic), and (3) a decrease in synaptic potential of neural assemblies surrounding the excitatory foci. "All systems are go;" we attend. Modification of the spontaneous or resting rhythm of the reticular system prior to alteration of cortical electrical activity suggests that the reticular system, not the cortex, instigates attention.[6] The reticulum also may contribute indirectly to the focus of attention by preventing the intrusion at the cortical level of information irrelevant to the task.[7]

[5] Lord Brain does not believe that the alpha rhythm of the adult is reached before the thirteenth year.—R. Brain, *Recent advances in neurology and psychiatry.* Boston: Little, Brown, 1962. Pp. 180–182. Others set maturation at 10 years.
[6] H. W. Magoun, *The waking brain.* Springfield, Ill.: Charles C Thomas, 1963. P. 188. M. Harder, S. Spong, and D. B. Lindsley, Attention, vigilance and cortical evoked-potentials in humans. *Science* (July 10, 1964), 145: 180–182.
[7] H. W. Magoun, *op. cit.*, pp. 103–104.

Other sources of feedback control via the classical primary route undoubtedly contribute to the attention-setting mechanism. Presynaptic inhibition, Eccles says, is entirely inhibitory.[8] In the classical experiment of simultaneous stimulation of two modalities in the cat, Hernandez-Peon found that cochlear potentials in response to sound were completely suppressed at the presynaptic level when more demanding retinal stimuli occurred.[9] Brazier emphasizes the importance of cortical contribution to the attention-setting mechanism through inhibition of activity in areas surrounding the main focus of excitation. Sensitized or aroused cortical fields normally exercise inhibition on surrounding areas.[10] Certain neural tracts in conjunction with endocrine activity also influence the set-to-attend mechanism either directly or indirectly. The limbic-thalamic tracts that receive fibers from the hypothalamus are instrumental in emotional reinforcement of attention. Marits and Denisenko, in independent contributions, describe the intimate connection of the reticular system with the endocrine system in attention setting. Marits stresses the tonic effect of thyroxin on the reticular formation which, in turn, intensifies the set-to-attend in cortical areas.[11] Denisenko finds that the reticular formation contains both cholinoreactive and adrenoreactive biochemical elements which ensure indirectly the activation and "attention" of the cortex.[12] The role of the reticular system in attention-setting is described in greater detail in the section devoted to this system (pp. 71–79).

Set-to-Attend and Language Impairment. The ability to exclude irrelevant stimuli from the field of attention is basic to language learning, or to any form of learning. In the individual with language disturbances, these blockades of certain receptors and enhancement of others often are absent. It is supposed that afferent and corticofugal influences interact in the reticular system and result either in interference or facilitation. If the interaction is moderate, it could lead to facilitation but if the bombardment is excessive, complete blocking may result, thus upsetting attention and awareness. The CNS which ordinarily integrates only those impulses concerned with the object of attention—a limited amount of information at best—now has been flooded with

[8] J. C. Eccles, Inhibitory controls on the flow of sensory information in the nervous system. In R. W. Gerard and J. W. Duyff, Eds., *Information processing in the nervous system III*. Amsterdam: Excerpta Medica Fdtn., 1964. P. 28.

[9] P. Hernandez-Peon, *et al., op. cit.*

[10] M. A. B. Brazier, The electrical activity of the nervous system. *Science* (December 11, 1964), 146: 1427.

[11] A. M. Marits, The relationship between reticular formation tone and the endocrine function of the thyroid gland. *Fiziol Zh SSSR Sechenov* (October 1961), 47: 1235–1240.

[12] P. P. Denisenko, Participation of the cholinergic and adrenergic reactive systems of the reticular formation of the midbrain in activation reaction of the cerebral cortex. *Fiziol Zh SSSR Sechenov* (October 1961), 47: 551–558.

disparate sensory bits. Like the operator of a traffic control system at a great airport, he has too much information to handle simultaneously so that he either reacts to an unimportant signal or he is frozen in a position of inactivity. The gating of incoming patterns of information is controlled jointly by indirect reticular and direct cortical brainstem networks (p. 36). Presumably the reticular system has lost its power to inhibit impulses not useful to the present behavioral response, or electrical activity around the cortical field of influence, which ordinarily declines with an increase in potential in the sensitized area, now exhibits increased activity. The cerebral-palsied child often tries to surmount this problem by shunting into the background sensations that are deleterious. Occasionally he is successful.

The aging mind suffers from an additional problem in paying attention to language. Like the child with an injured nervous system, he also is unable to shut out, to block those auditory, tactile-kinesthetic, and visual stimuli which are not useful in comprehending the immediate verbal pattern. But something else acts to destroy his capacity to attend. His set-to-attend mechanisms are weak or unpracticed. He no longer charges his mind to attend. It is the disease of poor listening which has afflicted him. As a result perception is diffuse and retention poor.

Feedback Mechanism

Purpose. Attention has been refocused recently on the principle of feedback as it applies to self-regulatory mechanisms. Attention has come chiefly from cyberneticists who have employed feedback circuits in the development of a servomechanism or slave system. The dominant feature of this system is a controlling device which "recognizes" the discrepancy between the state of the machine at any given moment and the final purpose assigned to it by its constructor. The error-detecting device possesses a feedback circuit which enables it to send back to the servomotor controlling the output the information coming to the error-detecting device. We said that attention has been *refocused* because such a mechanism actually was recognized by Claude Bernard (1865) when he enunciated the principle of homeostasis. Then in 1930 Cannon extended the idea of a calibrator of man's input to his own integrating machine.[13] Today the *feedback loop* has replaced the reflex arc as the functional unit of the nervous system (Figure 3-1).[14]

Feedback Loop. Since motor fibers have been found within the presumably sensory dorsal roots and sensory fibers have been found within the presumably motor roots (p. 82), the feedback loop must

[13] W. B. Cannon, *op. cit.,* pp. 268–286.
[14] J. M. Hunt, How children develop intellectually. *Children* (May–June 1964), 11: 83–91.

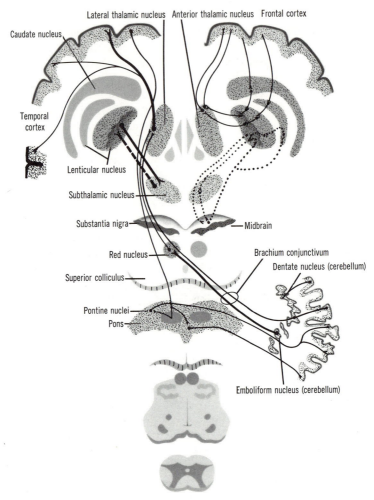

Caudate nucleus

Lateral thalamic nucleus Anterior thalamic nucleus Frontal cortex

Temporal cortex

Lenticular nucleus

Subthalamic nucleus

Substantia nigra

Red nucleus

Superior colliculus

Pontine nuclei

Pons

Midbrain

Brachium conjunctivum

Dentate nucleus (cerebellum)

Emboliform nucleus (cerebellum)

Figure 3-1. Diagram of four closed sensory-motor circuits.

SOURCE: Adapted from A. Brodal, Some data and perspectives on the anatomy of the so-called "extrapyramidal system." *Acta Neurol Scand*, 39 (4): 32, 1963. Copenhagen: Munksgaard Press. Used by permission.

operate as a sensory-motor unit. Very much like the thermostat or any apparatus operating with a compensator, the feedback mechanism in the central nervous system is able to control or monitor the input. It does so by setting the peripheral receptors through a central mechanism so that there is a special filtering, blocking, or acceleration of impulses proceeding to the cerebral cortex. Such a process must inevitably determine the quantitative and qualitative aspects of sensation. It makes possible a more refined analysis, not only by supplying information directed *to* the CNS, but also through centrifugal impulses in the feedback loops directed *from* the CNS to the peripheral organ. In Sniakin's words,

The higher analysis of external stimuli is not possible unless there is not only a flow of impulses from the receptor to the center, but also in the reverse direction to the receptor which seems to attune the latter to a certain level of sensitivity to stimulation.[15]

Fairbanks makes application of the servosystem and feedback to speech:

A servosystem . . . employs feedback of the output to the place of control, comparison of the output to the input, and such manipulation of the output-producing device as will cause the output to have the same functional form as the input. The system performs its task when, by these means, it produces an output that is equal to the input times a constant. . . . It seems evident that the speaking system has at least the rudiments of a servosystem.[16]

One should note the qualification made by Fairbanks, *viz.*, that input-output comparisons cause the output to have the *same functional form* as the input. Input and output are not matched, as they are in the thermostat of your house air conditioner. Indeed it is the business of feedback to impress modifications upon the coding process.

Although Brazier regards feedback as a very potent mechanism for introducing more information into the centrally directed pathways, she also believes that the feedback loops are instrumental in creating inhibitory surrounds for the excitatory cortical focus.

Control by descending systems modulating input have been identified for many sensory pathways as has the modulating influence of the ascending reticular system on the cortical response to a peripheral stimulus. In the somatic system a descending inhibitory action has been shown to act on the interneurone that lies between the incoming dorsal root fibers and the ascending fibers of the dorsal column in the spinal cord. There is strong evidence that this descending inhibitory influence may play a role in "editing" the flow of information by acting to suppress some of the input from the periphery of the receptive field and thereby producing an effective inhibitory surround to the main focus. Inhibitory surrounds to an excitatory focus have been demonstrated also in the retina, and evidence for centrifugal control of input has also been identified in the auditory system, the olfactory system, and in the efferent gamma fiber system innervating muscle spindles.[17]

Feedback Circuits and Language. All sensory-motor processes possess this mode of centrifugal control.[18] Feedback occurs at the level of the

[15] P. G. Sniakin, Central regulation of the activity of sensory systems. *Fiziol Zh SSSR Sechenov* (November 1961), 47: 1479–1487.

[16] G. Fairbanks, A theory of the speech mechanism as a servosystem. *J Speech Hearing Dis* (June 1954), 19: 135.

[17] M. A. B. Brazier, The electrical activity of the nervous system. *Science* (December 11, 1964), 146: 1427.

[18] Sensory and motor impulses should not be regarded as distinct processes inasmuch as no separation can be found between sensation and the motor end of the

receptor itself, at the first or second synapse, and in more centrally located stations along sensory-motor routes. The reticular system (p. 71) is one powerhouse of centrifugal control. In a sequential transaction such as speech, feedback determines the rate, precision, and progression of the response. Muscular coordination of the tongue, for example, is no better than its proprioceptive innervation. Feedback control in tongue movement modulates the emission of reticular-fugal and corticofugal impulses in a long loop; it is known as an *output-informed* feedback circuit. Other controls are made up of shorter loops connecting the motor cortex with the cerebellum or the reticular system. They do not include the peripheral output of the system, and hence may be called the *input-informed* circuits.

More familiar to the student of speech are the auditory feedback circuits which provide instant information to the CNS concerning the progress and bodily effects of the transmission of sound. The controller in the CNS, in turn, uses the information to direct subsequent speech and adjunctive activity. The cortex certainly enters into auditory feedback but the major job of calibration of centrifugal processes probably is accomplished by homeostats in the reticular system or in an axonal ring mechanism immediately subjacent to the nerve terminals in the cochlea. Galambos found that stimulation of the olivocochlear bundle on the floor of the medulla suppressed the activity of the auditory nerve.[19] The olivocochlear pathway belongs to the reticular complex, and through a "special system of centrifugally conducting dorsal root fibers" is capable of conditioning the auditory nerve endings. A receptor event, a speech syllable let us say, may be modified at any point from its reception to its expressive outlet. By the mechanism of feedback, events originating within the nervous system itself thus suppress, modify, or accelerate the sensory-motor operation.

In the learning of a complex function such as language, multiple feedback circuits are in operation. They must determine the priority, segregation, and integration of sensory-motor processes. Visual, tactile-kinesthetic, and auditory impulses must be conjoined and in the appropriate sequences with respect to time and space. Neuronal assemblies that mediate the retrieval of memory patterns of linguistic sequences, for example, may be suppressed or brought actively into the percept. Finally, if the muscle synergies are to be organized so that we "speak the speech" expertly, the feedback circuits governing the muscle spindles (gamma fibers) of the larynx, jaw, palate, tongue, and lips must operate in near-perfect synchrony. Else here we "miss or there exceed the mark." Feed-

process. See H-L. Teuber, Summation. In M. A. B. Brazier, Ed., *Brain and behavior, I.* Washington: Amer. Inst. Biol. Sci., 1961. Pp. 415–416.
   [19] R. Galambos, Suppression of auditory nerve activity by stimulation of efferent fibers to cochlea. *J Neurophysiol* (September 1956), 19: 424–437.

back begins at the periphery and operates throughout every phase of linguistic coding.

Feedback in Muscle Contraction. Feedback control also is present in all muscle spindles. Granit [20] found in the spindle special, large fibers with nuclear bag endings which responded to stretch. He called them gamma-efferent fibers. They represent a kind of loop control exerting an inhibitory effect upon the extensor muscles but an excitatory effect upon the opposed flexors. The control may be purely local at the level of the spinal reflex or it may be subject to a much more complex regulation by the reticular system. The effect in either case is to regulate proprioceptive input and, in this way, to "modify the alpha-motor discharge responsible for both the postural and phasic contraction of muscle." [21] Gamma-efferent fibers also are present in such fine intrinsic muscles as the tongue.

In the postural regulatory system, normal feedback "acts like time-continuous error-detecting devices that position the body in space by varying the output of the muscle to counteract changes in gravitational force." [22] Many cerebral-palsied children suffer from injury to this self-regulating system. There is little or no effective feedback regulation of the sequence of afferent impulses entering into posture possibly because the reticular system is out of commission. Sometimes the impairment produces a tonic postural response known as torticollis (deviation of head and neck to one side) with marked side effects upon speech. Ward postulates that

the lesions functionally denervate clusters of reticular cells in the rostral reticular formation. . . . Once denervated they become hypersensitive to acetylcholine liberated by neighboring cells of different function. Activation of the reticular formation by stress is then postulated to release sufficient acetylcholine to activate them, and the postural movement is accentuated.[23]

Two methods of control of righting responses are generally used: anticholinergic drugs and external conditioning of feedback. In the latter method external means are employed to establish certain basic body positions in space. Once the basic positions have been established, proprioceptive feedback loops will convey via the reticular-cerebellar complex the proper information for inhibiting postures. Speech then can be built upon acceptable motor patterning of the body.[24]

[20] R. Granit, *Receptors and sensory perception*. New Haven: Yale, 1962. Pp. 238–254.

[21] *Ibid.*, p. 276.

[22] J. Paillard, The patterning of skilled movements. In J. Field, Ed., *Handbook of physiology; sec. 1: Neurophysiology III*. Washington: Amer. Physiol. Soc., 1960. P. 1701f.

[23] A. A. Ward, Efferent functions of the reticular formation. In H. H. Jasper, et al, Eds., *Reticular formation of the brain*. Boston: Little, Brown, 1958. P. 265.

[24] K. Bobath and B. Bobath, A treatment of cerebral palsy, based on the analysis of the patient's motor behaviour. *Brit J Phys Med* (May 1952), 15: 1–11.

Less dramatic manifestations of distorted movement may disturb
oral expression. Ruch described a tremor that affects all voluntary movement and is caused by defective control of feedback loops in cortico-
cerebrellar or reticular-cerebellar pathways. He likens the tremor "to
the oscillation of an undamped servomechanism in which the feedback is
removed." [25]

Delayed Feedback. When time relations in coding verbal symbols
are disturbed by experimentally delayed auditory feedback the stable
milieu necessary for fluent speech and for the well-being of the individual usually is upset. Anyone who has subjected himself to this
laboratory experiment recognizes that his ongoing motor speech activity
has been altered in a way wholly unnatural. Sound pressure levels and
phonation duration are increased, repetitive errors occur; in short, the
temporal pattern of speech is completely disorganized.[26] Apparently we
learn speech in certain temporal relationships to hearing and perception
of our own sound sequences.[27] Is it possible that some children handicapped by neurological insult or deficit are unable to learn speech
because distortion in time, delayed feedback, is the modus operandi of
their nervous systems? We believe it is and suggest that feedback, not
from one but from several modalities employed in comprehension-use of
language, may be so delayed or so deficient in power that patterning in
brainstem and cortical organizers is completely decorrelated in the time
domain. As a consequence, organization and control of motor activity in
speech are seriously disturbed.

Precisely how great a delay in feedback may be incurred without
adverse effect we do not know. In experimental studies, the maximal
interference of speech occurs when feedback is delayed 180 msec.
(3/11 sec.).[28] Neither do we know exactly what aspects of perception
of oral language are mediated by auditory feedback, what aspects
by tactile-kinesthetic feedback. McCroskey concluded that auditory feedback was essential in monitoring duration and rate of speech, and tactile-
kinesthetic feedback was responsible for accuracy of articulation.[29]

[25] T. C. Ruch, Motor systems. In S. S. Stevens, Ed., *Handbook of experimental psychology.* New York: Wiley, 1951. P. 154.
[26] B. Milner, Brain mechanisms suggested by studies of temporal lobes. In F. L. Darley, Ed., *Brain mechanisms underlying speech and language.* New York: Grune & Stratton, 1967. Pp. 136–137. J. W. Black, Persistence of effects of delayed sidetone. *J Speech Hearing Dis* (March 1955), 20: 65–68. B. S. Lee, Artificial stutter. *J Speech Hearing Dis* (March 1951), 16: 53–55. R. A. Chase, S. Harvey, S. Standfast, and I. Rapin, Studies on sensory feedback: I. Effect of delayed auditory feedback on speech and keytapping. *Quart J Exp Psychol* (August 1961) (Part 3), 13: 141–152.
[27] C. Cherry, *On human communication.* New York: M. I. T. Press and Wiley, 1957. P. 294.
[28] J. W. Black, The effect of delayed side-tone upon vocal rate and intensity. *J Speech Hearing Dis* (March 1951), 16: 56–60.
[29] R. McCroskey, The relative contribution of auditory and tactile clues to certain aspects of speech. *Southern Speech J* (1958), 24(2): 84–90.

Coding Mechanism

Nature of Coding. Code is a new name for a very old concept—a concept as old as the pictographs in French caves or the stone inscriptions of the Hittites. In its present use it is as new as the binary-number pulses in a modern computing machine. Primitive man devised a code by which he could communicate his thoughts. Language, a system of symbols, a code, developed making possible the meeting of mind with mind. But the meeting is not a true contact. We can only cast our thoughts into symbols or signs and so communicate. William James once said, "It is the happy accident when we are understood," and a contemporary psychologist has reminded us that language is a danger to the individual because he becomes less able "to recognize and hence respond to important sense impressions." The result is that man's ambience is "a dream-like, loose-coupled reality." And Cohn asks finally, can language destroy its maker, Man, through imperfect communication? [30] We are not certain of the proper answer but we do not predict such dire consequences. Admittedly language is a poor vehicle, subject to all the ills that flesh is heir to, but until a speech synthesizer takes its place, man's mind must hobble along with its own language machine.

Unity of Coding Process. A code is "an agreed *transformation,* or set of unambiguous rules, whereby *messages* are converted from one representation to another." [31] The act and vehicle of transformation is called coding, and since the act is simultaneous, continuous, and inseparable, the division into *decoding* and *encoding* seems neurologically unsound. Feedback control is operative throughout the nervous system so the code must undergo constant modification from input until the final response. Response furthermore may not always be oral or written expression. The response may consist in the act of awareness or comprehension of meaning, of perception itself. It can be a response in inner language. On occasion it probably is only an internal emotional response. At other times the response does entail the transformation of the signal patterns into overt acts of the organism: writing, gesturing, speaking. Even in this last possibility, the code is continuously being altered or transformed by interpretation of data, both from the internal and external environment—by sensory data, stored and viable data of the CNS, and by constant modification through feedback of motor spindles. It would be more consistent with neurological principles to describe this process as one of coding and recoding all along the route in the CNS until one type of response is made.

Unity of the coding process is consistent with our knowledge of anatomical relations of the nervous system. We know that close topo-

[30] R. Cohn, Language and behavior. *Amer Sci* (March 1961), 49: 502–508.
[31] C. Cherry, *op. cit.,* p. 303.

graphical association and plurivalent or multimodal neurones of sensory-motor pathways preclude seriatim coding in nervous systems possessing homeostasis. And if it *were* possible, the chances are that seriatim coding would not result in a clear, complete percept—a response. A fusion of the temporal-spatial patterns of several modalities "engineered" in part by the reticular, limbic, and corticofugal pathways is one step in coding. Simple sequential mapping may be possible for physiological function but in gnostic spheres such as language, propositional programming involves continuous transformation of material from all neuronal assemblies and circuits, including those mediating memory storage.[32]

Unity of Coding and Neurological Function. Coding can best be explained in terms of neurological function if one conceives of it as a continuous process from input to output. If language learning is to be effective, the code must undergo continuous modification in analyzers of peripheral receptors, in primary sensory-motor trunk lines, multisensory convergences upon polyvalent neurones of reticular and limbic systems, in thalamo-strial-cortical bidirectional systems from integrative fields of cortex and subcortex, and in cortical projection tracts. In all these networks the process of coding must continue without a break. Where does one find in this process of decision-making a dividing point that marks the end of decoding and beginning of encoding? In pathological states there may be breaks, "disconnexion syndromes"; [33] in healthy states, coding, we believe, is an uninterrupted process.

Unity of Coding and Diagnostic Terminology. If coding is continuous we have meager scientific basis for such categorical divisions as *receptive* and *expressive* aphasia. Certainly no point marking the end of impression and beginning of expression has been determined by electronic investigations. On the contrary there is ample evidence that alterations of electric activity (by deficit or trauma) in one sector or subsystem is not discrete or self-contained. Their effects extend from peripheral analyzers to the final step in coding. In supporting this concept of the neurological integrity of communication, Macdonald Critchley said in his address to the International Congress in Neurology (1962), the terms, *motor* versus *sensory*, or *receptive* as opposed to *expressive* types of aphasia "have become just as vestigial as 'word deafness.' " [34] Hardy lends qualified support to this position when he says, "It is the intake-problems that are the major ones in all problems of children who do not normally, naturally, and readily learn language meanings and ulti-

[32] D. Denny-Brown, Cerebral dominance. In V. Mountcastle, Ed., *Interhemispheric relations and cerebral dominance.* Baltimore: Johns Hopkins, 1962. P. 252.
[33] N. Geschwind, Disconnexion syndromes in animals and man. *Brain* (June–September 1965), 88: 237–294; 585–644.
[34] M. Critchley, Aphasia at the 7th international congress in neurology. *Speech Path Ther* (London) (October 1962), 5: 53.

mately learn to talk." [35] Although Myklebust still uses the division of receptive and expressive aphasia, he concedes that "the involvements of the brain affecting areas for reception as contrasted with areas for expression, may be more basic to the total integration of experience." [36]

Some clinicians claim that adults suffer only from receptive aphasia, others only from expressive aphasia. A disturbance in electrical activity undoubtedly may affect certain networks more adversely than others but some measure of disability undoubtedly pervades the whole continuum of language comprehension and use. Feedback, for example, is a very sensitive thermostat and quickly becomes distorted, is delayed, or is intermittent in its control. Even the speech of a "normal" person becomes disturbed if he is compelled to listen to it after a short delay of 0.18–0.3 secs.[37] Those who have engaged in the laboratory experiment of speaking under conditions of delayed feedback know that input is as greatly disturbed as output.

In the child with a neurological developmental deficit the categorization of aphasia as receptive or expressive seems even less permissible. Lee, age 7 years, was referred to us with a diagnosis of receptive aphasia. His mother said frequently, "He seems to understand what I want him to do." Lee *does* understand very simple directions—if one uses many gestures and if one precedes directions with a demonstration. It is the understanding, however, of a child of 4 years, not 7. In studying and assessing his language behavior, comprehension and use were approximately equal. Both were seriously impaired. After a year of diagnostic teaching, both verbal understanding and speech have improved moderately. We know of no way to increase the competence of neural receptors and synaptic potentials, power of feedback controls, strength of synchronizing and segregating mechanisms, or the power and extent of cortical fields of influence and facility of motor outlets except through motivation, stimulation, and exercise in an environment conducive to learning. As comprehension improves, we expect verbal expression to improve.

Unity of Coding and Paradigms. Although Wepman and colleagues endorse current neurophysiological principles at the beginning of their provocative article, "Studies in Aphasia," [38] their paradigm of cognitive and perceptual levels seems to us to represent a return to theories of mechanical transmission of impulses and of functional divisions for which the neurologist finds no structural correlate. Clear-cut divisions

[35] W. G. Hardy, Differences in language disorders of children and adults. In H. G. Burr, Ed., *The Aphasic Adult.* Charlottesville, Va.: Wayside, 1964. P. 19.

[36] H. R. Myklebust, Psychoneurological learning disorders. *J Ontario Speech Hearing Assn* (January 1962), p. 4.

[37] R. Brain, *Speech disorders.* Washington, Butterworths, 1961. Pp. 56–57.

[38] J. Wepman, L. Jones, R. Bock, and D. Van Pelt, Studies in aphasia: Background and theoretical formulations. *J Speech Hearing Dis* (November 1960), 25: 323–332.

of input, integration, and output are made in the construct. Integration in this scheme is the exclusive function of the cortex, whereas the organization of a frequency code, the basis of sensory discrimination, and integration of incoming messages, is generally thought to be a continuous process from input to output.[39] As Lenneberg puts it, "We may be fairly certain that physiological processes of pattern perception are not confined to horizontal activity at the level of the cerebral cortex." [40] If feedback control (also included in the paradigm) is a constant modifier of the code, integration could scarcely be limited to a single level of the nervous system. Discrimination of auditory patterns in speech, for example, begins in the Organ of Corti; they may still be modified by feedback as one verbalizes.[41]

Stages of Coding. Exploration goes on in the heavy thickets of neurology, and yet many aspects of the coding mechanism have not been discovered. We do know that the nervous system has many signals to read, and probably the most important are those conveying the time and rhythmic (time-space) patterning of impulses. Here one must reckon both with short time spans and long time spans. In the former, frequency is determined by the time interval over which intervals between firing are averaged. Long time spans are the result of staggered firings from different patterns of stimulation of afferents and hence must employ both space and time. They are, in other words, rhythmic patterns.[42]

Initial Stage. The initial form of time-space patterns will be determined largely by the frequency, locus, and duration of firing of nerve cells. Their firing characteristics vary widely so some meshworks of cells will respond to stimuli more effectively than others. The hair cells in the Organ of Corti, for example, are an extremely effective mechanism for the transduction of pressure changes into electrochemical codes.[43] Yet some electrochemical codes initiated in the hair cells may not get off the launching pad because they have been suppressed by presynaptic inhibition. Perhaps this is the way rudimentary cochlear analysis takes place.

Intermediate Stage. Let us assume that a battery of impulses has arrived in Neurone Assembly A, ventral and dorsal cochlear nuclei in the

[39] J. Wepman, General discussion. In *Proceedings of the institute of childhood aphasia.* San Francisco: Calif. Soc. for Crippled Children and Adults (September 19, 1960). P. 44. R. Granit, *op. cit.,* pp. 277–302.

[40] E. H. Lenneberg, *Biological foundations of language.* New York: Wiley, 1967. P. 212.

[41] R. Granit, *op. cit.,* p. 294.

[42] A. Rapoport, Information processing in the nervous system. In R. W. Gerard and J. W. Duyff, Eds., *Information processing in the nervous system III.* Amsterdam: Excerpta Medica Fdtn., 1964. Pp. 20–21.

[43] R. A. Chase, Evolutionary aspects of language development and function. In F. Smith and G. A. Miller, Eds., *The genesis of language.* Cambridge, Mass.: M. I. T., 1966. P. 260.

medulla. The neuronal chains in Assembly A constitute a meshwork of multiple input-output feedback loops, each neurone receiving input in the same temporal-spatial form and contributing output to other neuronal assemblies. The fate of the temporal-spatial patterns initiated in the cochlea will hinge largely upon the number, power, and position of the synaptic junctions with which they make functional contact. Certain patterns in the network may be inhibited, others activated. Depending upon the position of synapses, feedback by the reticular and cortical pathways may augment or repress the continuance of certain patterns or of all patterns. New patterns may be imposed upon patterns similar in temporal-spatial form which have been laid down previously, with the result that earlier patterns are enhanced, modified, discriminated, or sometimes blocked completely by the later one. And since each synaptic junction concerned with the patterns under consideration may also be utilized by other modalities, the activity at the synapse may trigger temporal-spatial patterns in widely separated neuronal chains.[44] Thus neuronal assemblies in other brainstem areas may enter into production of the percept.

Final Stage. By the time the temporal-spatial patterns reach cortical circuits, the code may bear little relation to the original stimulus pattern.[45] Indeed perception may be so altered by the reticular system or by the earlier processes of coding that it represents a distortion of the actual nature of the stimulating world.[46] In the final steps of coding many systems must enter the ring: reticulocortical tracts, centrally directed classical pathways (auditory, tactile-kinesthetic lemniscal tracts), bidirectional corticofugal and limbic pathways, transcortical and pyramidal tracts. Here again patterning in time and space will form the basis of final discrimination or configuration of the code. Since many tracts from major projection systems of vision, hearing, and somesthesis converge in the temporoparietal fields, they are thought by some researchers to be essential for verbal comprehension and expression. The response may be the *act* of perception; or the modification and elaboration of the percept may continue through the stages of inner language and implicit or

[44] J. C. Eccles, *The neurophysiology of mind.* London: Oxford, 1953. P. 266. T. H. Bullock, The problem of recognition in an analyzer made of neurons. In W. A. Rosenblith, Ed., *Sensory communication.* Cambridge, Mass.: M. I. T., 1961. Pp. 722–723.

[45] Adey *et al.* found that the maximal transductive response in the reticular system has different latencies for different cortical areas so that certain patterns will be forced into association with specific cortical circuits on the basis of its latent period of response.—W. R. Adey, J. P. Segundo, and R. B. Livingston, Corticifugal influences on intrinsic brain stem conduction in cat and monkey. *J Neurophysiol* (January 1957), 20: 1–15.

[46] R. Livingston, Central control of afferent activity. In H. H. Jasper, *et al.*, Eds., *Reticular formation of the brain.* Boston: Little, Brown, 1958. P. 181.

explicit expression. At the last synaptic junction, and only then, can one predict the final form and substance of the code.

New Information and the Coding Process. We have discussed the mechanics of coding information that is not entirely new to the organism. It has been experienced in whole or in part before. There are times, however, in which wave fronts do not fit in with established patterns. The configuration may be significantly different from those which past experience has set the neurones to "expect." [47] Then how does an entirely new pattern evolve into a percept? Let us begin by assuming that the situation confronting the individual is entirely novel. There is no mystical parcel of engrams residing perhaps in the subcortical dendritic layer or in the limbic system with which the new stimuli can do business. Certainly the incoming impulses will arouse greater areas in the nervous system, beginning with the receptors. The electrochemical potentials, both for excitation and inhibition, will be vastly increased by the reticular system. The "new information" will be chipped, modified, enlarged as it goes along until it reaches final reticular pools where further discrimination takes place. To these pools, cortical and sub-cortical pathways make a contribution. The pattern, in both a temporal and a spatial sense, finds no correlative neuronic arcs; it must make its own arc. If it can do so, the individual has learned something new.

What Makes the Difference? Variables in Neural Function. We do not know all the specific neurological variables operative in language learning. We have suggested several in the discussion of neural processes of coding. The basic difference among individuals, of course, resides in the dynamic plasticity of the nervous system, but this is a very general answer. Among the recognized specific variables are the following: (1) competence of neural receptors; (2) strength of spontaneous rhythms in neuronal assemblies; (3) strength and speed of transmission of neural patterns; (4) form and competence of synaptic potentials; (5) power of feedback controls; (6) alerting power of the reticular system (arousal, set-to-respond mechanism); (7) strength of segregating, synchronizing, and fixation mechanisms (especially in reticular, limbic, and cortical fields); (8) power and extent of fields of influence, (sensitized areas of cortex and subcortex); and (9) integrity, power, and speed of motor outlets.[48]

Coding and Language Disorders. When we review these nine variables, any one of which could produce disruptions in coding, we marvel that normal development of communication is the rule, not the exception. Success in organizing and modifying the simplest temporo-

---

[47] M. A. B. Brazier, The electric activity of the nervous system. *Science* (December 11, 1964), 146: 1428.

[48] R. W. Gerard, Neurophysiology: An integration. In J. Field, Ed., *Handbook of physiology, sec. 1: Neurophysiology III.* Washington: Amer. Physiol. Soc., 1960. P. 1949.

spatial patterns of verbal sequences that were initiated in visual, haptic, and auditory receptors may be blighted at any one of these critical junctures in coding. In the prelingual stage the young child acquires a repertoire of sounds, some of which may *not* be the phonemes of the language which he later must learn. Can he modify these prelingual sequences to fit into developing more complex temporospatial patterns or will they be forced into later developing patterns and so distort them? Or will he employ atypical phonemic patterns in "first words and phrases" but modify them in later learned speech patterns? Kim at 2 years used [w] for [l] in "little boy," [wɪtə bɔɪ]. Now one year later she says, "that's ex*cell*ent!", but she persists in saying [wɪtə bɔɪ]. We presume that Kim's nervous system is sufficiently plastic so that these atypical, prelingual phonemes soon will be modified in all sound sequences.

But what will the child do who has a slight neural deficit at any one of the critical points listed above? Does his communication homeostasis demand that the original temporospatial patterns making sound sequences remain unmodified? Perhaps the demand of homeostasis is one factor in the language behavior of a child who suffers from "minimal neurological disturbance." [49]

Synaptic Deficits. It is impossible to chart all the effects upon language learning of neural deficits for each of the nine causes noted above. If we should select one crucial variable in language disorders it probably would be the form and competence of synaptic potentials. The question at this point is, "What is happening at the synapses when language is impaired?" Two hypothetical answers come to mind: (1) The synaptic junctions may possess so high a threshold that the input frequency, let us say, of several hundred per second may be reduced to an output frequency of two, a reduction great enough to cause the input to peter out "like spilt milk over stone." This hypothesis might apply particularly to the child with a language deficit caused by mental retardation. (2) The synaptic thresholds are so low that excessive input overpowers gating, and the analyzers or coders, particularly in reticular, limbic, and corticofugal systems, are unable to process the information. The nervous system is overloaded and fails to filter out and discard unimportant informational bits and hence cannot synthesize essential material. The result is diffusion, not synthesis of patterns, either within a modality or among modalities. How much information must be dropped or modified or elaborated from the incoming load is anyone's guess. Gerard estimates that

the inflow of information is in the millions of bits (binary digits) per second, but the amount that can be handled is only in the tens. . . . Problems of input load are met everywhere. . . . Sophisticated problem-solvers often become

---

[49] B. Boshes and H. R. Myklebust, A neurological and behavior study of children with learning disorders. *Neurology* (Minneap) (January 1964), 14: 12.

entrapped in an hypothesis more inextricably than do naive ones; the trees may blot out the woods for anyone. . . . What is omitted in perception, memory and reason is of the highest moment.[50]

A breakdown in coding induced by low synaptic thresholds may be illustrated in hypothetical fashion in auditory imperception. As the centrally directed auditory impulses enter the brainstem, they make either diffuse connections or the wrong connections with neuronal assemblies. The resultant patterns are atypical and diffuse in form. Their central organizers—reticular, limbic, cortical—attempt to continue processing the information but they are unable to do so because they neither can fit in these bizarre bits of information, atypical wave patterns, with bits coming simultaneously from visuoceptors and hapticeptors, nor can they impress the resulting disparate patterns upon previously acquired patterns. Discrimination fails; perception is distorted. This is one possible explanation of auditory imperception in children handicapped by neural insult or deficit.

Diffusion in Neural Circuits. Although language learning in these children and language deterioration in the aged are not strictly analogous, excessive diffusion in neural circuits seems to occur in both groups. The aged person, for example, cannot grasp the significance of the subtle passages or sophisticated cartoons in his favorite journal. In thinking about a specific problem he fails to cut out irrelevant information and effect convergence of essential neural circuits. The same problem, excessive diffusion, continues throughout the coding process, even in motor expression. The aging person leaves off the beginning or end of the noun; he substitutes closely related words—*breakfast* for *dinner;* or words, not *related,* which sound alike—*avaricious* for *voracious.* The steps in the progression of language in the child, he takes in reverse order. As a child does in learning language, he now attacks the "salient" words leaving out the "little words"—*and, to, the, from.* When asked to define a common noun, *house,* he says repeatedly, "My house is *in* Oak Drive," just as a child, also unable to abstract qualities, to generalize, insists, "You know what fire is; we like a bonfire." This must be the "Seventh age of Man," the return to second childhood. Yes, man is as young as his synapses.

Deficits in Final Coding Stage. There are more discrete perceptual disorders of children that seem to be connected with the final stages of coding, with deficits in cortical analyzers and synchronizers, (variables 7 and 8 above). If visual discrimination is distorted or weak, for example, we do not form accurate concepts of form and size. The child who has normal visual discrimination and recognizes one square generally will

[50] R. W. Gerard, Neurophysiology: An integration. In J. Field, Ed., *Handbook of physiology, sec. 1: Neurophysiology III.* Washington: Amer. Physiol. Soc., 1960. P. 1939.

perceive other forms as "squares" although they may vary in size. The concept of bigness, in the same way, is attained by comparison of various concepts of size. Discrimination, both of form and size, is based on generalizations presumably made in the final stages of coding. Recently in the press there was an account of four members of one family in Italy, blind since birth, who acquired sight through surgical intervention. The adolescent boys were astonished to find that an elephant was not "as big as a house," and did not have the "shape of a house."

The child with a CNS deficit and the adult aphasic often have similar problems in making accurate perceptual discriminations and generalizations. Janet, 7 years old, who recently suffered a cerebral injury, has been engaged in matching shades of colors. A navy-blue ribbon is blue, she says, but the light-blue ribbon does not fit into her concept of "blueness" (generalization). Is it possible that cortical fields are unable to modify the previously laid down engram of navy blue so as to accommodate other patterns of "blueness?" Rex, an adult aphasic, cannot perceive the significance of accounts he reads of military action in Viet Nam, although he served in World War II. He makes no discrimination or generalization on the basis of his own military experience. Why cannot he do so? Is it because the memory circuits laid down in his premorbid years have been interrupted (disconnected), or are the new circuits of learning organized into temporospatial patterns that do not coincide with residual circuits? Or is it possible that new patterns cannot be discriminated because the reticular system is unable to alert and sensitize ailing cortical fields? The answer, in any case, can logically be connected with the final stages of coding.

Fixation Mechanism: Memory

Nature of Fixation. Halstead defines memory as a "process whereby organized time-space events are carried forward in time." [51] These events, represented in the nervous system as substantive memory traces, constitute the time-bind feature of the brain. Establishment of a memory trace presumably depends upon the ability of the organism to retain in its neural organization a skeletal relationship among neurone assemblies that have responded together in earlier time-space events and to reproduce it when needed.[52] The exact processes by which such a relationship is established we do not know. Electrochemical precursors, special circuits,

[51] W. C. Halstead, Thinking, imagery and memory. In J. Field, Ed., *Handbook of physiology, sec. 1: Neurophysiology III*. Washington: Amer. Physiol. Soc., 1960. P. 1675.
[52] W. K. Estes, Information storage in behavior. In R. W. Gerard and J. W. Duyff, Eds., *Information processing in the nervous system: III*. Amsterdam: Excerpta Medica Fdtn., 1964. Pp. 282–283.

and "storage bins" in the medial and superior temporal-parietal areas of the brain have been attached to the rubric, memory mechanism. They could be attached equally well to the learning mechanism. We know, for instance, that electrochemical activity rises sharply as the learning curve rises and continues for some time afterward. The functional relations among neurone assemblies established in learning could be stabilized by the ongoing electrochemical activity. Does this stabilization account for memory? [53]

The electrochemical basis of memory also seems to parallel that for learning. Both rely on some combination of chemical agents, plastic interaction of the neuronal-glial "couplet," and relatively permanent alteration of potentials at synaptic junctions. Among the probable chemical precursors are ribonucleic acid (RNA), and/or other proteins, and acetylcholine.[54] Pribram postulates that RNA is the power mechanism in establishing memory loops. RNA metabolism is maintained, he believes, by the interaction between neurones and their surrounding glial cells (connective tissue element in which neurones are embedded). During excitation RNA builds up in the neurone as it falls in the glia; "after excitation ceases the glia in turn increase their RNA production while that of adjacent neurons diminishes." [55] The pattern or configuration of time-space events is established by these ordered sequences in nucleoprotein activity. By synthesis, breakdown, and resynthesis, the RNA organizer maintains a state of quasi-permanent repetitive firing, a sustained depolarization that induces pre- and postsynaptic changes. "These are the so-called plastic changes (memory trace) which manifest themselves either in long persistence of frequency variations, or in prolonged alterations of transmissive potentialities." [56] The result is that the same pattern of polarized molecular configurations which were initially present in the neurone network have been perpetuated or regenerated.[57] The period of fixation is variable, of course, but Gerard believes that some hundred thousand repetitions are possible in the fixation time—

[53] R. John, Chemical and electrophysiological studies of memory. In R. W. Gerard and J. W. Duyff, Eds., *Information processing in the nervous system: III.* Amsterdam: Excerpta Medica Fdtn., 1964. Pp. 288–298.

[54] B. W. Agranoff, Memory and protein synthesis. *Sci Amer* (June 1967), 216: 115–121.

[55] K. H. Pribram, Proposal for a structural pragmatism: Some neuropsychological considerations of problems in philosophy. In B. B. Wolman, Ed., *Scientific psychology*. New York: Basic Books, 1965. Pp. 433–438.

[56] A. Fessard, The role of neuronal networks in sensory communication within the brain. In W. A. Rosenblith, Ed., *Sensory communication*. Cambridge, Mass.: M. I. T., 1961. P. 592.

[57] K. Rodahl, Nerve as a tissue. *Science* (January 22, 1965) 147: 413–414. F. Morrell, Lasting changes in synaptic organization produced by continuous neuronal bombardment. In J. F. Delafresnaye, Ed., *Brain mechanisms and learning*. Oxford: Blackwell. 1961. Pp. 385–389.

certainly enough to leave a relatively enduring trace.[58] An ancillary action in fixation also should be noted at this point: As the potentiation increases (with each replay of the circuit), it induces an incremental inter-action among neurones in the same area so that the original memory pattern is elaborated and more firmly established. So memories of verbal sequences, for example, continue to grow and crystallize in definite patterns after the initial memory loops have been set.

"Storage" of Memory Patterns. We are reluctant to use the term storage, because it implies a specific section of the CNS in which memories are kept. Such a concept runs counter to present-day hypotheses of engram-setting. If the circuits of learning and recall are continuous throughout the CNS, all sectors must be involved. It is reasonable to assume for language learning that bidirectional cortical tracts, particularly those in temperoparietal fields are included among the components of engram-setting. But one must remember that these bidirectional tracts handle traffic within and between the cortices, to and from basal nuclei, thalamus, reticular formation, cerebellum, and other brainstem structures. Whether the limbic complex (p. 79) makes a direct contribution to the fixation mechanism has not been substantiated. In laboratory studies memory fixation appears to be blocked when the organism is in an environment of stimulation so high that it exceeds the bounds of homeo-static control.[59] Results of experimental lesions suggest that recall of recent events may be affected by damage to any one of the structures of this complex.[60] Adey, Penfield, and others suggest that hippocampal structures (part of the limbic system) "may play an essential part in laying down of the record elsewhere." [61] Since the limbic complex is supposed to mediate emotional reinforcement, it could aid learning and retention in this way.

Localization of memory patterns in temporoparietal fields usually has been predicated upon the site of lesions in cerebral accidents. One must remember, however, that a lesion in a locus where *countless neuronal assemblies* converge will affect many sectors; at another site there may be relatively few active neuronal assemblies to be impaired by a lesion. Memory is the retention of patterns of perception, and these patterns are laid down in a continuous process that may extend from receptors through motor expression. If temporoparietal areas seem to be involved in retention, it may be because these areas are extremely active in language comprehension-use.[62] Memory patterns cannot be

[58] R. W. Gerard, *op. cit.,* p. 1947.

[59] B. W. Agranoff, *op. cit.,* pp. 115–122.

[60] P. D. MacLean, Psychosomatics. In J. Field, Ed., *Handbook of physiology I: Neurophysiology III.* Washington: Amer. Physiol. Soc., 1960. P. 1741.

[61] W. R. Adey, Brain mechanisms and the learning process. *Fed Proc* (July 1961), 20: 617–627. W. Penfield, *Res Publ Assn Res Nerv Ment Dis* (1958), 36: 210–226.

[62] R. L. Masland, Discussion: Brain mechanisms suggested by neurophysiologic

contained in a "store" or be allocated to levels or specific areas of the CNS.

Long- and Short-Term Retention. Some neuropsychologists hold that there is a difference between long- and short-term memory. Both Hebb and Konorski think that reverberating chains, developed among neurones with short axons, account for short-term or immediate memory.[63] A view more consistent with current thinking is presented by Eccles. He reasons that if frequency variations in wave-patterns persist so that there are prolonged alterations of transmissive potentialities, one must conclude that a permanent change in the nucleoprotein configuration at the synapses has taken place, and long-term retention is the result. Whether memory endures or is only a short-term trace will be determined by the permanence of these plastic changes at synaptic junctions.[64]

Retention and Language Impairment. If memory is defective, either genetically or adventitiously, it goes almost without saying that language learning and relearning also will be impaired. Reports are now appearing on experiments to increase the amount of ribonuclease (RNA) in the nervous system of aging individuals. Undoubtedly attempts will be made to increase synaptic power by ribonuclease infusion in mentally retarded children and in children handicapped by specific neural deficits or injuries.

The problem of retention pervades every facet of language impairment. Alex is a child of 9 years who recently suffered a cerebral lesion as the result of a fall. If we ask him to repeat four numbers in series, which we have said very slowly, he forgets the first number; he is unable to hold the information as a unit for "immediate playback." When we say them at a rapid rate, he repeats them correctly. In learning again to read, he finds that he must read at a certain pace or he cannot recall how the sentence began. If he reads slowly he gets nothing at all from the printed page. His behavior is puzzling, however, because the optimum rate does not seem to be the same from day to day. We have attempted to stretch his memory span in oral language by emphasizing pivotal words through rate and pitch changes. We try to highlight verbal cues of perception to be retained. He thinks this technique is helpful because in ordinary conversation he seems only to remember a blur of sounds, a sink from which he cannot pull out the meaningful patterns. [65]

studies. In F. L. Darley, Ed., *Brain mechanisms underlying speech and language.* New York: Grune & Stratton, 1967. P. 202.

[63] D. C. Hebb, *The organization of behavior.* New York: Wiley 1949. Pp. 61–62. J. Konorski, The physiological approach to the problem of recent memory. In J. F. Delafresnaye, Ed., *Brain mechanisms and learning.* Oxford: Blackwell, 1961. Pp. 115–133; 349.

[64] J. C. Eccles, *op. cit.,* pp. 225–226.

[65] Wootton observes that children with developmental language delay remember the most heavily stressed word or "only a few 'mountain peaks' of accented syllables."— M. M. Wootton, Some aberrations of language function in children. *VIIIth International Congress of Neurology.* New York: Excerpta Medica, 1961. Pp. 49–50.

Unlike the adult aphasic, Alex has little ability to search his memory; his scanning sphere is limited. The adult aphasic often retrieves the word by purposeful activation of allied neural circuits. Alex attempts to scan, looks frustrated, bursts into tears and says, "I knew it once." When the missing word is supplied, he does not say, "Oh, yes, that's it," as the adult aphasic often does. It seems to be an entirely new word to Alex; he must learn it as though he had never encountered it before. Is it possible that the adult aphasic is more successful because he has long-established language patterns, whereas Alex was still developing language when he suffered the cerebral accident? Neither vocabulary nor syntax was securely set in the CNS, and as a consequence his scanning comes to nought.

An adult aphasic in our Center who suffers from mild aphasia does not show these extreme memory deficits because he tries a series of language circuits in speaking. Sometimes the maze of circumlocutions in which he engages, however, finally entraps him. He cannot extricate himself from the labyrinth and lapses into defeat and silence. A subjective impression of retrieval is dramatically recorded by another aphasic who had suffered a cerebral accident as the result of a motor-cycle accident:

. . . my memory or repository-for-past-impressions (learnings), I'll call my "revolving cardfile of experience." In order that I recall something, this card-file must revolve, so to speak, until a pattern or image at least begins to take form. . . . In order to know what to say, I must first "get a clear signal." [66]

His success in retrieving the pattern probably will depend on the electro-chemical dynamics of neurones and their synapses in patterned, stable relationships extending to many parts of the nervous system.

The Summing Up

The new look at neural function in language learning which we have presented in these chapters might be called a *transactional* view. Neural activity is an intercommunication or a transaction among cell assemblies or polysynaptic systems by means of functional circuits. The original components of the action cannot be recovered after the "trans-action" because they have been modified by the activity. Impulses are contained in circle networks, providing interchanges for ingress and egress but at no point on the circle can one point to the final direction of the neural assemblies. Rather we think of it as a continuous circular process and interaction in which a whole series of neural events takes

[66] L. F. Sies and R. Butler, A personal account of dysphasia. *J Speech Hearing Dis* (August 1963), 28: 261–266.

place in a definite time sequence and during which the original elements undergo alteration. In the transactional view the message undergoes constant modification and elaboration from receptor to response, in which process a vast company of neuronal assemblies "with collaterals unlimited" mediate and modify the code. The transaction begins in the peripheral receptive systems where the code first may be altered; and it continues in classical sensory-motor routes, in multisensory convergences upon polyvalent neurones of reticular, limbic, subcortical, and cortical bidirectional systems, through specific and nonspecific sensory-motor and motor-sensory fields in cortex and subcortex (Figure 2-6). The transaction is completed in the response, i.e., in the act of perception, inner language, or explicit expression. In the transaction, the cortex has not "abdicated," although it no longer holds exclusive rights over language learning. Its new role may be described as a merger, a cooperative movement, in which its circuits participate with all sectors of the CNS. Contributing to the success of the transaction are homeostatic (controlled lability), alerting or set-to-attend, feedback, and fixation mechanisms.

II

Language and Learning

4

Psychological Parameters of Language Learning

In the preceding chapters we described the neurophysiological bases upon which oral language is built. This chapter deals with psycholinguistic correlates of language learning and their application to language disorders. Auditory and tactile-kinesthetic perceptual processes, for example, which we considered from a neurophysiological point of view in preceding chapters, also have psycholinguistic parameters which shall be discussed. Mental growth will not be treated extensively because we have excluded from consideration children whose language retardation stems from severe and general deficits in mental ability.

We begin with an overview of learning theories and their application to language learning. Next we consider the psychology of auditory and haptic (tactile-kinesthetic) perception, and the types of learned responses one makes to verbal stimuli. The consideration of psycholinguistic components of language—phonology, syntax, and semantics— follow. Some psychosocial determinants, for which neurological correlates also were posed in preceding chapters, conclude the discussion.

Learning Theories and Language Learning

Unfortunately for our area of interest much of the research on learning has been conducted on that noble animal, the laboratory rat. Yet if the mastery of oral language follows the rules of all learning, general principles may be applied to the problems of language learning of children.

The central concept in learning is conditioning. Pavlov's theory of *classical conditioning* concerns itself only with the temporal association of events and will not be discussed in detail. One valuable tenet advanced by Pavlov, particularly applicable to speech, is the tendency of a conditioned response to spread, to generalize, so that it pervades all behavior. We borrow a colleague's story as illustration: A teenager was recalled for the fourth time to register for clinical study because his speech was marked by what seemed to be an irremediable distortion of the s-phoneme. "Look," he said to his clinician, "I've worked at this thing for four years and nothing's happened. I'm going to be stuck with it for the rest of my life. It's my badge. You might as well say I am an S!" He had generalized so well that the defective sound had taken over the person.

Instrumental conditioning is the general method endorsed by two learning theorists, Mowrer and Skinner, although their mode of attack and interpretation of the process differ. In instrumental conditioning new patterns of learning are acquired by associating them with systematically applied rewards and punishment. Mowrer has applied his theory of conditioned learning specifically to oral language learning.[1] He focuses upon the reinforcing power of the verbal *context*. When the parent utters repeatedly the word sound, "hello", in a *pleasant, agreeable context,* the speech of the parent produces a "good feeling" in the baby. Subsequently in verbal play when a baby makes—and hears and feels (kinesthetic feedback)—sounds somewhat like the word or phrase, the built-in pleasure reinforcer operates to stimulate the child to repeat the word or phrase. He now transfers this pleasurable feeling to the stimulus word or phrase as made by the parent, to the stimulus that he, the baby, now provides. Now the reward of pleasure attends his own speech-making efforts. Note that both motor-proprioceptive and auditory feedback are concerned in the child's first "imitations." Note, too, that it is the baby's *covert, emotional reaction of pleasure and hope* that is conditioned, not his overt action of word or phrase repetition. Soon he employs his mother's sounds or a meaningful word in order to represent or recall his mother. He no longer needs to rely upon his autistic satisfactions which indeed would be worn out quickly were it not for the social approval of others. He is able to command the reward from his environment. He can use speech not only to comfort or satisfy himself directly but also to interest, satisfy, and control mother, father, and others in his immediate environment. As the child apprehends the power of the word he advances beyond the phonological aspects of language and charges himself with the responsibility of developing his own grammatical system and lexical content.

[1] O. Mowrer, Hearing and speaking: An analysis of language learning. *J Speech Hearing Dis* (May 1958), 23: 143–152. O. Mowrer, *Learning theory and the symbolic processes.* New York: Wiley, 1960.

Mowrer's theory of language development has been summarized by Mysak. In condensed form (1) the teacher (mother) represents positive emotional connotations for the child by providing pleasure sensations for the child; (2) the mother produces a specific spoken word-pattern just before and as he confronts the child; (3) the mother evokes positive emotional feelings within the child by his word pattern alone; (4) during random vocalization the child will experience a positive emotional feedback (self-stimulation) when he approximates the mother's word pattern; (5) the child repeats the word approximation and refines it because his satisfaction increases as he produces the word pattern more accurately; and (6) the child retains the learned word pattern because of the feedback received from social approval of his speech.[2]

A somewhat different concept of instrumental conditioning has been developed by Skinner.[3] He calls activities that operate upon the environment *operant behavior*. Speech obviously is such an operant, and if it is to acquire strength and long-term stability, Skinner says it must be followed by immediate reinforcement. In a normal family environment these spontaneous reinforcers are always present. A baby's copy of an intonational pattern of the mother is reinforced instantly by her expression of delight or her action in picking up and cuddling the baby. The copy may be a remote facsimile, but in the beginning any verbal behavior that is part of the final pattern will be immediately reinforced. As speech develops only closer approximations or matches of the speech in the baby's environment will be rewarded. With systematically applied rewards, the child tends to repeat the word or phrase. He learns also to associate a particular response with a specific stimulus (stimulus discrimination). In the first stage of learning speech, Baby Kim returned our greeting, "Hi, Kim," with the same words. Such fragmentary echoic behavior also occurs sometimes among adults. If you use whispered speech for a few minutes in conversation your interlocutors very soon also resort to whispered response.

As the baby matures, stimulus discrimination and response begin to sharpen. He learns to facilitate certain stimulus-response patterns that bring him into command of his environment and to inhibit those that are not rewarding. Operant conditioning, then, is primarily a *systematic* and *immediate* application of rewards at every *forward step* in learning a language. The form of reward in operant conditioning varies considerably. In groups of very young children with language handicaps, such primary reinforcers as edible rewards (candy, sweet cereal) are preceded by verbal conditioned reinforcers: *good girl, fine*. In one class observed by the writer both sweets and brightly colored tokens were

[2] E. Mysak, *Speech pathology and feedback theory*. Springfield, Ill.: Charles C Thomas, 1966. Pp. 41–42.

[3] B. F. Skinner, *Verbal behavior*. New York: Appleton-Century-Crofts, 1957.

immediate reinforcers. Words of praise, hand clapping, pats, and hugs were used in a slightly older group.

The essential difference between these two views on instrumental conditioning seems to be that in one the *act* of repetition and *external reinforcement* or reward are essential conditioning agents, whereas in the other a built-in reinforcer, *viz.,* the covert emotional reactions of pleasure and hope in the baby, and not the *act* of imitating the speech of others is the prime conditioner.

Both types of conditioning, classical and instrumental, provoke questions about teaching methods currently employed in speech clinics and public school programs of speech rehabilitation. What hope, do you think, has been inspired in the "I am an S" fellow? What fears have been regularly inculcated in the child handicapped in language? Does not the child pulled out of a classroom to go to a remedial speech class often experience demoralizing embarrassment? What effect has the drab physical environment of the proverbial basement speech clinic on great expectations and feelings of pleasure about learning speech? A former student, whose "laugh doeth good like a medicine," wrote us about her new clinical assignment as a graduate student: "Larry is eleven years old and has been in the clinic for five years because of a defective /r/ sound. What can I do to motivate him to learn? I've tried everything I know." The advice was sent by return post: "Take Larry to the drug store next door. Sit at the soda bar—if they still have one—and treat him. Tell him the good news. You're giving him a long vacation from the clinic." There has been no further word about Larry.

Sensory-Motor Correlates of Speech Perception

A great portion of human utterance still belongs to that fundamental stratum of speech: the language of the emotions. The child's early perception of intonational patterns is an emotional response and quite logically could follow the pleasure principle advocated by Mowrer. But as the child advances in speech learning, his perception as sensation and as ideation seems to follow the principle of reality. That is to say, the child recognizes the essential stability or veridicality of the sensation or the idea.[4]

Kinesthetic Perception: Its Role in Language Learning. Our faith in the auditory route as the chief modality in the perception of speech has been shaken by research reports that a child perceives sound sequences in terms of his own motor reactions. This is not to say that acoustic events are unimportant; they are, but they are linked in time with the equally

[4] O. Mowrer, *Learning theory and the symbolic processes.* New York: Wiley, 1960. P. 200.

important articulatory events. Liberman would give priority to the motokinesthetic feedback loops in the comprehension-use of language. "Perception of speech sounds," he says, "is somehow more closely related to the articulation than to the acoustic stimulus. The proprioceptive return (feedback) from a mediating articulation is most important. . . . Speech is perceived by the articulatory movements, and their sensory effects mediate between the acoustic stimulus and the event we call perception. . . . We believe that a speaker (and listener) learns to connect speech sounds with their appropriate articulations, and that the sensory feedback from these movements (or, more likely, the corresponding neurological processes) comes to mediate between the acoustic stimulus and its perception." [5] Twaddell agrees with Liberman and goes on to suggest that listeners classify sound sequences on the basis of motor articulation rather than acoustic properties. It is the motor-proprioceptive activity, not the acoustic character, they maintain, which dominates perception.[6] If there is an order in acoustic and articulatory events, both Cherry and MacNeilage would say that we perceive the sound sequences only *after* the neuromuscular patterns of articulation have been mediated.[7] We conclude that taction-kinesthesis must be the coequal of audition at least in the baby's first attempts to speak. Later he may be more dependent on acoustic signals, but it is doubtful if he ever relies entirely or even mainly upon them.

Sound Sequences and Kinesthesis. Two principles emerge from the researches we have reviewed: (1) Movement patterns are highly significant in our ability to perceive sequences, and (2) movement patterns of greatest significance in the perception of linguistic units probably are the shifts in muscular action *between* phonemic and morphemic sequences. Theoretical support of these principles has been reviewed in detail in the discussion of proprioception in a preceding chapter (p. 50).

Limited attention has been paid to these principles of tactile-kinesthetic perception in testing and training the speech-handicapped child. Stimulation of the sound-in-isolation seems to be the current practice in speech clinics and public schools. In a few areas, however, the winds of change are blowing. McCroskey,[8] Ringel and Steer,[9] and

---

[5] A. M. Liberman, Some results of research on speech perception. *J Acoust Soc Amer* (January 1957), 29: 117–123.

[6] W. Twaddell, Phonemes and allophones in speech analysis. *J Acoust Soc Amer* (November 1952), 24: 607–611.

[7] C. Cherry, *On human communication.* New York: M. I. T. and Wiley, 1957. Pp. 293–295. P. F. MacNeilage, Electromyographic and acoustic study of the production of certain final clusters. *J Acoust Soc Amer* (April 1963), 35: 461.

[8] R. McCroskey, The relative contribution of auditory and tactile clues to certain aspects of speech. *Southern Speech J* (1958), 24: 84–90.

[9] R. Ringel and M. Steer, Some effects of tactile and auditory alterations on speech output. *J Speech Hearing Res* (December 1963), 6: 369–378.

Klein [10] in separate studies have found that speech is adversely affected by auditory and tactile-kinesthetic interruption. In one study, motor speech seemed to be more greatly disturbed by anesthetization of the articulators than by auditory masking. Using both topical anesthesis and a masking noise, Ringel and Steer report that the resulting interference has a cumulative adverse effect on speech performance. The writer has experienced the effects of single sensory interruption of feedback from anesthetization of the articulators by the dentist. On two occasions she observed an additional effect on which these researchers have not commented, *viz.*, that the speech of those about one also did not seem to be as intelligible as it was before anesthetization. Can the disturbance of tactile-kinesthesis *alone* also affect audition?

Standardized tests of general motor skills based on tactile-kinesthetic perception are available (p. 292). Assessment of this ability in motor speech has only begun. Usually a plastic form of abstract design is placed in the child's mouth without his seeing it. After palpation of the form in his mouth, he is asked to select a matching form from the designs in the frame before him. Presumably the test measures only taction, but if muscular activity is involved it must perforce stimulate proprioceptive end organs. Attempts to reinforce tactile-kinesthetic feedback have been made in special areas of speech. McDonald's first objective in articulation therapy is "to heighten the child's responsiveness to the patterns of auditory, proprioceptive, and tactile sensations associated with the overlapping, ballistic movements of articulation." [11] His method entails practice with bisyllables and trisyllables. Speech training of cerebral-palsied youngsters in some centers here and in England rests indirectly upon motokinesthetic reinforcement. Both Bobath, whose work has been reviewed elsewhere in this book (p. 57) and Kabat [12] emphasize proprioceptive control of posture as precursor to proprioceptive control of phonatory and articulatory muscle groups. In addition to postural training, Kabat employs techniques of maximal resistance and successive induction in order to facilitate motor sequencing in a pattern. The assumption is that once fundamental postural patterns are corrected, articulatory postures will improve. One wishes, however, for some reliable technique for training synergies engaged in sequencing articulation. If one could place external guides on the tongue, for example, which would direct it smoothly from one articulatory position to the next, the intact supply of proprioceptive fibers eventually might perform correctly without the guide. A

[10] D. Klein, An experimental study of selected speech disturbances and adaptation effects under conditions of auditory, tactile, and auditory-tactile feedback interference. Unpublished master's thesis, Cornell University, 1963.

[11] E. McDonald, *Articulation testing and treatment: A sensory-motor approach.* Pittsburgh: Stanwix House, 1964. P. 138.

[12] H. Kabat, Proprioceptive facilitation in therapeutic exercise. In E. Licht, Ed., *Therapeutic Exercise.* (2nd ed.) New Haven: Licht, 1961.

possible alternative is tactile stimulation of motor units, a method employed by Young and Hawk.[13] If their methods were applied, not to articulation alone, but to all motor synergies engaged in speech the principle would seem to be on sounder ground. Since fine movement patterns are a part of larger synergies, the patterning of proper postural shifts that precede or accompany movement patterns of articulation and exercise of fine gestural patterns of head and hands should prove an excellent reinforcement to speech. One observes, for example, that exercise of proper postural and gestural patterns frequently serves as a stimulus to verbal recall. A renowned actor falters over a line but recovers it quickly by increasing the vigor of the established gestural pattern. Teachers of the deaf, who also employ motokinesthetic methods, are emphasizing the practice of facial and hand gestures in teaching oral communication. Perhaps the "tip of the tongue" phenomenon, prompting near recall, could be pushed to complete recall by gestural reinforcement.[14] The winds of change indeed are blowing. When will they ruffle the research papers in our speech clinics?

Auditory Perception. Temporal Variables. Auditory cues consist of sound sequences in which phonemes are combined in an interactive relationship so that the resulting pattern constitutes a dynamic unit of language. The sound sequences depend, in turn, on an elaborate multiple set of codes transmitting information concerning their differences in frequency, amplitude and duration (p. 66). The most important of these cues in perceiving *sequences* of acoustic events probably is duration, a *temporal dimension.* Unlike visual cues, perceived mainly by spatial relations, auditory events are primarily analyzed by their time patterns.

Psychoacousticians tell us that the auditory system has a differential sensitivity for sounds of different duration. Vowels in sequences may be discriminated almost entirely by their duration. The distinction between [bɑ] and [wɑ], for example, is determined principally in the ears of the listener by the rate at which the energy changes from one concentration to another, even though the two concentrations in *frequency* location are identical.[15] In other words, one perceives the sound sequence by recognition of the rate at which changes occur between sounds. In other sound combinations one may recognize not only durational shifts but also changes in frequency or intensity; time, however, is their common denominator. Some plosive consonants, notably [p-b], [t-d], and

[13] E. H. Young and S. Hawk, *Moto-kinesthetic speech training.* Stanford: Stanford Univ. Press, 1938.

[14] R. Brown and D. McNeill, The "tip of the tongue" phenomenon. *J Verbal Learn Verbal Behav* (August 1966), 5: 325–337.

[15] I. J. Hirsh, Audition in relation to perception of speech. In E. C. Carterette, Ed., *Brain function III: Speech, language, and communication.* Berkeley: University of California Press, 1966. P. 103.

[k-g], when placed in certain contexts may reflect other differences, but sounds in sequence are distinguished mainly by time factors.

Another perceptual variable in the temporal dimension is the ability of the listener to distinguish the *order* of occurrence of sound sequences in speech. Children who habitually say *lips* for *lisp, gavry* for *gravy,* or *lebow* for *elbow* are rarely cognizant of their errors in sequencing sounds or syllables. The critical denominator again is time. Hirsch finds that normally more than one millisecond must separate two acoustic events if their order of occurrence is to be judged correctly.[16] Perhaps in these children a much wider separation is necessary. Equally important in the perceptual process are the temporal aspects of intonational contours and basic rhythmic patterns. The *auditory* component of these cues, fundamental in a baby's perceptual repertoire of contextual speech, is the product of frequency shift and duration.

Other Variables of Auditory Perception. Studies of speech intelligibility suggest other determinants of auditory perception, *viz.,* the noise level of the surround, binaural as opposed to monaural reception, the presentation of the word or phrase in context as opposed to the isolated word, the redundancy of cues, and the influence of certain vocal and feeling attributes of speech. Finally memory must be a consideration in the auditory perception of speech, for certainly a child who has a reservoir of words and phrases against which incoming auditory patterns may be compared has a tremendous advantage over one who holds few words in memory.

Auditory Perception and Language Learning. We have been observing closely a little girl of 15 months who distinguishes clearly between "Want to go bye-bye?" and "No, you can't go bye-bye." Her responses are unmistakable. The intonational contour or melody pattern is the first differential. The second is the discrimination of syllables, morphemes, and combinations of morphemes in order. She does not add one sound to another and yet to another in an attempt to perceive meaning, as linguistically handicapped children are wont to do. To the average child learning language, the syllable becomes the irreducible acoustic unit, and there is reason for it.[17] The critical cues are the transitions between phonemes and morphemes. They are not there, as Liberman says, "to avoid 'clicks and thumps;' they are not merely the incidental acoustic accompaniments of the movements that a speaker must make when he goes from 'consonant' to 'vowel.' They are authentic perceptual cues." [18] By

[16] *Ibid.,* p. 104.
[17] A. M. Liberman, F. Ingemann, L. Lisker, P. Delattre, and F. S. Cooper, Minimal rules for synthesizing speech. *J Acoust Soc Amer* (November 1959), 31: 1496.
[18] A. M. Liberman, K. Harris, J. Kinney, and H. Lane, The discrimination of relative onset-time of the components of certain speech and non-speech patterns. *J Exp Psych* (1961), 61: 379. A. M. Liberman, Some results of research on speech perception. *J Acoust Soc Amer* (January 1957), 29: 117–123. A. M. Liberman, F. S. Cooper, K. S. Harris and P. F. MacNeilage, A motor theory of speech perception. Speech communication seminar. Stockholm: Proceedings, Royal Inst of Technol, 1963.

the time the child is an adolescent he has built up a vast stock of morphemic sequences and melodic patterns. Indeed they are so deeply set that when he begins the mastery of a second language, he is loathe to give them up. To a great extent, even the adult seems unable to discriminate new auditory cues to syllabic sequences and intonational contours. Generally he continues to use the perceptual patterns of his native tongue in learning a foreign language.[19]

Speech cues are highly redundant so a baby very early learns to select peak cues and disregard others, just as the adult in his daily rounds disregards many cues and selects only peaks at random from much of what he hears. As a result he interprets only partially perceived patterns and integrates them into a meaningful whole. Cherry estimates that the informational capacity of the ear actually may be measurable in tens of thousands of bits per second, but of course the adult cannot comprehend at this rate.[20] Indeed he does not need to for most of these bits are redundant. Because he has learned extensive patterns of sound sequences he rejects much of what assaults his ears. He perceives information at a much slower rate, perhaps 25–50 bits per second. In terms of words per minute, it has been found that comprehension of verbal material is much better at the rate of 175 words per minute than at 275 w.p.m. In one comparative study nonhandicapped children made the same number of mistakes as cerebral-palsied groups at the faster rate.[21]

In children handicapped by language disorders, the disturbance in perception frequently is demonstrable. They attempt to select or discriminate particular phonemes, but they do not join these isolated sounds in a sequence. Hence they do not use the important cue, that contained in the transitional phases of sounds. Sometimes they attempt an even more difficult task: They try to comprehend and recall a succession of single sounds in a "beads-on-a-string" fashion. They select each sound in a syllable as a peak sound, not peak syllables or words in a sentence. Obviously they cannot attend to and recall all sounds in a sequence so they usually center their attention on the initial sounds, much as they attend to a button on the clinician's jacket but rarely recognize the clinician. Sometimes, when they find no meaning "in the piece" they try to get rid of it. The adult aphasic's problem is similar in some respects. "Why can't I learn that sentence again? I knew it once," he complains. He too is unable to respond to the sequence of sounds; like the language-handicapped child he does not focus on peak cues to meaning. Other linguistically handicapped children might learn to select peak cues and reject redundant ones if informational bits came at a slower rate, much

---

[19] A. M. Liberman, Some results of research on speech perception. *J Acoust Soc Amer* (January 1957), 29: 117–123.

[20] C. Cherry, *op. cit.*, p. 289.

[21] W. de Hoop, Listening comprehension of cerebral palsied and other crippled children as a function of two speaking rates. *Exceptional Child* (January 1965), 31: 233–240.

slower than the normal rate of 25–50 bits per second. In the neurologically handicapped child we have witnessed all too often his inability to perceive meaning in contextual speech, although he may snatch every cue available to him. He either tries to receive too many bits of information, much of which will be redundant, or he may not be able to order sequences of information at the usual rate of reception. Sometimes he gambles on the meaning; frequently he is wrong.[22] Perhaps one day we will devise individual time-modality scales for the optimum perception of oral language.

Delayed Auditory Feedback. We can perceive only those acoustic units that are presented within our range of reaction-time, and this range varies widely among individuals. Some children with language delay may need 75 msec. in contrast to a normal child's reaction time of 5 msec. in order to perceive a syllable-sequence at the acoustic level.[23] Skinner suggests that in young children whose verbal behavior is weak because it still is in the process of being acquired, delays of the order of minutes are sometimes observed.[24] These abnormally long reaction intervals may be caused by delayed feedback. The neurophysiological basis of interruption of this monitor in the nervous system has been explored in an earlier chapter (p. 96).

We know the effect on speech of experimentally delayed feedback in individuals, but we can only hypothesize from knowledge of neural function how neural delays in feedback might affect the language handicapped child. When the speech is "returned" 250–300 msec. after vocalization has begun, the subject's speech becomes hesitant and cluttered. Articulatory disturbance is primary but one is also disturbed by a noticeable increase in intensity and pitch. One is also confused and unable to pursue his ideas. In this case the confusion in feedback may arise from a conflict between the delayed return of speech and synchronous *auditory and proprioceptive* feedback associated with the same vocalization. In other words the subject must attend both to synchronous and delayed feedback in the same instant. In the language-retarded child comprehension may be disturbed because auditory impulses are delayed whereas visual and tactile-kinesthetic cues to the phonemic sequence have *not* been delayed. The impulses cannot be organized in a pattern because they have not arrived in the same temporal order in the CNS. As in cases of experimental delay in feedback, so in the language-retarded child one notes the effect in motor response. Perceptual disorganization may produce hesitant, cluttered, partially blocked responses.

[22] R. Tiffany and S. L. Kates, Concept attainment and lip reading ability among deaf adolescents. *J Speech Hearing Dis* (August 1962), 27: 265. I. Hirsh and C. E. Sherrick, Perceived order in different sense modalities. *J Exp Psychol* (November 1961), 62: 423–432.
[23] W. G. Hardy, Hearing in children—Panel discussion (Sixth International Congress on Audiology). *Laryngoscope* (March 1958), 68: 224–228.
[24] B. F. Skinner, *op. cit.,* p. 24.

Tests of Auditory Perception of Speech.   Since auditory perception of language is posited on discrimination, not of single phonemes but of a series of phonemes in a prescribed order, we doubt the value of tests of recognition of isolated sounds. They go a very short way, it seems to us, in assessing the child's perception of the speech continuum.

The development of deep tests of articulation by McDonald and his colleagues at Pennsylvania State University reinforce this conclusion.[25] They found that traditional tests of articulation were not related to the child's consistency of articulation. Other workers in the field have developed tests of auditory perception employing *words in context.*[26] *The Michigan Language Inventory* (p. 258), *The Illinois Test of Psycholinguistic Abilities* (p. 255), and the *Ohio State University Test for Identifying Misarticulations* include sections on sentence discrimination but the *content* is meager. Moreover no attempt is made to measure perception of other phonological components (intonation and speech melody) or to assess auditory perception of syntactic and semantic information. They are not measures of the auditory perception of the *continuum of speech.*

Interdependence of Modalities in Perception.   Study of a "simple case of auditory agnosia" recently referred to us proved not to be simple and not exclusively or even mainly a disturbance of auditory perception. The whole sensory-motor continuum of this young man's speech was impaired. We have known children, on the other hand, who were handicapped primarily by visuomotor deficiencies. And it is possible, as Myklebust points out, for an aphasic child to have normal auditory perception.[27] In general, we may say, children with learning disabilities customarily exhibit disorganization of some degree in all modalities.

The disorganization frequently extends to motokinesthetic feedback. The resulting disturbance in effector mechanisms leading to motor speech, in turn, may adversely affect all other systems contributing to the response just as sensory behavior affects motor speech. Children with perceptual loss or deficit, for example, usually do not gesture.[28] The

[25] E. T. McDonald, *Articulation testing and treatment: A sensory-motor approach.* Pittsburgh: Stanwix House, 1964. C. V. Mange, A study of speech sound discrimination within words and within sentences. Unpublished master's thesis, Penn. State University, 1959. H. Dorsey, The relationship between performance of kindergarten children on a three-position and a deep test of articulation. Unpublished doctoral dissertation, Penn. State University, 1959. L. F. Aungst and J. V. Frick, Auditory discrimination ability and consistency of articulation of /r/. *J Speech Hearing Dis* (February 1964), 29: 76–85.

[26] G. N. Traul and J. W. Black, The effect of context on aural perception of words. *J Speech Hearing Res* (December 1965), 8: 363–369.

[27] H. R. Myklebust, Speech, language development and language disorders. Address at International Convention, Council for Exceptional Children, Chicago, April 3, 1964.

[28] H. R. Myklebust, Psychoneurological learning disorders. *J Ontario Speech Hearing Assn* (January 1962), pp. 1–11.

functional unity of the entire organism seems to be upset when one
modality is impaired.[29]

Unisensory vs. Multisensory Training. If modalities are interdependent, should we employ the unisensory or multisensory approach
in teaching the child who is severely handicapped in language learning?
Some educators argue that the child learns best through a unisensory
approach, and some neurological support could be advanced for this
position. We know that neural assemblies in several receptor systems may
use the same routes; a child with CNS injury or deficit may be able to
accommodate only impulses from one modality in a unit of time. In the
normal child, on the other hand, the same neurones can participate
in countless specific patterns of activity.[30] The reticular system of the
neurologically handicapped child may be impaired so that he is unable
to inhibit or to integrate the flow of sensory information from several
modalities. Damage to neural assemblies in this and other integrative
and projection systems probably results in lowered threshold at the
synapses so that they are no longer selective. The result is diffuse perception, exaggerated response, and feeble retention of the percept. One
frequently sees a kind of catastrophic response in language-disturbed
children when too many bits of information must be handled by an inadequate nervous system.[31]

Teachers who support unisensory training claim that sensitivity of
the auditory channel can be heightened by blocking visual receptors with
an ordinary blindfold. Or the auditory channels may be blocked and
visual-proprioceptive stimulation emphasized. On the other side of the
coin we have clinical reports of the salutary effect of multisensory training in language learning. We know that certain kinds of multisensory
training aid language learning in the child with subtle perceptual deficits.
It seems reasonable to assume that mutual reinforcement promotes the
establishment and recall of patterns of speech. Successive steps of unisensory, bisensory, and multisensory training probably should be taken
in accordance with the child's developing abilities to handle neural
traffic.[32]

[29] J. L. Olson, A comparison of sensory aphasic, expressive aphasic, and deaf
children on the Illinois test of language ability. Ann Arbor: University Microfilms,
61–81; 1964. P. 46.

[30] J. C. Eccles, General discussion. In J. F. Delafresnaye, Ed., *Brain mechanisms
and learning.* Oxford: Blackwell, 1961. P. 657.

[31] B. Buser and A. Rougeul, Observations sur le conditionnement instrumental
alimentaire chez le chat. In J. F. Delafresnaye, Ed., *Brain mechanisms and learning.*
Oxford: Blackwell, 1961. P. 553. R. W. Gerard, Neurophysiology: An integration. In
J. Field, Ed., *Handbook of physiology, sec. 1: Neurophysiology III.* Washington: Amer.
Physiol. Soc., 1960. P. 1936.

[32] T. H. Eames, Association pathways in language disabilities. *J Educ Psychol*
(January 1956), 47: 8–10.

Responses in Language Learning

Perception an Act. Perception and discrimination are regarded as synonymous terms in this book.[33] Perception and inner language are responses. Perception must be regarded as an *act* in itself, for "perception involves doing . . . doing involves perception."[34] Neural processes in which stimuli from our internal and external environment are adapted and organized into a percept are behavioral phenomena. They constitute action, a response. The difference between an individual's perceiving and not perceiving rests, in part, with the *action* at synaptic junctions. The cortex too is aroused to action by the interruption of its alpha wave. In the same way, kinesthetic feedback is a response to movement. And when the individual perceives, he is prepared to respond to the percept.[35]

Inner Language. Sometimes the individual responds to the percept by further action resulting in *inner language*. This term has had various interpretations. It has been defined as "speech minus sound," "implicit speech," or as "subvocal speech." Chesni describes it as a manifestation of subliminal or overt acts of speech.[36] Inner language, it is generally agreed, is abbreviated in form and substance. Some describe it as condensed external speech, a brief predication with highly simplified syntax. Although we cannot agree with Vygotsky that "inner speech is speech almost without words," we concede that when syntax and speech sequences are reduced to a minimum, the sense (dynamic, fluid, holistic interpretation) of a single word or a saturated phrase may constitute inner speech.[37] Certainly overt (oral expression) and inner language involve much the same central processes.[38] Sometimes oral expression may precede inner speech. This is Vygotsky's view, who describes the egocentric monologues of the child as manifestations of symbolic thought processes (percepts) *before* the processes are finally converted into inner speech.[39]

Inner language probably is developing rapidly as egocentric speech declines but it seems likely that the *rudiments* of inner language probably were established with the first bits of comprehension in the baby's brain. Myklebust believes, for example, that the baby cannot understand what is

[33] See H-L. Teuber's support of this point of view in his chapter on Perception. In J. Field, Ed., *Handbook of physiology, sec. 1: Neurophysiology III*. Washington: Amer. Physiol. Soc. 1960. P. 1601f. Others may wish to adopt Lindsley's view: "Discrimination and recognition amount to perception."—D. Lindsley, Basic perceptual processes and the EEG. *Psychiat Res Rep Amer Psychiat Assn* (October 1956), 6: 170.

[34] O. Mowrer, *op. cit.,* p. 181.

[35] R. W. Sperry, Neurology and the mind-brain problem. In R. I. Isaacson, Ed., *Basic readings in neuropsychology*. New York: Harper & Row, 1964. P. 415.

[36] Y. Chesni, La parole intérieure. *Confin Neurol* (1963), 23: 192.

[37] L. S. Vygotsky, *Thought and language*. Cambridge, Mass.: M. I. T., 1962. Pp. 145–146.

[38] T. K. Landauer, Rate of implicit speech. *Percept Motor Skills* (1962), 15: 646.

[39] L. S. Vygotsky, *op. cit.,* p. 133f.

said to him until he has acquired a minimum of inner language.[40] In a sense Vygotsky acknowledges these rudiments when he describes the child's early speech as sociocentric, not egocentric. The young child's monologues, he believes, are first manifestations of embryonic thought processes before these processes are finally suppressed and converted into inner speech.[41] In the monologue the child regards the word as a live attribute or property of the object rather than as a mere sign, a referent. So lights wink, knives bite, and flowers sleep (wilt). The baby's verbalizations are signals (labels of action) rather than symbols.[42] They are embryonic thought processes indeed, and considerable time will elapse before the child thinks words rather than pronounces them. The relation of inner language to the time schedule of language development is discussed in Chapter 5.

We find no neurological or psychological support for the position taken by some workers in the field that neural deficit or injury may affect only inner language. The very nature of the continuity of neural events controverts such a view. The results of electromyographic studies indicate that the same circuits that are employed in oral expression also mediate inner language, although in inner language they exhibit a lessened intensity and are consequently accompanied by incomplete phonatory and articulatory movements.[43]

Tactile-kinesthetic feedback apparently is a main instigator of internal language. During "subliminal speech" potentials of phonatory and articulatory muscles, for example, show a definite increase. When a subject *mentally* performs various experimental speech tasks, tongue and lip potentials reflect their activity.[44] It seems to Chesni that internal speech is largely the result of feedback control which has its triggering point in the proprioceptors of the phonatory and articulatory musculature.[45] Deaf children, it is thought, acquire inner language entirely by proprioceptive feedback. This group regularly exhibits increased neural potentials during such mental operations as memorizing words and figures, and solving arithmetic problems.[46] From his study of young deaf children Wooden comes to the same conclusion. He maintains that when

[40] H. Myklebust, *Auditory disorders in children*. New York: Grune & Stratton, 1954. P. 12.

[41] L. S. Vygotsky, *op. cit.*, p. 28f.

[42] A. A. Strauss and E. N. McCarus, A linguist looks at aphasia in children. *J Speech Hearing Dis* (February 1958), 23: 54–58.

[43] Y. Chesni, *op. cit.*, pp. 189–196.

[44] F. V. Bassin and E. S. Bain, Application of electro-myography to the study of speech. In N. O'Connor, Ed., *Recent Soviet psychology*. New York: Liveright, 1961. Pp. 195–209. L. A. Novikova, Electrophysiological investigation of speech. In N. O'Connor, Ed., *Recent Soviet psychology*. New York: Liveright, 1961. P. 213.

[45] "La parole intérieure est soumise à un contrôle rétractif ou feed-back à point de départ des propriocepteurs de la musculature phonatoire et articulatoire, et donne prise de cette façon aux méthodes de la cybernétique."—Y. Chesni, *op. cit.*, p. 195.

[46] L. A. Novikova, *op. cit.*, p. 219.

speech reading (visuoproprioceptive feedback) is taught from infancy, the young child inevitably develops inner language.[47]

Oral Expression. Speech is a response that entails more than the muscle synergies of respiration, phonation, resonation, and articulation. As we have said in preceding paragraphs, it embraces essentially the same central processes that one employs in perception and inner language. Just as in other behavioral responses, sensory-motor fields and their circuits must be engaged in oral expression. Effector pathways may receive more intense facilitation and reinforcement through feedback from the receptive systems (visual, proprioceptive, auditory), and from reticular and limbic systems but the basic neural processes remain the same. The action is reciprocal. As peripheral impairment of projection pathways mutes or disturbs inner language, so perceptual distortion will affect markedly the speech production of the child.[48]

Speech, as in all learned motor activities, employs synergies, sequences of movement patterns that once learned may be activated by feedback from a single sector of the pattern. Subglottal, laryngeal, and supraglottal muscles engaged in phonation contract in an established sequence. In such a relatively simple synergy of movements as those employed in articulation of the nursery rhyme, "Peter, Peter, Pumpkin Eater," lips and tongue, velopharyngeal sphincter, mandible and hyoid, and the muscles of facial expression must move in synchrony. These synergies are often very unstable in children with language handicaps. Lips or tongue may approach the proper articulatory position but voice may not be initiated. Or the velopharyngeal sphincter may fail to close. Sometimes the child begins speech very well, and then as synergic relationships break down, speech deteriorates. As de Hirsch says, one can almost detect the fading features of the word or phrase.[49]

Many variables operate in motor speech. External feedback of noise, affecting not only volume but one's total speech behavior, is a powerful determinant.[50] Observe supposedly normal people in their attempt to carry on a conversation above cocktail clatter, and you will note peculiar changes in facial expression, bodily movement, pitch, quality, and volume of voice. Articulation patterns generally become more definite in first efforts, and then they slowly deteriorate as the noise level increases and communication reaches a dead end. When children with poor neural gating power are subjected to unusual noise levels, the response frequently is catastrophic. Internal environment also is a variable in motor speech. Personality deviations and internal emo-

---

[47] H. Z. Wooden, Dramatized language for the deaf. *Exceptional child* (December 1962), 29: 155–163.

[48] Y. Chesni, *op. cit.*, pp. 189–196.

[49] K. de Hirsch, Plasticity and language disabilities. In J. Hellmuth, Ed., *Learning disorders I*. Seattle: Special Child Publications, 1965. P. 247.

[50] J. W. Black, The loudness of sidetone. *Speech Monogr* (1954), 21: 301–305.

tional disturbances may produce disorganization of speech, or if intense, interrupt completely the operation of motor synergies of speech. Children who suffer prolonged or chronic illnesses are often so low in physical strength that they do not possess the energy requirements for stable motor patterns. Suppurative otitis media in a high percentage of Eskimo children in the Arctic Circle (Point Barrow, Alaska) seemed to this writer to be sufficient cause in itself for their very poor speech, although auditory loss admittedly is another contributing factor. Maturational decrements affect motor speech. The 6-year-old child who reaches out with his whole body, clenches his fists when he hops, exhibits ill-defined laterality and primitive patterning. His nervous system is not sufficiently mature to effect the lightning-like shifts of motor patterns required in speech. We observe these variables in operation but we have no way of determining whether central or peripheral processes, internal or external environmental factors, are the more significant in production of atypical motor speech. We assess proficiency in motor speech by its performance; we only speculate on the *causes* of poor performance.

Psycholinguistic Components of Oral Language

Phonology

In the first months of life, a baby employs intonational signals. They usually are annunciatory or interjectional responses, meaningful only in the sense that they have physiological reference. Shortly the baby will copy those pleasurable intonational patterns of speech he hears in his immediate environment. As he matures he uses these intonational contours as primary speech signals. Later he will impose upon them morphemes and more elaborate sound sequences. And as language learning proceeds, syntactic and semantic patterns will be impressed upon those early melodic patterns.

Prosodic Elements of Speech. Prosody, the music of our speech, is the earliest dimension of phonology to be employed in the comprehension-use of language. From infancy to old age it will continue to be the critical marking that makes one's speech peculiarly his own. Yet it is flexible varying with one's bodily state, mood, thoughts, and with his psychosocial environment. Because the melody of speech is complex, all characteristics of tone—pitch, quality, loudness, and duration—must enter into its making.[51] But precisely what shifts in elements occur to produce

---

[51] *Pitch* is determined primarily by the frequency of the sound.

Quality of a tone is its color (timbre) and is determined by overtones derived from the complexity of the wave pattern.

Loudness (strength) is related to the amount of energy or power of speech sequences and measured by the amplitude of the wave pattern.

Duration applies to three determinants of rate or timing of speech: syllable length, pause, and overall rate of speech.

For further discussion of these attributes of tone, see J. Carrell and W. Tiffany,

the features of prosody we do not know. To what degree is each responsible for *intonation*, the contour of melody, and for *rhythmic* and *nuance patterns* which characterize a child's developing speech melody?

Intonation. Some authorities believe that frequency or pitch changes are the primary characteristics of intonation.[52] Lieberman hypothesizes the basis for these changes in fundamental frequency. An infant's first cries, he says, are dictated by the normal breath-group,* and all subsequent modification of the intonational pattern will be fashioned on the same innately determined organization of the respiratory and phonatory mucles. As these intonational contours develop with speech, their most stable characteristic is the "fall in fundamental frequency that always occurs at the end of the normal breath group."[53] Some psycholinguists would add shifts in loudness, duration, and stress to pitch as determinants of intonational patterns.

Rhythm. Speech rhythm is sometimes regarded as synonymous with intonation. We know that intonational contours influence rhythm as do syntactic and semantic patterns, yet speech rhythm has an identity of its own. The characteristic rhythms of speech are difficult to describe. Those familiar with dialectical Danish language recognize immediately its staccato rhythm. This speech is peppered with glottal stops, a time-space factor, but other factors undoubtedly contribute to the sharply punctuated rhythm. Some of these factors are highly subjective, some objective. Speech rhythm is the result of a total bodily response and hence is determined by kinesthetic feedback from great and small muscle synergies. In psychoacoustic analysis of rhythmic speech, elementary beats (pulse movements) or syllables are differentiated from each other. Some are short, some long; some are stressed, some unstressed.[54] Some are released quickly; others are arrested. Some may be characterized by crescendo, others by diminuendo.[55] It is, in short, the temporal-spatial patterning of syllables, words and phrases, and the play of stress which account for the rhythmic patterns of speech.

Nuance Patterns. The *nuances* of one's speech melody are heavily dependent on vocal quality. They convey subtleties of meaning and seem

Phonetics. New York: McGraw-Hill, 1960. Pp. 259–273; and P. Ladefoged, *Elements of acoustic phonetics.* Chicago: The University of Chicago Press, 1962. Pp. 13–33.

[52] J. Carrell and W. Tiffany, *op. cit.,* p. 261. E. Fischer-Jorgensen, What can the new techniques of acoustic phonetics contribute to linguistics. In S. Saporta, Ed., *Psycholinguistics.* New York: Holt, Rinehart and Winston, 1961. P. 132. P. Lieberman, *Intonation, perception, and language.* Cambridge, Mass.: M. I. T., 1967. Pp. 38–47.

[53] P. Lieberman, *op. cit.,* p. 39.

[54] Stress apparently is determined, not by intensity, as one might suppose, but by pitch prominence in the morpheme or larger speech unit.—D. L. Bolinger, A theory of pitch accent in English. *Word* (August–December 1958). 14: 110–149.

[55] R. H. Stetson, *Bases of phonology.* Oberlin, Ohio: Oberlin College Publication, 1949. Pp. 38–42.

* The normal breath-group is an innately determined, synchronized standard pattern of activity wherein the respiratory and laryngeal muscles act to produce phonation on the flow of expiratory air.

to be largely independent of pitch, loudness, and duration. As overtones develop in a child's voice, quality makes this important contribution of color to prosody and speech perception. Some children as late as adolescence possess thin, tired voices. Others develop overtones producing nasal, guttural, or harsh voice qualities. Such undesirable qualities invariably distort perceptual cues.

Prosody and Learning a Second Language. In learning to speak foreign languages today a fundament of the aural-oral approach is prosodic training. Pronunciation and vocabulary exercises have been deemphasized and the melodic pattern of the new language is stressed. The adult who attempts to master a second language is told that he must discard his overlearned patterns of prosody peculiar to his native tongue—but he rarely does. The young members of his family, who have not overlearned their native language and whose nervous systems still are plastic, acquire the second language quite easily. The adult finally learns to speak the foreign tongue fairly well—"after his fashion." But here is the rub—"after his fashion." He is more comfortable conversing with other Americans who also speak the second language as he does, with American prosodic patterns. He understands them more easily than native speakers. And he is in special trouble when he wrestles with a language in which sound-length differentiates meaning. In Norwegian, for example, *bønner* is the word for *beans* and for *farmers*. The length of the [n:] phoneme determines the meaning. Sounds, however, may be in correct order and have proper duration, yet perception may be difficult because the melodic patterns of Norwegian speech do not accord with ours. Several times in a foreign speech center the same sentences spoken both by the American and native teachers were recorded and analyzed. The rhythmic patterns varied only slightly but sufficiently to obscure meaning. Another experience with language comprehension comes to mind, that of listening to foreign speech in the United Nations Assembly through translator headphones. The translator, in an unfamiliar speech melody, repeats detached phrases without intonation or rhythmic cues. The translator is not communicating meaning; he is saying words. The prosodic cues are so few that we, too, give up the struggle to comprehend. Cherry suggests that such a translator "is almost in the situation of a parrot which had been taught to speak and could say, 'Wipe your feet!' or 'Go to hell!' without having thoughts of dirty shoes or of damnation." [56]

Prosodic Disturbances. A few years ago an adult aphasic, whom the writer had known previous to the friend's cerebral accident, was entered in our Center. The man had lived in the United States since early childhood and spoke English without a trace of his native Swedish tongue. His associates, both business and social, did not know Swedish, so he had no occasion to use it. His wife was English by descent. The

[56] C. Cherry, *op. cit.*, p. 279.

results of the accident which we could not explain were these: (1) His speech bore unmistakable patterns of Swedish intonation and stress; and (2) there was a marked loss of comprehension of English, the language that he had used for fifty-five years, but a less severe loss when he was addressed in Swedish, a language that he had used only up to the age of nine years. We have no clear explanation of the greater loss in his comprehension and use of English. We surmise that Swedish prosodic patterns remained the more basic ones in the neural networks mediating language. Perhaps the cues of intonation and rhythm which he learned in early childhood triggered perception of Swedish phrases and sentences.

A Scandinavian neurologist was among the first to study these prosodic disturbances in neurologically handicapped children and adults.[57] He found that a sentence spoken with a certain intonation pattern often had no ideational connections in the child's mind with the very same sentence, spoken with a different intonation. Monrad-Krohn recalls also an aphasic adult, a Norwegian, whose altered prosodic quality of speech following cerebral injury in a bomb explosion, caused her to be mistaken for a Norwegian-speaking German. In Nazi-occupied Oslo (1940–1945), the strange prosody of her speech was a source of constant embarrassment. In working with the adult aphasic we have noticed that if he can *initiate* a familiar rhythmic sentence pattern, he is usually able to complete the sentence. Ettore Bocca (Milan) found in testing the deterioration of auditory perception in the aged that rhythm was of paramount importance in the correct recognition and repetition of sentences. When the rhythm was altered by "varying irregularly the output velocity of speech" or "by shifting the accent of words to wrong places," the old-age group dropped in perception from 50 to 0 percent.[58] Teachers of language-handicapped children regularly report that when they employ marked variations in intonation and rhythm, comprehension of language is increased.

Morphemic Unit: Perceptual Basis of Sound Sequences. The baby's elementary intonational patterns gradually give way to keener analysis of phonological components. He begins to perceive the free morphemic unit, composed perhaps of a single syllable or of several syllables. The morpheme, as defined by Mario Pei, is a minimal unit of speech that is recurrent and meaningful; it may be a word or part of a word (un-friend-ly); it is a free morpheme if it can stand alone (friend), a bound morpheme if it cannot be used by itself (un-, -ly).[59] Morphemes are

[57] G. A. Monrad-Krohn, The prosodic quality of speech and its disorders. *Acta Psychiat Neurol* (1947), 22 (3–4): 255–260.

[58] E. Bocca, Clinical aspects of cortical deafness (Sixth International Congress on Audiology). *Laryngoscope* (March 1958), 68: 305–308.

[59] M. Pei, *Glossary of linguistic terminology.* New York: Columbia University Press, 1966. P. 167.

characterized by a specific distribution. Compounds, phrases, clauses, and finally, sentences all are higher order constructions composed of morphemes.[60] Physiologically they correlate most closely with the breath pulse and acoustically with the intensity curve.[61] They are true message units and are composed of phonemic sequences that are meaningful *only* in their sequential combination. The single acoustic event, the sound in isolation, is not important in the perceptual process. What is important is the identification and discrimination of *sequences* of acoustic events, and the smallest sequence with which meaning can be associated is the *morpheme*. Lieberman calls this sequence the "phonemic phrase." [62] The acoustic-kinesthetic cues to the morpheme actually are the auditory and movement patterns occurring as *transitional sounds* within and between sequences. "These transitions," Liberman says, "are not merely the incidental acoustic accompaniments of the movements that a speaker must make when he goes from 'consonant' to 'vowel.' Rather they are perceptual cues, and it is difficult to exaggerate their importance." [63]

Another argument for the morpheme as a perceptual unit relates to scanning and feedback (p. 91). In perceiving language, the "scanners" in the nervous system cannot review every phoneme. There are cues, highlights, which the feedback mechanism sets upon as significant. So a sound in isolation may bear little resemblance proprioceptively and auditorially to the sound in a phrase. In books devoted to articulation therapy, it is assumed that the teaching of the correct production of individual phonemes is the logical way to proceed. The very nature of the feedback process, however, controverts such teaching. By scanning, the circuits mediating feedback must light upon those cues, those language bits, which transmit the essential information most readily. The bit may be a single morpheme; it may be two or three syllables; it could be an entire phrase. In terms of economy in time and in the preemption of pathways, the scanner could not attend to a serial review, phoneme by phoneme. Yet an idea often persists long after the brains have been knocked out of it. Some day perhaps we will witness the demise of the sound-in-isolation approach to language learning.

Syntactic Structure

Noam Chomsky [64] was among the first to call attention to the importance of syntactic structure in developing language. He and his

[60] J. Lotz, Linguistics: Symbols make man. In S. Saporta, Ed., *Psycholinguistics.* New York: Holt, Rinehart and Winston, 1961. Pp. 7–8.

[61] R. H. Stetson, *Motor phonetics.* Amsterdam: North Holland Publishing Company, 1951. Pp. 1–5. P. Lieberman, *Intonation, perception, and language.* Cambridge, Mass.: M. I. T., 1967. Pp. 104–105.

[62] P. Lieberman, *ibid.,* p. 108f.

[63] A. M. Liberman, Some results of research on speech perception. *J Acoust Soc Amer* (January 1957), 19: 120.

[64] N. Chomsky, *Syntactic structures.* (The Hague: Mouton, 1957). N. Chomsky,

fellow linguists have attempted to find universal rules which generate functional grammars. These universal features of grammar, Chomsky believes, are innate in the human being for they vary little from language to language. Hence a child has internalized a set of rules for forming, using, and understanding sentences. It is the business of the linguist to discover these rules.

Speech scientists have been concerned primarily with developmental schedules for certain features of language. We have age indices for the acquisition of phonemes and words, vocabulary studies detailing comprehension, word count, frequency, and length. Phrase, sentence length, and complexity have been measured. What we have not determined seems more basic to language, *viz.*, the age at which children develop a generative grammar, the kind of grammar children use, and the modifications they make in grammar as they mature. Our principal knowledge on this subject is borrowed from scholars in psycholinguistics.

Quite early the child develops a sense of word order: subject, verb, direct object. At 18 months he reduces the number of words when he imitates adult speech but preserves the syntax. Brown and Bellugi believe that he makes the reduction because he cannot store more than four morphemes at that age or because he is able to program only a specific length of utterance.[65] Another explanation is that he only *perceives* the stressed, semantically strong words; nouns, verbs, adjectives. The "little words" belong to syntactic classes, called *closed functors* in psycholinguistic terminology, which are unimportant in terms of semantic content. In fact he may not hear the weakly stressed functors. And if the word is polysyllabic he retains and repeats only the stressed part. So at 2½ years, Lisa says "nocer-nose" (rhinoceros) and "kan-roo" (kangaroo). The telegraphic speech of the young child may be considered to be syntactical just as is the telegraphic speech of the adult who is under constraint of time or of the adult handicapped by aphasia.

By 2½ years the child has advanced a good way in developing syntactic structure. Now he identifies phrase structure in a "string of words." He learns that noun-phrases include the articles *a, an, the*. He understands the difference between an imperative and a declarative sentence. Since only certain classes of words, both from a semantic and grammatic point of view, can be placed in the various phrases, he limits his selection to specific classes of words. Words, however, often have multiple meanings; here the child must establish from the context, which often extends beyond the sentence, the appropriate meaning. By combining semantic and syntactic knowledge in this process, he is able to limit further the set

The formal nature of language. In E. Lenneberg, Ed., *Biological foundations of language*. New York: Wiley, 1967. Pp. 397–443.

[65] R. Brown and U. Bellugi, Three processes in the child acquisition of syntax. In E. Lenneberg, Ed., *New directions in the study of language*. Cambridge, Mass.: M. I. T., 1964. Pp. 131–163.

of alternative words from which he makes his perceptual choices.[66] Finally he comprehends semantic rules involving multiple meanings of words and fine discriminations within a context. He emerges in free-wheeling fashion to construct his own sentences, but that is a part of the chapter which follows.

The child with a language impairment often does not perceive the "natural phrase structures" inherent in the string of words of the sentence. Since he does not understand noun and verb phrases he does not know which words belong in each class. As a result he must canvass an un-classified vocabulary, attempting by trial and error to select appropriate words. At 7 or 8 years he still may omit the closed functors: conjunctions, prepositions, auxiliary verbs, and articles. He regularly confuses the order of words in a simple sentence: noun, verb, object. He seems un-able to discover the latent structure in the imitated sentences and, there-fore, he cannot construct independently his own sentences. Sometimes he tries to memorize a related group of sentences on which he can draw. His language is markedly defective.

Articulatory Defects and Syntactic Imperception. In several recent reports the link between articulatory defects and aspects of language retardation has been explored.[67] Menyuk connects articulatory defects specifically with retardation in syntactical form.[68] Articulation ap-parently is poor for the same reason that sentence structure is poor—because the child's perception of the structure of the speech *continuum* is undefined. He is not skilled, he may never be skilled in the perception of grammar and syntax.

Semology: Perception of Linguistic Information [69]

Syncretism: "Perception of the Whole and Nothing First." The child learning language comprehends it as a whole, whether that whole be a two-word phrase or pivot words that stand for the whole. He comprehends it in its total frame including background, although there

[66] In a study of auditory perception involving grammatical, anomalous, and ungrammatic sentences, it was found that "both syntactic and semantic rules are normally involved in the perception of sentences."—G. A. Miller and S. Isard, Some per-ceptual consequences of linguistic rules. *J Verbal Learn Verbal Behav* (September 1963), 2: 226.

[67] C. V. Mange, Relationships between selected auditory perceptual factors and articulation ability. *J Speech Hearing Res* (September 1960), 3: 67–73. K. de Hirsch, J. Jansky, and W. Langford, The oral language performance of premature children and controls. *J Speech Hearing Dis* (February 1964), 29: 64. E. K. Monsees, Aphasia in children. *J Speech Hearing Dis* (February 1961), 26: 83–86.

[68] P. Menyuk, Comparison of grammar of children with functionally deviant and normal speech. *J Speech Hearing Res* (June 1964), 7: 109–121.

[69] *Semology:* For interpretation of term see H. Gleason, The organization of language: A stratificational view. In C. Stuart, Ed., *Language and linguistics: Mono-graph series 17.* Washington: Georgetown University Press, 1964. P. 81.

may be diverse elements in the frame. Claparède called this stage of comprehension syncretism, and applied it particularly to the development of language and thought in the child.[70] Just as the child perceives objects, people, experiences as part of the setting in which they are found, so he comprehends language in a matrix that includes bodily postures, facial expression, gestures, and background noises. Adults frequently engage in the same kind of syncretic perception. The playwright demonstrated in *Arsenic and Old Lace* that gesture, intonation, facial expression, and dulcet tones may veil completely the meaning of the words, "May I put a tiny pinch of arsenic in your tea?" Generally we do not divorce the symbols of speech from man's gestures, his facial expressions, or from the physical surround. Sometimes we are fooled by gestural accompaniment, for gestures do not possess universal meaning. In Ankara, Turkey, the writer approached a bus driver to ask if he were going her way. "Kavakledere, Efendim?" she inquired. The driver raised his head quickly in assent—or so the writer thought—and gurgled something like "Yok" in his throat. The writer attempted to board the bus but twenty Turks, who also nodded their heads, protested her entrance most vigorously. In Turkey the gesture we associate with *yes* means *no*.

The child, like the adult, does not analyze the meaning of individual words when he is learning to comprehend and use language. The child comprehends meaning, at least in the elementary stages, in terms of complete units, of phrases or sentences. Much later (3 to 4 years), he may attend occasionally to recurrent smaller acoustic units, occasionally to phonemes, but only after he has developed a closed and structured repertory of utterances.[71] He may not be able to explain word meanings in his closed repertory but undoubtedly he understands them. The writer reads a foreign newspaper, sometimes aloud. When asked to explain the meaning of specific phrases, however, she is completely at a loss. Others have reported another experience which the writer can corroborate. Once several languages, in the Indo-European group, for example, have been mastered, the individual may understand the meaning of a language with which he has had no real experience. He perceives the sense of the speech although he cannot repeat a single word. If one speaks and reads Scandinavian languages, for instance, he can get the sense of a paragraph in German or, at least, follow the oral directions of the hotel doorman in Bonn. If he flies from Helsinki to Leningrad, however, his knowledge of all the Indo-European languages may not help him unless perchance he wishes to order cucumbers (modifications of the word, *agurk*, are found in many Indo-European languages and in Russian). A diet of cucumbers palls on one quickly, particularly for breakfast.

[70] M. Claparède, Exemples de perception syncrétique chez un enfant. *Arch Psychol* (July 1907), 7: 195–198.

[71] C. F. Hockett, *Modern linguistics.* New York: Macmillan, 1958. P. 358.

So the child in early language learning comprehends meaning in the total context. He perceives the word *ball* in the sentence *Find the large, red ball* more easily than when the word is taken out of context and he is asked to respond to *ball*. If the principle of all-or-nothing perception is the basis of learning in the young child, it seems reasonable to assume that teaching of language to children handicapped by linguistic disorders should proceed by wholes, or at least by substantial linguistic units. One cue *in context* is far more valuable than many isolated ones.

A child *uses* oral language in the same syncretic manner. The symbols of speech are one with his gestures, his facial expression, his total action. In talking over the telephone, Kim accompanies her speech with very explicit gestures. One day she telephoned the writer to show her how she had learned to wink in nursery school. Speech and gestures are learned as "one piece." Sometimes words do not agree with Kim's understanding of the gestural pattern. "It's spitting snow," the writer said to her. "Spitting?" she said aloud but to herself, "like this," and then proceeded to demonstrate spitting of saliva. A physically handicapped child suffers disadvantage at the outset in speaking because he is unable to command the total pattern of expression, including gestures, facial expression and the prosodic elements.

Syncretism and Figure-Ground. Perception of the whole does not mean the whole of all verbal stimuli surrounding the child. Rather syncretistic perception suggests that he comprehends all significant cues belonging to the percept as a whole. Implicit in syncretism is the ability to distinguish these cues from the welter of speech noises in the surround. Very early in language learning the average child recognizes the figure-ground structure, i.e., the organization of a salient central feature which is separate and distinct from its surrounding background.[72] So the salient features or cues to speech belonging to the whole are perceived against a background of other sounds just as a visual cue of a figure is perceived against a background of other visual stimuli. In language learning these peaks or cues in sound sequences emerge from the general sink of sounds in the surround and coalesce in a melodic pattern which they possess in common. It is this pattern which the baby perceives as a whole and which accounts for his first verbal responses.

Reversals and confusion in figure-ground perception are a frequent experience of every child in a learning situation. It takes maturity to hold a cue against a tendency to reverse it. As our perceptive tracks develop, we gradually fix cues in the proper matrix. So learning skills advance. In children with language delay or disturbance, maturation without special training does little to improve their skill in perception of foreground. They must be taught how to find the cues and to fix

---

[72] H. Grey, M. D'Asaro, and M. Sklar, Auditory perceptual threshold in brain-injured children. *J Speech Hearing Dis* (March 1965), 8: 49.

them. Some children find it difficult to perceive foreground cues because their attention fluctuates just at that second when the cue significant to meaning appears. Nancy, aged 6 years, seriously handicapped in language learning, cannot hold the auditory foreground against any change in the background of sound. Words and phrases are mixed in Nancy's perception with the clang of the Coke machine down the hall, the class bell, the drone of an airplane, and her sister's chatter in the lounge. As a result, she frequently responds with "pieces of recall," disordered verbal fragments. Steven, a cerebral-palsied boy, now 15 years of age, recognizes his problem and talks about it. In the welter of speech and other noises assaulting his ears, he says that he cannot select the ones he is "supposed to hear." Because he cannot separate foreground from background he is unable to structure his auditory world. For him no *patterns* of sound can be clearly differentiated. After five years of instruction, he has improved his skill in this area but only in controlled clinical situations. He tried out his abilities at a school party six months ago. The following morning he could not recall for us a single remark made to him. He vows he will not go again. Steve's problem is not a unique one. There are many children with language disabilities who cannot select meaningful auditory cues. Steve is *not* like the majority in this group in one respect: he still has an interest in acoustic phenomena. Some children who cannot separate foreground from background sounds reject completely the world of sound. They feel more secure when they shut out the auditory field they cannot structure.[73]

Syncretism and Closure. Closure, in a sense, is so closely related to discrimination of figure-ground that it scarcely can be discussed as a psychological entity. It might be best conceived as the tool of figure-ground perception. The figure or form of a sentence, for example, is set in a ground or a "frame of expectation in which the sentence occurs." [74] Even a child of 3 years, knowing what to expect, can predict much of what he hears *before* he hears it. An adult, relying upon realized expectations in the past, predicts much, even without paying rapt attention. Notice, however, how difficult is the comprehension of language when it is not one's native tongue. Although one responds in his native language to minimal cues, supplying missing words and completing unfinished sentences himself, now he must hang breathlessly on every syllable, sure that if he misses a single one he will understand nothing. In part he does not comprehend because he has no frame of expectation. Parenthetically we might add that one will be more successful if he does not try to attend in this way. When he attends only to the peaks

[73] H. Myklebust, *Auditory disorders in children.* New York: Grune & Stratton, 1954. Pp. 165–166. J. Reichstein and J. Rosenstein, Differential diagnosis of auditory defects. *Exceptional Child* (October 1964), 31: 64–82.
[74] A. Strauss and N. C. Kephart, *Psychopathology and education of the brain-injured child, II.* New York: Grune & Stratton, 1955. P. 110.

of meaning the figure will emerge more clearly and speedily from the background.

Some neurologically handicapped children with language disorders do very poorly on tests of closure (p. 288). They are not able to complete such simple sentences as: *May I have some bread and* _____?; *We go to church on* _____.; *Put the shoes and* _____ *on the dolly.* They do not know what to expect but behind their failure lie more profound deficits in comprehension of phonologic, grammatic, and semantic patterns of language. They have no frame on which to hang their expectations.

Categorization. The young child takes another step in perception of meaning of oral language when he begins to categorize words and word sequences. In the beginning he may select from pivotal phrases the word *don't,* for example, and combine it inaccurately but meaningfully in his own pivotal phrases. Two-year-old Kim understands *don't eat that* and many similar *don't* phrases so is it not quite sensible for her to say, *don't look me; don't sit down me* (I don't want to sit down). Her phrases belong to the general group of *don't* activities. Often she makes semantic mistakes in her transfer of "pivot words," demonstrating the instability of the syncretic phrase. She says that the hot stove "will bite" or the knife "will bite" just as she says "that dog will bite."

Very soon the child drops this form of differentiation and recombination, although he will return to it in a more sophisticated form in a later stage of synthesis. Now he begins to categorize by the perception of *differences.* According to Claparède's principle of awareness, the normal child perceives differences before he is able to detect similarities.[75] Binet also acknowledged this principle in the construction of the intelligence test. At 4½ years, the child is asked to determine in what way two objects are different whereas he is 7 years old before he is asked to detect similarities between two things. Claparède reasons that differences produce maladaptation and upset the internal equilibrium of the child; hence he is made aware of differences very early in his life whereas similarities create no such state of internal unrest. Vygotsky disagrees with Claparède's reasoning although he agrees with the premise: "The child becomes aware of differences earlier than of likenesses, not because differences lead to malfunctioning, but because awareness of similarity requires a more advanced structure of generalization and conceptualization than awareness of dissimilarity." [76]

As Vygotsky has said, categorization must become more advanced before both processes, *differences and similarities,* enter the structure of perception. We frequently see language-handicapped children with perceptual deficits who cannot reach this stage of categorization. Given

[75] L. S. Vygotsky, *op. cit.,* p. 88.
[76] *Ibid.*

a matching problem which demands that he find what goes with what, as in the Leiter International Test of Intelligence, the 4-year-old child with language delay frequently displays the kind of syncretism typical of the first stage of learning. He places the blocks in the order in which he finds them. He simply reproduces the pattern presented to him. In block assembly based on color, he heaps block upon block; he does not recognize the direction to assemble by color. In some instances children with language delay adopt a bizarre plan of categorization. For example, a cerebral-palsied lad, faced with an array of blocks of many shapes and colors, used neither shape nor color as the basis of grouping. He attempted to make designs composed of circles, squares, triangles, and rectangles. He could not abstract the features which these blocks had in common and thus failed to perceive the usual mode of categorization.

Synthesis. The perception of similarities and differences leads to synthesis, a stage generally accompanied by increasing language facility. Perhaps language growth precedes this stage of synthesis, for we know that young children *use* language to assist them in finding relations. The perceived object or experience becomes related to a definite category through words. "Under the influence of the word, the young child's perception . . . acquires new features; by allowing him to distinguish the essential features of an object, the word makes his perception of objects generalized and constant." [77] So a young child verbalizes, or talks aloud to himself as he discriminates differences. A child working on a puzzle and talking aloud—to himself—says, "No, that's not the way; that color doesn't belong there; it must go this way." Finally he announces to no one in particular, but with a sense of elation, "Now, that's right!" The verbal signals have aided him in differentiating color and form, and in stabilizing the percept. Language has a definite function in developing perception.

Another child, Lynn, has had instruction since 3 years of age when he was entered in the Center because he had no speech. Now at age 6, he is repeating kindergarten but the report of the teacher is indicative of a spurt in mental development which is almost phenomenal:

> He talks about everything now, although much of his speech is incomprehensible. But the singular growth is in all activities of the class. He understands what is wanted in construction, design, games, colors, numbers, and enters into every activity with zest. At last we can assure the parents that he will be ready shortly for the first grade.

Language motivation and group training in speech and language may have been but two factors in his progress. The chances are that they were significant ones.

---

[77] A. R. Luria and F. Ia. Yudovich, *Speech and the development of mental processes in the child.* London: Staples, 1959. P. 17.

The basic processes of categorization and synthesis become a major problem in teaching the adult aphasic. The day following a presidential inauguration the writer asked Sina, "Did you see the inaugural ceremony on television?" "Yes," Sina replied, and belatedly added "Johnson." "Johnson and Humphrey," the writer continued, "What will they do?" The question was filled with fearful implications for some people, but the writer was moving on to the idea, "What have *they* in common?" "Johnson," she began and then added "Humphrey," but the writer came in with a hasty, "No; *they*: What can you say about the two together?" The writer wrote their names and tied them together with "they." "Oh, I see," said Sina. But she did not *see;* she did not perceive the meaning of the pronoun, *they,* as the next session proved.

Laura Lee, in her illuminating paper, "Two Kinds of Disturbed Communication," [78] tells in greater detail of the need to help the aphasic to see similarities and differences, and so to develop generalization or abstraction. Here is her account of the problem of an aphasic who also is unable to comprehend and use the word, *they:*

The lady whom I wish to tell about had a stroke when she was fifty and lost much of her former language skill. At one of our meetings she pointed to an unfamiliar word on the page and said,

"Mrs. Lee, this . . . what, please?"

"Mrs. Lee, this . . . what, please?"

"That's the word *they,*" I said. "Do you understand *they?*"

"They? they? I never, never . . . *they.*"

"I'll show you *they,*" I said. "Tell me something about Tom and Mary."

I knew they were friends of hers.

"Well, Tom—Mary—dinner—Saturday night."

I supplied the missing abstract words and wrote it on a paper—"Tom and Mary are coming for dinner Saturday night." Then I circled the words *Tom* and *Mary,* crossed them out, and wrote *t-h-e-y* above them. "*They* are coming for dinner Saturday night."

"Oh, *they* . . . they. Yes, you. *They* . . ."

And she seemed to understand. She even said,

"Funny thing. Always, always, I speak . . . names, names, names. Never, never *they*." And this was true. In fact, she very seldom used pronouns at all.

Just as some adult aphasics must be taught to ascend the ladder of abstraction toward synthesis so others begin with a generalized construction, the top of the ladder, and must be taught how to descend. Sten, who at 45 suffered a serious cerebral injury, told the writer that he gave flowers to his wife on their wedding anniversary. ("My wife . . . wedding . . . flowers.") "What kind of flowers?" He ponders for a while and then says, "red flowers." Sten is a gardening buff and grows

[78] L. L. Lee, Two kinds of disturbed communication. *Gen Semantics Bull* (1958), 22–23: 49.

red roses. Yet he could not go down the ladder of abstraction to the concept of red roses. It remained a weak generalization. The adult aphasic, like many language-handicapped children, cannot discover in an experience those factors that are common and those that are different— or if he can, he is unable to verbalize them.

Perceptual Elaboration: Thinking. The neural circuits mediating perception, inner language, and motor speech may be extended by their continued exercise and excitement of neighboring circuits so that finally they have taken into their company many engrams that were not represented in the initial response. The continuance of the process of correlation and integration results in ideas, in *thought.* Apparently the neurological events (coding processes) are the same as for other types of behavior. They are the same, Halstead says, "whether *the prevailing set of the system* be predominantly for perception, learning, emotion or thinking." [79]

Language and Thinking. Can we think without the implement of symbols? *Do* we think without symbols? The dialogue on both questions has been recurring since the seventeenth century. Yeas and nays on the first question seem to be tied. Vygotsky,[80] Koehler,[81]and Buehler [82] contend that there is a "prespeech nonsymbolic phase of thought development" in childhood. Vygotsky says on this point: "When the child approaches his second birthday . . . the curves of development of thought and speech, 'til then separate, meet and join to initiate a new form of behavior . . . the child makes the greatest discovery of his life that everything has its name." [83] Stewart would agree that nouns mark the advent of real language because they alone make sentences possible, but he does not say that thinking and rudimentary symbolic expression have not occurred before the advent of "real language." [84]

The current of the argument advanced by Lewis,[85] Chesni,[86] Whorf,[87] and Luria [88] takes this direction: In the early "preoperational stage" of thought there may be no outward expression but the child nonetheless may be using linguistic symbols in responses of perception and inner

[79] W. C. Halstead, Thinking, imagery and memory. In J. Field, Ed., *Handbook of physiology, sec. 1: Neurophysiology III.* Washington: Amer. Physiol. Soc., 1960. Pp. 1669–1670.

[80] L. S. Vygotsky, *op. cit.*

[81] W. Koehler, *Cerebral mechanisms in behavior.* New York: Wiley, 1951.

[82] K. Buehler, *The intellectual development of children.* Stuttgart: Gustav Fischer Verlag KG, 1927.

[83] L. S. Vygotsky, *op. cit.,* p. 43.

[84] G. R. Stewart, *Man, an autobiography.* New York: Random House, 1946.

[85] M. M. Lewis, *Language, thought and personality.* London: Harrap, 1963.

[86] Y. Chesni, *op. cit.,* pp. 189–196.

[87] B. L. Whorf, Language, thought and reality. In J. B. Carroll, Ed., *Selected writings of Benjamin Lee Whorf.* New York: Wiley, 1956. Pp. 213–215.

[88] A. R. Luria and F. Ia. Yudovich, *Speech and the development of mental processes in the child.* London: Staples, 1959. Pp. 7–24.

language. Moreover, symbolic expression is not always linguistic. Perhaps linguistic symbols are not employed, for example, in the use of tools or in operations requiring "practical intellect." Of course we have no evidence that they were not used in internal language before or during praxic operations. Whorf's study of the Hopi and Shawnee Indians supports the language-thought bond. The linguistic system (grammar) in our minds, Whorf contends, organizes our percepts, our ideas. If the linguistic system does not permit, for example, the pluralization of nouns—and this is the case in the Hopi language—categorization or generalization of a concept perforce is limited. So language can scarcely be called a *reproducing instrument* for voicing ideas but rather is itself the shaper of ideas, the program and guide of the individual's mental activity, for his analysis of impressions, for his synthesis of his mental stock in trade. Whorf does not say that we cannot think *unless* we have a symbol system; what he does say is that thought without the tool of symbolization cannot be organized, elaborated, or directed. Luria would go one step further to suggest that the acquisition of a language system is the tool which *forms and incites mental activity.* "In the beginning there was the word," and continuously there has been the word which abstracts, isolates the necessary signals, and generalizes perceived signals.

The questions pertaining to thought and verbal symbols are perennials, flourishing in each new spring of thought. We cannot accept Chomsky's recent statement: "I am quite convinced that thinking can proceed perfectly well without language"; [89] neither are we willing to say with Whorf that "if we have no word for it we do not perceive it." Thought and language development in the young child undoubtedly are bound in close valence. Occasionally he may use cruder tools in his intellectual processes. Verbal symbols, we think, are his *best* tool, and if auditory and visual modalities are intact, assuredly he is not going to rely upon less skillful tools very long. As he becomes more skillful in verbalization, perceptual organization, elaboration, and direction advance. The vast problem of training perception of deaf children is convincing proof that the symbols of language are the prime tool in perceptual development—in thinking.

Evaluation of Meaning. Words, phrases, sentences are not immutable, set in cement with the object or idea they represent. They are dynamic, not static formations. As thought changes, so expression changes. Thought and expression embrace a continual movement from thought to verbal sequences and verbal sequences to thought, and as they move back and forth, each changed. Language has a form, a morphology that provokes new ideas; new ideas stimulate a new vocabulary, which in turn

[89] N. Chomsky, The general properties of language. In F. Darley, Ed., *Brain mechanisms underlying speech and language.* New York: Grune & Stratton, 1967. P. 85.

stimulates language development. So language develops; so thought develops.

Language Disturbances, Thought, and Intelligence. The development of thought and language does not proceed at the same pace in all children. In some children oral expression apparently lags behind thought; in others the converse seems to be the case. In a sizeable group, both thought and language are substandard. They are the mental retardates, children whose perceptual ability is poor because their genetic maturational index is low.[90] The neural assemblies, possessing synaptic connections that are sparse in number and low in potential, have insufficient numbers and lack power to transform, to organize the sensory experiences into meaningful concepts. As a consequence both implicit and explicit speech is meager, and correlatively, thought, too, is a starveling.

After we have pondered all these relations between thought and language, there are still "marbles left in the ring." The "secret sits in the middle and knows." Perhaps the secret of the agate may be posed in this form: Does a disturbance of language entail a disorder of intellect either on a quantitative or qualitative basis? If language is the tool of thought, the answer must be yes; if language and thought are reciprocally related, still the answer is in the affirmative. The secret lies in the variable nature of the loss in mental ability. The CNS deficit may be molecular or molar in its effect, but in either case, there is a diminution in mental power. It may be so subtle that the individual is able to conceal it from everyone except himself.

Although Critchley was writing about adult aphasia, his remarks apply to the intellectual deficits associated with neurological learning disorders of children. He approaches the secret of the remaining marbles in the ring:

> Eventually there will surely emerge proof of some affection of intellect . . . running like a scarlet thread through the pattern of all the aphasics. As Marcus Victoria said, "aphasic patients do not see or hear the other world like the rest of mankind. Their defects are deeper than the language defects and comprise functions correlated with the manipulation of symbols." . . . Aphasia must therefore constitute an aberration in the pattern of total behavior rather than a scotoma within the field of language behavior.

The primary defect in symbolization must cut deep into the entire process of coding and so affects perception, critical discrimination and evaluation (judgment), and the retention of ideas.[91]

[90] E. Maccoby, Developmental psychology. In P. R. Farnsworth, Ed., *Annual review of psychology.* Palo Alto: Annual Reviews, 1964. 15: 208.
[91] M. Critchley, Jacksonian ideas and the future. *Brit Med J* (July 2, 1960), 2: 10–11.

Motivation, Attention, and Retention in Language Learning

We shall consider motivation, attention, and retention separately although they scarcely can be called independent operants. Motivation and attention interact in learning. Whatever motivates one also commands his attention, and the effect of attention is to heighten motivation. The principal conditioners of motivation and attention, *viz.*, inner drives and external forces, also seem to be the same. If there is priority in these two operants in learning, attention might be considered the result of motivation. Retention or memory also belongs in this ring, for whatever facilitates motivation and attention enhances learning, and thereby increases retention.

Motivation. The purpose of motivation "is to arouse; to cause the organism to attend more closely to his environment. To motivate is also to influence the direction of the organism's attention; to increase the probability that the organism will respond to one class of stimuli rather than other classes of stimuli." [92] Both primary and secondary motivators (*push* and *pull* forces) cause the individual to exercise drive in order to achieve specific goals. Among these goals are: (1) identity, (2) self-worth, (3) competence, and (4) control of his environment.

Primary motivation is predicated upon a basic genetic drive, a kind of built-in force that varies with physical and neural potentials. In the push-pull theory of motivation, dynamic drive supplies the push producing a phase of discomfiture that is followed by action to reduce the tension. Some authorities describe this action as a biased homeostat, building up tension and restoring homeostasis when the act of learning has been accomplished.[93] So a child learning language resolves his needs and thereby reduces his tension states which are manifested in increased activity.[94]

Physical, psychical, and emotional factors also act to increase or decrease effectiveness of the built-in drive. Children with constitutional predispositions to physical or mental debility regularly exhibit low-powered drive. Prolonged emotional disturbances likewise upset the biased homeostat of innate drive. Emotion, properly controlled, is a powerful accessory to, if not an integral part of, genetic drive. Ordinarily frustration and fear produce an increase of drive; [95] hope results in drive

[92] R. C. Johnson, Linguistic structure as related to concept formation and to concept context. *Psychol Bull* (November 1962), 59: 468.

[93] K. H. Pribram, Reinforcement revisited: A structural view. In M. Jones, Ed., *Nebraska symposium on motivation.* Lincoln, Nebr.: University of Nebraska Press, 1963. Pp. 121; 124.

[94] R. L. Shelton, W. B. Arndt, and J. B. Miller, Learning principles and teaching of speech language. *J Speech Hearing Dis* (November 1961), 26: 368.

[95] "The existence of strong behavior which cannot be executed or if executed, is repeatedly ineffective, generates the familiar pattern called 'frustration.'"—B. F. Skinner, *Verbal behavior.* New York: Appleton-Century-Crofts, 1957. P. 214.

reduction. And when hope wins out over fear and frustration, learning is facilitated. Hopefulness supplies the probability of success and becomes an adjuster of homeostasis. A master teacher in any field is constantly aware of the need to keep hope going by intermittent reinforcement. Sometimes the teacher is sorely tried to find reinforcers. *The New Yorker* recently depicted in a cartoon a muscular camp director towering over a skinny bedraggled moppet as he confers with the father. "Mr. Poster," assures the director, "I never met a boy who accepted defeat as gracefully as your Borden." [96] If hope cannot be kept going—by a somewhat better reinforcer than the camp director's—the expectation of failure quickly brings motivation to a halt.

Secondary drives come from the pull side of motivation. They are external forces controlling and guiding action as it occurs.[97] Very early in life a child learns to respond to these secondary drives of reward and punishment in his environment. A baby's tensions and frustrations are reduced by rewards of pleasurable sounds and stimuli, by comfort and security. Between 4 and 5 years, the child becomes selective in his rewards, responding particularly to nurturance, praise, and recognition by his model, the *significant other person.* He is further rewarded and motivated as he increases his similarity to the model, for here is the image of what he wants to be. If he achieves identity like that significant other person, he too will enjoy the reward of self-worth, competence, and control of his environment.[98]

A master teacher uses this tool of facilitation by significant others in many ways. Especially among young children the act of taking one's cue from others and successfully imitating another's response is a great reward. They learn to do what they see and hear others are doing. The importance of an excellent model in a stimulating physical environment cannot be exaggerated. Both the environment and the people in that environment constitute powerful secondary drives in children's learning. In lower socioeconomic classes children generally lack motivation despite the fact that they have been told, warned, and admonished by their models to do well in school. But if their adult models, the parents, do not behave as if they valued intellective skills, they can scarcely expect the child to be motivated to acquire them.

Motivation and Language Learning. A baby learning to talk normally receives both immediate and intermittent reinforcement for his effort. The act of speaking, in itself, produces pleasurable responses within him and these internal responses are further reinforced by pleasur-

[96] *The New Yorker,* August 26, 1967, p. 21.

[97] O. Mowrer, *Learning theory and the symbolic processes.* New York: Wiley, 1960. P. 180.

[98] W. F. Hill, *Learning.* San Francisco: Chandler Pub., 1963. P. 82. J. Kagan, Motivational and attitudinal factors in receptivity to learning. In J. Bruner, Ed., *Learning about learning.* Washington: Bur. of Res., U. S. Office of Educ., 1966. Pp. 34–36.

able or satisfying responses from his environment: food, clean clothing, fondling, and pleasant sounds. As speech develops any language behavior that is part of the final pattern is accepted and praised. Hope replaces discomfiture and with the successful activity of language learning, self-reinforcement increases. Olver likens intermittent reinforcement to the continuous feedback of "getting warmer" or "getting colder" which children employ in guessing games.[99] But unlike the guessing games one does not finally say, "you're right"; to do so would mean complete homeostasis, a deterrent to new learning. It is the mild uncertainty that spurs one at any age to mastery. Untermeyer recognized this goad to achievement when he wrote,

> From compromise and things half-done
> Keep me, with stern and stubborn pride.
> And when, at last, the fight is won,
> God keep me still unsatisfied.[100]

By the age of 4 years self-reinforcement becomes a dominant means of learning. The child is eager to learn more language. In its practice, either overtly or implicitly, he internalizes both the substance and the linguistic form of a conversation with the parent, and then runs it off for himself. The child is his own paymaster, which is to say that by his mastery he provides his own continuing motivation and reinforcement.[101] This kind of activity is not random behavior produced by an overflow of energy. It is directed, selective, and persistent, and it continues because it satisfies an intrinsic need to establish his identity as a person and to deal competently with his environment.[102] The writer surrounded by 4- and 5-year-olds on a trip is under perpetual bombardment: "What's that?" or "What do you call it?" They will do it at home, too, but there the attack seems less concentrated. More frequently at home or in the nursery school, the child may not ask questions of others, but he still is asking himself, "What is that thing?" He contemplates it; he scans independently; he is searching for the cue.[103] As a result of this activity, the child establishes learned expectancies. He is becoming a real person in the sense that he knows what to expect from himself and his environment.

Motivation and Language Disorders. A major problem in teaching

[99] R. Olver, Tutor and learner. In J. Bruner, Ed., *Learning about learning.* Washington, D.C.: Bur. of Res., U. S. Office of Educ., 1966. P. 97.
[100] From *Prayer* in *Long Feud* by Louis Untermeyer. Copyright 1962 by Harcourt, Brace & World and Louis Untermeyer. P. 76.
[101] J. S. Bruner, The act of discovery. In J. P. DeCecco, Ed., *Human learning in the school.* Holt, Rinehart and Winston, 1963. P. 264f.
[102] R. W. White, Motivation reconsidered: The concept of competence. *Psychol Rev* (September 1959), 66: 297–333.
[103] J. S. Bruner, On perceptual readiness in perception. *Psychol Rev* (February 1957), 64: 123–152.

children with severe language handicaps is that many of them do not have the sense of identity to which we have just alluded. Lacking minimal competence in language, they seem to live in an existential vacuum, unable to say who they are, or worse, unable to *know* who they are. Perhaps the autistic child knows who he really is but he will not reveal his identity, at least to significant others. The nonautistic language-handicapped group so frequently seems to lack the built-in drive, inherent in neural potential and organization, which is necessary for perceptual readiness. Consequently they do not expect to hear what they hear, see what they see, feel what they feel. And the less their readiness, the greater must be the input or redundancy of auditory, visual, and tactile-kinesthetic cues if they are to learn at all. Some of these faceless children enter our resident summer Speech Center. As hope develops and fears and frustration diminish with speech training, we have watched them emerge as children with distinct identities and with some competence in dealing with their environment.

Specific reinforcers employed in teaching these speech and language-handicapped children follow the general pattern for all learning but with some modifications. For young language-handicapped children food (sugared cereals or sweets) seems to be the most effective operant conditioner. Plastic tallies and other tangible rewards also are used. Somewhat later the teacher's verbal praise ("That's a good try"; "Good boy,") and the approval of others outside the circle of significant others may become effective reinforcers. One wishes that the child might develop early the potent impetus that comes with a favorable feedback from the task accomplished, but in the severely handicapped the achievement may not meet the requisites even of early subgoals. If the child does attain a modicum of competence in speech, this achievement becomes a motivating force with several supplementary benefits. He gains a sense of self-worth, he is able to exercise some control over his environment, and most importantly, he assumes responsibility for his own learning. All too frequently speech teachers fail to recognize this transfer of responsibility from teacher to child. Ringing in the teacher's ears is the parent's injunction to "fix up" the youngster's speech, a responsibility the teacher cannot and should not assume. Rarely does the teacher ask the child for ideas on how he could fix up his own speech, yet this is one way of getting the child to realize his responsibility.

Some older children, preadolescent and adolescent, seem to be singularly resistant to any form of reinforcement. The replacement of hope by expectation of failure has practically eliminated motivation for language learning. Social rewards such as special privileges may constitute immediate positive reinforcement. In some instances such negative reinforcers as withdrawal of social reward following self-defeating language behavior or the use of imaginary, threat-inducing situations, for the purpose of enabling the individual to reduce anxiety by increased learning efforts, may work. And if the adolescent has been in a special speech class for three or four years, a semester's holiday could be a remarkable reinforcer.

Reinforcement gained by matching a model sometimes is not possible at any stage of language learning. Severely handicapped children, for example, very early in life appreciate the fact that they cannot hope to become like those significant others in their home environment. What motivation can a cerebral-palsied lad substitute for the drive to emulate his handsome father-model? What model will this 9-year-old girl find who is handicapped by cleft palate, and who cried out recently, "Who would want a kid with this ugly face and speech?" Our best hope as teachers may be to have them model after the leader in their group.

Motivation of a stimulating and pleasurable environment is much more important to language-handicapped children than to the normal child. The writer visited two institutions of child care in the Middle East. The children there, from infancy to 4 years, were left lying supinely in their cribs until they could pull themselves into a sitting position. When they could sit alone, they were placed on a linoleum strip covering a cement floor. There were no toys, no picture books, no children's furniture except cribs. Silent attendants took care of only minimal physical needs of the children. Gestural language was largely absent. One could detect few incentives to speech in blank walls, equally blank countenances, and silent aides. When the directors of the institutions were asked about the language development of these children, the reply was, "Retarded, of course, but you must realize that many homeless children are mentally retarded."

Deprivation of stimulation also had its effect upon the language development of a group of cerebral-palsied children in another country, and they were not seriously retarded in intelligence. These youngsters with many sensory-motor handicaps had little language, in part, because they had been deprived of stimulation. They were true perceptual retardates. When they were given opportunities to participate in the excitement of living which usually surrounds nonhandicapped children, they made notable advances in speech.

Contrast these environments with a school for mentally retarded children in this country where the writer served briefly as consultant. As we walked into a sunny corridor we noted "talk" placards everywhere, and we heard speech and laughter of children and staff. The goal clearly was "Get them to talk and respond to their talk." In a leaflet for the staff, reinforcement techniques are described—e.g., praise, reward of a toy, and oral demonstrations to others. Motivation seemed to be a primary operant throughout the school. In an advanced group learning to read, instructors used a special motivating device: linking the familiar with the unfamiliar. These children knew colors so a primary color was associated with letters of a single phonetic value. So the letters *u* in *cup* and *o* in *love,* both phonetically represented by [ʌ], were printed in yellow. Motivation becomes stronger when the material to be learned is reinforced by percepts already in one's command.

Attention. The neurological correlate of attention, the set-to-attend or perceptual set, has been discussed in the preceding chapter (p. 89). Its maturation may be accounted for by the developing wave patterns of the nervous system. In the very young infant attention is absent except for the crudest form of orientation response. He may react to stimulation but the response is not selective.[104] Attention is described in psychological terms as the directive process that exerts a selective influence on perception and derives its direction from the motivation of the learner and the nature of the materials to be learned.[105] Note in this description, as in the introduction to this section, that motivation and attention are interactive forces in learning (p. 144). Focus and span are aspects of attention but again we cannot have one without the other. A child must learn *what* to attend to, but he cannot do this if he is unable to focus over a time period or span. In other words, a focus demands temporal extensity as well as intensity.

Attention and Language Learning. The average child learns early how to focus on prosodic or melody patterns and on the peak phonological sequences of language. This is speech pared to the bone. He does not attend to single phonemes because such attention interferes with comprehension. When he is adult he will not attend to every dialectal variation or mispronunciation for the same reason. A little later in the learning period, the child will focus on syntactic cues that will subsume phonological sequences. Yet even in this stage of perception of phrase and sentence structure, he does not attend to every word or even to every phrase. If he attends proficiently, he picks out phrasal cues embedded in sentences or even groups of sentences. Much later he probably will focus his attention on the relation of semantic cues in context. The normal child sometimes can attend to two messages simultaneously, if the information is simple and response is immediate. If there are melodic differences and spatial separation of voices presenting the information, he even may succeed with more complex messages.

Attention and Language Disorders. We cannot account for all the vagaries of attention which we meet in teaching children with language disorders. We have coped with children who are highly distractible, who manifest a fleeting attention to the task at hand. Both focus and span of attention are very limited. Some in this group probably

[104] M. M. Lewis, *How children learn to speak.* London: Harrap, 1957. Pp. 34–36.
[105] M. Henle, Cognitive skills. In J. Bruner, Ed., *Learning about learning.* Washington: Bur. of Res., U. S. Office of Educ., 1966. P. 54.

have a neurological incapacity to maintain attentional intensity (focus) or a consistent level of extensity (span). All stimuli seem to affect them; almost compulsively they must respond to sights and sounds which intrude upon or are tangential to their environment. Consequently there are few foci of attention. Other linguistically handicapped children *seem* to attend, to listen to speech. They watch the teacher's face as she speaks. Their bodily tension and mimesis of articulatory movements simulate those of attention, yet if we judge by immediate recall, they have not focussed on the critical cues. Like the radar operator, they may suffer from peripheral or central distractions which make it impossible for them to pick up the blip on their screens. Rosenberg and Edwards suggest that their attention on the foreground fluctuates just at that second when the cue significant to meaning appears.[106]

We have tried various ways of establishing a consistent level of attention in language-handicapped children. We know, for instance, that a pleasing pitch pattern and vibrant quality are far more potent in holding this level than is the intensity or loudness of voice. We know that rhythmic speech acts as a carrier for syntactic and semantic elements and hence has a better chance of holding attention than nonrhythmic speech. More important, perhaps, are the quality of materials and the process of working with them. Endless drill can never compete with the attention manifested in a "talking commission" with the supervisor, principal, or significant others in the child's environment. Both focus and span of attention improve as the child *does* something with materials, particularly if the doing links his old skills with new skills to be learned. The writer asked a colleague to teach an acoustically handicapped group of preadolescent boys whose progress had been minimal in two preceding sessions. The instructor decided to center his teaching in electronic experiments and filled his classroom with hardware. He maintained the attention of these boys who could work with the equipment only if they responded to his directions as they worked. Neither closing time nor bells impinged upon their attention. And their gains in language proficiency were three times as great, in a single session, as the gains made in two previous sessions.

Another group of children with language disturbances is troubled by abnormal fixation of attention. They cannot shift attention to the next syllable, phrase, or sentence. John, 12 years old, is seriously retarded in speech. In reading a sentence aloud, he pulls letters out of the word, words out of phrases until meaning has disappeared in the sink. He attends over and over again to the same cue. Sometimes the fixation takes a different turn. With great effort and often accompanied

[106] R. Rosenberg and A. Edwards, The performance of aphasics on three automated perceptual discrimination programs. *J Speech Hearing Res* (September 1964), 7: 295–298.

by manifest anxiety, the child tries to attend to every word he hears, and in recall will attempt to repeat the passage word by word. Obviously he cannot do so. He must be taught to attend to the cues, the peaks of language.

Retention (Memory). The neurological correlate for memory, the fixation mechanism, has been discussed in the preceding chapter (p. 105). Because whatever increases the effectiveness of speech learning increases retention, we would expect motivation and attention to be prime effectors of memory. The aged frequently complain that their great problem in speech is failure of recall but, in reality, motivation and attention also are declining in strength. One must be motivated to remember. One also must remain an attentive listener; as Carlyle said, it is the disease of not listening which afflicts us all.

The baby developing speech remembers peak cues and hence unconsciously engages in economical and proficient learning. He saves on the costs in energy by developing a perceptual repertoire of cues, just as we save on the financial cost of sending a cable by eliminating all unnecessary words. In the initial stage of language development the child is able to recall a few word-sentences because he has a very limited repertoire. But as his acquisition grows he has little chance of remembering all contextual interpretations even of a few word-sentences. To hold in memory a record of every word or phrase in every conceivable context (holophrastic dictionary) is out of the question. Instead he develops a word-dictionary of cues which follows phonological, syntactic, and semantic rules.[107] He will remember, for example, the intonation contour or the syntactic order of a phrase because these patterns will carry the words in a sequence. In building this dictionary he is dependent, as he is in all language learning, upon the correlated power of auditory, visual, and tactile-kinesthetic feedback. When he cannot hear himself speak because of a noisy surround, for example, he may continue speaking because he remembers the movement patterns. The exercise of these movement patterns with auditory and visual patterns is essential if the correlated neural circuits are to remain potentially active and subject to ready recall. Such an exercise involves all the sensory-motor routes mediating language. An indirect bit of proof of this point comes from a longitudinal study of verbal behavior and intelligence by Bayley and colleagues, who report that noisy, active, vocalizing infants have higher intelligence ratings when they reach adulthood than do quiet ones.[108] Memory span has been tested generally by the recall of single phonemes or nonsense syllables. If a child remembers cues on phonological, syntactic, and semantic carriers, recall of

[107] D. McNeill, Developmental psycholinguistics. In F. Smith and G. Miller, Eds., *The genesis of language.* Cambridge, Mass.: M. I. T., 1966. Pp. 62–65.
[108] J. Cameron, N. Livson, and N. Bayley, Infant vocalizations and their relation to mature intelligence. *Science* (July 21, 1967), 157: 331–333.

meaningful sentences and short stories would seem to be a more valid assessment of a child's competence.

The child with a severe language impairment often tries to do what the normal child knows he cannot do. Unable to select the peak cues, he attempts the impossible job of constructing a holophrastic dictionary, which means that he must "record" the word in all contextual cues. The frequent complaint of their parents that these children say only words and will not attempt sentences is indicative of this basic deficiency in the coding process. Sometimes the child attempts to develop a set of sentences in one syntactic pattern. This, too, is a fruitless task because it allows him no freedom to develop a flexible grammatical system. Some workers in the field believe that short-term memory deficits are the primary cause of a child's inability to master sentence structure. He is unable, for example, to repeat a sentence that includes a subordinate clause. How does one measure short-term memory for sentence form? The test of memory for digits is scarcely analogous to the recall of a complex sentence. We can infer, perhaps, that short-term memory is deficient if a child does less well in the immediate repetition of speech samples in which he must adhere to a syntactic pattern than in spontaneous speech. The first step in training these children seems to be the strengthening of peak cues, and this may best be achieved by reauditorizing, revisualizing, and rekinesthesizing patterns of melody, syntax, and semology.[109]

These three aspects of language learning—motivation, attention, and retention—belong to a ring of interacting operants. Although psychologists today may pay scant attention to them, the special language teacher finds that they are powerful forces in language learning.

Cultural and Social Factors: Their Influence on Language Learning

The language retardation of children reared in foundlings' homes or orphanages is indicative of the effects of cultural and social deprivation. Even when the chronological and mental ages among institutional and control groups have been equated, the orphanage group is still markedly retarded in all measures of language.[110] Silence among adults in any group, family or institutional, is a particular drawback because children learn language more quickly from adults than from other children.[111] If further proof is needed, it can be found in the reports of acceleration in language maturation of children who have been placed in

---

[109] D. J. Johnson and H. R. Myklebust, Dyslexia in childhood. In J. Hellmuth, Ed., *Learning disorders I*. Seattle: Special Child Publications, 1965. Pp. 259–292.

[110] J. K. Moore, Speech content of selected groups of orphanage and non-orphanage pre-school children. *J Exp Educ* (December 1947), 14: 122–123.

[111] G. M. Siegel, Adult verbal behavior in play therapy. *J Speech Hearing Dis* (January 1963), Monograph supplement, No. 10: 34–39.

foster and adoptive homes after a period of two to three years in an institution.[112] Under the stimulation and affectionate relationships of the normal family environment in the new home, they usually make rapid advances in communication skills.

Family size. In the preceding paragraph we have noted that children need adult stimulation and models in learning language. In large families in which the children presumably learn their language from other children, linguistic retardation is common. In an investigation in Scotland of more than 5,000 children between 11 and 12 years old, Lewis reports that the "environment of the large family constitutes a handicap to verbal development and . . . this verbal development also affects general mental development." He ascribes the retardation in language to the association of children only with children and concludes that if children are to realize their cognitive potentialities, they will need constant communication with adults.[113] Although he recognizes that other factors such as lowered intelligence, lack of books, and restricted experiences handicap verbal development among those in the lower socioeconomic group (where large families were found in his study), "the much profounder and more permeative influence upon the children (is) the everyday language of family life." [114] McCarthy too believes that family size generally influences language learning. An only child, she says, matures much faster in language than a child with several siblings. She ascribes this superiority to an environment "affording greater association with adults, broader experience, and greater opportunities for practice in the use of language under optimum conditions." [115]

Social Relation of Twins and Language Development. Numerous studies [116] have established that language retardation is common among monozygotic twins, and the cause has been generally assigned to the development of "twin patois," an idioglossia used by the two children. Although the close social milieu of twins may be a plausible reason for their handicap in language, it may not be the only reason. We would place greater credence in a genetic factor which results in an atypical neural organization and thus may account not only for the high incidence of language delay and language disorders among twins, but also for the incidence of other neurogenic defects.[117] Willerman and Churchill also

[112] W. Goldfarb, Effects of psychological deprivation in infancy and subsequent stimulation. *Amer J Psychiat* (July 1945), 102: 18–33.

[113] M. M. Lewis, *Language, thought and personality in infancy and childhood.* London: Harrap, 1963. P. 198.

[114] *Ibid.,* pp. 199–201.

[115] D. McCarthy, Language development in children. In L. Carmichael, Ed., *Manual of child psychology* (2nd ed.) New York: Wiley, 1954. P. 589.

[116] N. Hirsch, *Twins: Heredity and environment.* Boston: Harvard, 1930. E. J. Day, The development of language in twins. In W. Dennis, Ed., *Readings in child psychology.* Englewood Cliffs, N. J.: Prentice-Hall, 1963. Pp. 179–201.

[117] M. F. Berry, Twinning in stuttering families. *Hum Biol* (September 1937), 9:

question close social milieu of twins as a cause of delayed language development and suggest that "depressed Verbal IQ, at least to some extent, is related to congenital factors." [118]

Ethnic Patterns. The pattern of family life, often conditioned by ethnic customs, must be considered in its relation to language. In certain ethnic groups, for example, the environment is one of talk. Children and adults talk at the dining table; they plan their entertainment as a family; the home is the communication center. No one can question the beneficial effects of this opportunity for practice upon developing speech and language patterns. In the resident summer Speech Center conducted by the writer, a large part of the program was a conscious direction of talking activities under the guidance of adults. The practice of oral language in the dormitory playrooms, the dining room (not a cafeteria), in crafts, rhythmics, and organized play, and in excursions to farm, zoo, and park was consciously motivated by adults. An environment of talk among children and adults pays large dividends in language maturation. Templin remarks on the great loquacity and linguistic maturity of present-day children in all sectors of American society.[119] Increased practice with linguistic tools inevitably must advance not only the use of language but also intellectual development with which it is linked.

In many ethnic groups, children must learn two languages simultaneously. The bearing of bilingualism upon language maturation still is an unsettled question. Although the consensus, based on research, seems to be that the children from monolingual homes tend to surpass children from polylingual environments,[120] it remains doubtful that proper consideration has been given to socioeconomic and intellectual differentials of the two groups. In our experience the simultaneous learning of two languages is advantageous for a child of high normal intelligence. He possesses two codes which he usually has mastered without difficulty. He transfers easily from one communication pattern to another. The problem arises with the child who has difficulty coding one language. If he cannot learn the linguistic form and vocabulary of one language, a second language will undoubtedly confuse and retard him further in learning his native tongue.

Other Cultural Influences. Some reports link the type of occupa-

---

329–346. R. West, S. Nelson, and M. F. Berry, The heredity of stuttering. *Quart J Speech* (February 1939), 25: 23–30.

[118] L. Willerman and J. Churchill, Intelligence and birth weight in identical twins. *Child Devel* (September 1967) 38: 629.

[119] M. Templin, *Certain language skills in children.* Minneapolis: University of Minnesota Press, 1957. Pp. 150–151.

[120] W. Wolski, Some variables in speech and language development in children. *Med Times* (September 1964), 92: 868–871. Sister M. A. Carrow, Linguistic functioning of bilingual and monolingual children. *J Speech Hearing Dis* (September 1957), 22: 371–380.

tion of the father with the language development of his children. Probably the socioeconomic status resulting from occupational level relates more basically to language development. The total experiential enrichment that should follow upon the acquisition of financial and social status must have a positive effect upon language learning.

A child's linguistic development may be conditioned by many things that we have not considered. The authority of parents and teachers, the patois of group-language, and the language of television may affect the child's learning, either positively or negatively. Climate undoubtedly has some bearing upon one's propensities for communication. The possibilities of research in this area have not been exhausted.

5

The Child Develops Language

Purpose of Language

A baby learning to talk reminds one of Samuel Johnson's story of women on the platform. A woman preaching, said Johnson, is like a dog walking on its hind legs. Not that it's done well; the surprise is that it is done at all. The remarkable feat for our civilization is that so many people talk so well. The miracle of language learning appeared late in the evolutionary history of *Homo sapiens*. By extrapolation linguists estimate that man possessed the mental capacity and the physical equipment of speech for 40,000 years before he experimented with the rudiments of verbal language. Only within the short span of 8,000 years has he developed an oral language for the purposes of communication.[1] Is it proper to speak of language as a developing process in the race? Historical linguists would reject the concept of development; they tell us that "the earliest reconstructible stage for any language family shows all the complexities and flexibilities of the language of today."[2] No primitive language has been found. "The lowliest South African Bushman speaks in the forms of a rich symbolic system that is in essence perfectly comparable to the speech of the cultivated Frenchman."[3] Man speaks fairly well and frequently. Indeed he speaks so frequently that language may mean the end of us all, for it produces tension between groups which are similar in culture.[4] It becomes the primary determinant

[1] R. Cohn, Language and behavior. *Amer Sci* (March 1961), 49: 502–508.
[2] C. F. Hockett, The origin of speech. *Sci Amer* (September 1960), 203: 89.
[3] *Ibid.*
[4] R. Cohn, *op. cit.*

of man's action, and unless his language accurately translates his observations, based on sense impressions and concepts, he creates misunderstanding and tension. The disparity between observation and impressions and concepts finally may become so great that he will live in a dream-like world. Despite these dire predictions, we continue our efforts to develop a host of different systems of communication. Basic among all these systems is human language—although it may finally become an hypertrophied attribute of man. We shall not discuss systems of communication among animals. We are cognizant of current research in this area but we do not believe that the signals and emotional cries of chimpanzees,[5] dolphins, or crows [6] provide a satisfactory precursory system to human language. The speech of man—or woman—has not yet been reduced to the clucking of hens.

Of what use, language? In the presence of the great realities of life we are dumb; we cannot speak. Admittedly language is a poor vehicle of communication. Its physical mechanism is subject to every ill wind that blows. The rules of its phonemic system defy complete analysis. There are not enough different words to express the subtleties of thought so that "one word has to serve functions for which a hundred would not be too many." [7] Yet language endures as man's hope for adaptation and understanding, so we had best accept it for ill or good. It has survival value and we are not likely to give it up.

The baby will learn to use language in order to communicate with others but in the beginning it is either an emotional response or it is annunciatory, proclaiming his needs for biological and psychological satisfaction. He uses gestural and verbal responses to intervene in his environment to secure what he wants or to fend off what he dislikes. Language is an adaptive mechanism which he must employ in order to stabilize his environment, both internally and externally. By the instrument of language, he attempts to establish an equilibrium between assimilation and accommodation, but it is never fully realized, never quite successful despite his struggle for homeostasis.[8] He proceeds from one stage of development to the next, although his progress is not uniform or even. Periods of relative continuity alternate with phases of discontinuity, and between stages disequilibrium often is marked. Although the child does not inherit a language, he does inherit the *capacity* to acquire a language, and probably also a strong drive toward such acquisition. The capacity and the

[5] J. Goodall, My life among wild chimpanzees. *Nat Geog Mag* (August 1963), pp. 272–308.

[6] H. Frings and M. Frings, The language of crows. *Sci Amer* (November 1959), 201: 119–131.

[7] C. K. Ogden and I. A. Richards, *The meaning of meaning*. London: Routledge, 1949. P. 130.

[8] J. Piaget, Comments on Vygotsky's critical remarks concerning *The language and thought of the child*. Cambridge, Mass.: M. I. T., 1962. Pp. 2–4.

motivation of the child to comprehend and use language are primary concerns of the speech and language scientist.

Building Blocks of Language: Phone, Phoneme, Morpheme

Just as words never say "all about anything" so we would admit that definitions also fail to say all that should be said about the characteristics of language. "Language," states Carroll, "is a structured system of arbitrary vocal sounds and sequences of sounds which is used in interpersonal communication and which rather exhaustively catalogs the things, events and processes of human experience." [9] It should be noted, as Carroll pointed out in a later work, that "the *system* inherent in a language derives essentially and primarily from the sequence of articulated, heard sounds in *spoken* utterances or messages." [10] Since the child learning to read derives the written message from a reconstruction of the spoken message, both activities, learning to speak and learning to read, require a high order of perception. Language, from another point of view, is a system of symbols containing socially shared meanings which must be learned, and providing categories for classifying experience. The words are the signs which have significance by *convention*. They are empirical signs denoting a referent but not to be confused with the referent.[11] In the analysis of language problems whether of the child or adult, the central concept which we must bear in mind is the structure of the language. Structure concerns, however, much more than form and syntax. It embraces "the ordered or patterned set of contrasts or oppositions which are presumed to be discoverable in a language, whether in the units of sound, the grammatical inflections, the syntactical arrangements, or even the meanings of linguistic forms." [12] Encompassed in this definition are the dimensions of language—phonology, syntactic forms, and semology—which we shall trace in the baby's learning of language.

Phonetics. The speech scientist must delineate clearly phonetics, phonemics, and morphemics if he is to analyze successfully either normal or atypical oral expression. Formerly he was limited almost entirely to an analysis based on phonetics. Indeed in many of the early studies of the development of infant language, no distinction was made between the

[9] J. B. Carroll, Language development. In C. Harris, Ed., *Encyclopedia of educational research*. New York: Macmillan, 1960. P. 745.

[10] J. B. Carroll, The analysis of reading instruction: Perspectives from psychology and linguistics. In E. R. Hilgard, Ed., *Theories of learning and instruction*. Chicago: University of Chicago Press, 1964. P. 337.

[11] C. Cherry, *On human communication*. New York: M. I. T. and Wiley, 1957. P. 67.

[12] J. B. Carroll, *The study of language*. Boston: Harvard University Press, 1953. P. 14.

phonetic and phonemic levels of analysis.[13] The speech scientist paid attention almost exclusively to the *phone,* a sound represented by an arbitrary symbol and identifiable either by a definite adjustment of the organs of speech or by acoustic phenomena. So according to the standard classification of phonetics, he grouped the distorted, missing, or substituted sounds as vowels, semivowels, consonants; pitches or tones; stresses and junctures.

Phoneme. The speech scientist came slowly but inevitably to the realization that although the phonetic substance may be the raw material of language, it must be organized "into a finite set of mutually exclusive classes," if it is to be an instrument of analysis of the speech continuum.[14] Each class possesses a set of features and is called a *phoneme.* These features vary with the position of the phoneme in the sound sequence. Consider the final phoneme in the word *pays* in these sentences: *It pays to advertise* and *Honesty pays.* In the first sentence the phoneme (under the influence of the voiceless *t* which follows) probably belongs to the *s* family; in the second, it most generally joins the *z* phoneme. Considered alone, the phoneme possesses what someone has called a bundle of simultaneous, distinctive features: binary, two-valued oppositions or contrasts, such as high/low; rounded/unrounded; voiced/unvoiced. When it appears in a constellation of sounds in the speech continuum, it has added features of loudness, pitch, rhythm, duration, and juncture. Phonemes probably are acquired by the child in a definite, developmental sequence [15] and are grouped together into larger units according to definite rules of sequence so that all possible phonemic shapes can be predicted. *Phonemic sequences,* then, constitute linguistic units which possess characteristic distributions and interrelationships. Their precise features will be determined, in part, by such factors as intonation patterns, vocal modifiers, sentence types, and bodily gestures. Phonemics, in sum, is a branch of linguistics, dealing with phonemes, sound families that occur in a particular language.[16]

Morpheme. A parameter of language more closely related to language learning and language retardation is morphology, the *form* of language. More specifically it concerns the *morpheme* which is composed of phonemes, and is the definitive structural unit embodying lexical and grammatical meanings. In other words, it is the minimal acoustic unit that can convey meaning, *the minimal unit of perception of meaning.*

[13] O. C. Irwin, Research on speech sounds for the first six months of life. *Psychol Bull* (May 1941), 38: 277–285. O. C. Irwin, Development of speech during infancy: Curve of phonemic frequencies. *J Exp Psychol* (April 1947), 37: 187–193.
[14] W. Miller and S. Ervin, The development of grammar in child language. *Monogr Soc Res Child Devel* (1964), 29: 9–34.
[15] R. Jakobson, *Kindersprache, aphasie und allgemeine lautgesetze.* Stockholm: Almquist and Wiksell, 1949.
[16] R. H. Stetson, *Motor phonetics.* Amsterdam: North Holland Publishing Company, 1951. P. 166.

In studying this perceptual unit we must consider the morphemic changes which accompany changes in sentence construction and the manner in which morphemes designate relations among nouns, verbs, adjectives, and concrete adverbs. Some linguists group morphemes into two classes: *lexical* (nouns, verbs, and adjectives) and *functional* (prepositions, interrogatives, conjunctions, auxiliaries, and noun determiners). They also consider morphemes as *bound* or *free*. If a morpheme can stand alone in speech, it is free; if not, it is bound. *Fine* is free but the morpheme *er* in *finer* is bound, as is *un* in *undress* and *'s* in *cat's paw*. Since morphological lag and articulatory lag appear together in speech development, it behooves the speech scientist to reassess his understanding of certain kinds of articulatory problems. The linkage between articulation and morphology is additional evidence of the perceptual basis of many so-called functional articulatory defects.

An integral aspect of morphology is *syntax,* the way in which sentences are constructed out of morphemic substance. Syntactical modes, in fact, determine the morphological building blocks of language. A child first masters *phrase-wholes,* sequences of words in grammatical patterns as single entities, and somewhat later he may learn to differentiate the morphemic units. Although some linguists regard syntax as a separate aspect of language, it bears an intimate relation to morphology. In our view, syntax is neither adjunct nor subjunct; it is central to the theme of morphology.

The Baby Learns to Comprehend Language

A baby will not begin to use language until he *understands* language—a cliché. It is largely disregarded by those who work with the language-handicapped because their attention is centered on the child's *production* of speech, not upon his ability to understand speech. Yet it is as important to determine what the child *understands* as to record what the childs *says*. Furthermore we must be aware both of the *quality* and the *quantity* of his speech. Only recently have we recognized the paucity of language, for example, in children handicapped by cleft palate. Their speech generally is unintelligible, but more important is the fact that they talk so infrequently, and when they do talk they typically employ meager vocabularies, poor syntax, and atypical intonation patterns. Quantity cannot be equated entirely with comprehension, but they are related dimensions of speech.

Cognition of Signs, Symbols, and Prosody. Vocal behavior during the first months of infancy is so unstable as to defy analysis. The speech-like sounds that occur show extreme vocal fluctuations that cannot be analyzed by the usual means of phonetic study. Following the first months the baby demonstrates an increasing control over volume and pitch, and a repertory of sounds, some of which *resemble* the sounds of speech. That feedback reinforces and refines the repertory is evident from the fact that the nonhearing baby indulges in prelinguistic vocalization but, securing no reinforcement from feedback, soon becomes a silent child.[17] Between the eighth and tenth month most babies first evidence some understanding and recognition of certain symbolic gestures, intonations, words, and phrase structures. This is the critical period for the development of comprehension, a fact not always recognized by parents who are primarily responsible for the creation of a favorable linguistic environment. The "silent rationale" in feeding and handling infants, for example, which was advocated by some psychologists in the previous decade has been exploded, yet its effects still can be noted in child guidance clinics. Even with the deaf baby, the knowledgeable in this area would encourage parents to bombard the child with the sights, sounds, and feelings of speech. The deaf baby's world may be auditorially void but the visual and tactile-kinesthetic responses of language can and should inhabit his domain.

Verbal Syncretism: Intonation and Words (see pp. 128–141). In terms of understanding verbal signals, the child's linguistic experience before the age of 1 year is comparatively simple. We know that he understands commands, not in terms of single sounds or syllables but in terms of larger linguistic units. He comprehends phrases and perhaps single words, which are sentences to him, but he makes no fine discriminations on the basis of morphemes.[18] He perceives instead a bundle of elementary morphemic relationships carried on intonational contours, an insight essential for the understanding of language. So strongly set are these relationships in sound sequences that very small children are unable to reverse the sequence of words which belong in a certain order; they also are unable to separate sequences into word units. When asked to say a word in reverse, for example, they do not comprehend the single word. Like the Liberians who speak the Galsh language, separate words are not recognized.[19] An unknown word, consequently, may not be recognized by the child. He simply incorporates it into his general scheme of the percept—a practice which he will continue throughout his second and third years of life. In fact the child up to the age of 10 years rarely tries to understand every word. What he comprehends merely excites analogous ideas already existing in his mind; the result may not be understanding but a convergence of acquired schemes

[17] S. M. Ervin and W. R. Miller, Language development. In H. W. Stevenson, Ed., *Child psychology*. Chicago: University of Chicago Press, 1963. Pp. 109–110.

[18] J. Piaget, *The language and thought of the child*. London: Routledge, 1959. Pp. 127–161.

[19] J. Huttenlocher, Children's language: Word-phrase relationship. *Science* (January 17, 1964), 143: 264–265.

of thought. As commands are repeated, the child selects cue words, pivot words in a sentence, by which he comprehends the whole. Thus he develops "functional equivalents of comprehension" although he does not understand the specific words.[20] Comprehension of the whole probably is characteristic of the egocentric behavior of the child through the fifth year: "Egocentric thought ignores isolated words and deals with whole sentences, understanding them or altering them as they stand without analyzing them." [21] In other words, the baby treats a polymorphemic sequence of the model language as a monomorphemic unit which he may segment at some later stage of development into its parts. This kind of comprehension, to which we have alluded earlier (p. 134), is predicated on *verbal syncretism* (the whole is understood before the parts are analyzed).

Syncretism and Phonemes. If the child does not distinguish separate words in a phrase or sentence until his third year, then certainly he does not distinguish closely similar words on the basis of minimal phonemic differences until his fourth or fifth year. At this moment two 5-year-olds are in an argument. "I didn't say, 'he's late'; I said, 'he's eight!'" shouts one to the other. As Hockett says, "Human children learn their language . . . by learning some utterances as whole units, in due time testing various blends, based on that repertory, and finally adjusting their patterns of blending until the bulk of what they say matches what adults would say and is therefore understood." [22] In comprehending a foreign language, adults rarely attend to minimal phonemic differences. Indeed we usually do not attempt to comprehend the meaning of every word, no more frequently than the child does.

Because neither the young child nor the adult (learning a second language) attends to phonemic units or to such phonemic sequences as /seɪ/, /siː/, /saɪ/, /soʊ/, /su/, we question the general practice of teaching language to children by auditory stimulation and exercises of isolated sounds or nonsense syllables. The practice might possibly assist the child in perceiving phonemic and grammatic relationships, the bundle of characteristics which tie together sequences of sounds,[23] but we find no neurophysiological or psychological data to support this belief. In preceding chapters we have presented evidence to the contrary.

The Baby Begins to Use Language

Purpose. In terms of the elementary purposes of oral language, the young baby uses speech, in the first place, not to communicate mean-

[20] R. G. Natadze, Studies on thought and speech problems by psychologists of the Georgian S. S. R. In N. O'Connor, Ed., *Recent Soviet psychology*. New York: Liveright, 1961. Pp. 313–322.

[21] J. Piaget, *op. cit.*, p. 122.

[22] C. F. Hockett, The origin of speech. *Sci Amer* (September 1960), 203: 95.

[23] K. de Hirsch, Gestalt psychology as applied to language disturbances. *J Nerv Ment Dis* (September–October, 1954), 120: 259.

ing but as an enjoyable activity associated with the satisfaction of his physiological needs and feeling states. His gurgles and gargles act as self-reinforcement of more vocalization; the activity plays a motivational role in the child's behavior. These interjectional or emotional vocalizations are not invariably associated with a specific person or object. *Mama,* for example, may not be connected with the mother, but with diffuse states of dissatisfaction or satisfaction associated with the stimulus. As the mother brings the bottle, the child may stop crying and say *mama.* The writer's baby granddaughter calls our housekeeper *Cookie;* she makes no differentiation between the object of her biological satisfaction and the person presenting the object. In the second place, the baby uses oral language in this period in order to explore his environment. At 2 years he begins to investigate, not only the objects around him but also his relations with people. It is, in a sense, a global communication in which he names or describes something and usually accompanies his action with pointing. "He likes what'ere he looks on, and his looks go everywhere." Skinner has called this verbal expression the language of *reference.*[24] Shortly the baby takes the next step to the *primary perceptual stage,* the stage of direction. The child now is learning to ask questions about persons and things in his environment. If a child of 3 years asks no questions or demands no response from others, it should be cause for concern. The final stage is that of *responsive discourse.* He now enters a two-way street: he expects either to give or receive informational responses. These are the reasons why the baby speaks; the adult may have more sophisticated and subtle motives for his oral discourse.

Prelinguistic Vocalization. The first vocalizations of the infant probably have little connection with language use. Sounds of pleasure, comfort, or distress may represent a prelinguistic stage but one cannot assume that such noises make up his later repertoire of speech sounds. The early cries have constituents of the vowels /ɑ/, /æ/, /ɛ/, /eɪ/, and /ə/, but they bear little resemblance to speech sounds because of their nasal overtones. And similarly the consonants or consonantal combinations /g/, /k/, /əl/, and /əŋ/ may not be overnasalized but they are poorly defined in quality.[25] When the baby assumes a sitting position, the whole phonemic vocabulary changes because of the relational shifts in position of the resonating and articulating organs. Now the labial and alveolar nasal phonemes of /m/ and /n/, respectively, and of the labial plosives /p/ and /b/ appear. The consonants which appeared earlier, however, may drop out of his vocalizations at this point.

Whether *babbling,* which follows closely upon the very early vocalizations, should be considered a stage in the evolution of the child's speech also is debatable. There are linguists who believe that babbling is done

[24] B. F. Skinner, *Verbal behavior.* New York: Appleton-Century-Crofts, 1957. Pp. 114–118.
[25] M. M. Lewis, *Infant speech.* New York: Harcourt, Brace, 1936. Pp. 24–26.

in play and has no connection with expression; others view it in a double role, random play and expression. Between the second and third month the baby usually engages in this activity as a kind of purposeless play. The babbling that occurs later and has intonational form is quite different. Bayley calls it *jargon speech* [26] and Lewis describes it as play with the medium of language in order to secure satisfaction of the baby's wants and to portray *aesthetic emotion* (the beginning of the child's aesthetic use of words).[27] Contemporary linguists have cast considerable doubt on Lewis' conclusions. They find that the sounds of babbling may have value as a secondary reward but apparently they are unrelated to later phonemes. The sounds have no semantic distinctiveness and probably do not make up the repertoire from which the child later develops the phonemes of speech. Babbling, nonetheless, may be valuable as a tuning up and integrating process for the phonating, resonating, and articulating organs later to be employed in speech.

Imitation of Speech Melody. Between the fourth and sixth month the child usually makes some response to the speech of others, particularly when the speaker portrays the pleasurable gestural accompaniments of speech. The response is usually a rough copy of the intonational pattern of the speaker's interjection or expression of delight. It can scarcely be regarded, however, as a meaningful oral response to a specific stimulus. It is, instead, a general, all pervasive emotional sign of his enjoyment of the speaker's presence (p. 114). He also enjoys imitating his own noises: *oohs, ahs, ba-bas,* and *da-das.* Quite noticeably these imitative responses decline after the sixth month. One surmises that the baby is too busy acquiring a kind of implicit speech, a rudimentary understanding of the world of sounds around him to proceed with random vocalization and response. Shortly before or after his first year, however, the average child begins once again, and this time avidly, to copy the cues of oral expression.[28] He copies the cues that are serviceable to him, those which are reinforced by conditioning, repetition, and reward. Intonation and rhythm are vastly important because they will act as a carrier or basic pattern into which the child will fit sound sequences and syntactic structures (p. 128). Consequently he copies these cues, not as single words (although they may only be words) but as units of meaning with all the intonational and rhythmic accompaniments which he has heard. He recognizes, for example, rising and falling intonation and the range within the intonational contour. Extreme ranges will connote

[26] J. Cameron, N. Livson, and N. Bayley, Infant vocalizations and their relation to mature intelligence. *Science* (July 21, 1967), 157: 331–333.

[27] Lewis, *op. cit.,* pp. 65–69.

[28] F. Darley and H. Winitz, Age of first word. *J Speech Hearing Dis* (August 1961), 26: 272–290.

to him fear or excitement; and narrow ranges, quietness or sadness. Later (from 2.2 to 2.4 [29]) he will use the rising intonation in yes-no questions. By 2.8 the child normally will imitate the parent's frequent use of interrogative inversion. A baby is crying, for instance, because his ball has rolled out of sight so another youngster, 2.6 years old, questions: "D'you want ball, you do? O. K.," and he proceeds to get it for him. When Kim was 2.8 she was told to sit in her chair at the table. She promptly climbed into the host's chair and said in an unmistakable melody pattern, albeit the phonemic quality was poor, "I'm the master in this house." Television's blessings are mixed!

First Sounds and First Words. So far we have said little about the exact month at which specific first sounds or first words appear. We do not think such reports are highly significant for several reasons. First there is a wide age range in the acquisition of specific phones and of words among normal children. Secondly, as we have suggested, such data may have little bearing on the development of language or speech. The child of 6 months may have a vast repertoire of sounds, but as we have pointed out, these sounds bear little resemblance to the sounds in a speech repertoire which he will acquire later. Perhaps "through processes of conditioning the repertoire (of early sounds) is chiseled to contain the sounds necessary in his language"; [30] but very few traces of early repertoires can be identified in later development of words. Thirdly, many reports of first words are based on parental memory and conditioned by parental pride; they scarcely can be reliable. Finally a list of first sounds or first words tells us very little about the actual development of the child's speech. It is an uncertain quantitative, not a qualitative assessment, of *one aspect* of growth.

Phonemic development has been studied exhaustively by Templin who has transcribed the speech of 480 children, between 3 and 8 years of age.[31] She has been concerned specifically with the child's use of phonemes in meaningful speech. Her delineation of the use of speech sounds in various positions in the word underscores the fact that a child does not use a sound in all positions in a word or use it consistently in that word during one age level. The two charts of phonemic development (Table 5-1 and Figure 5-1) do not provide data on the competence of the child in articulating these phonemes in oral expression. Articulatory competence, we believe, is more significant in the growth of language than the appearance of phonemes at a particular age in the child's speech.

[29] Age is indicated by year and month—2.2, for example, means 2 years, 2 months.
[30] S. S. Osborn, Concepts of speech development. *J Speech Hearing Dis* (November 1961), 26: 392.
[31] M. Templin, *Certain language skills in children.* Minneapolis: University of Minnesota Press, 1957. Pp. 19–60.

Table 5-1. Table of phonemic development.

CA	Phonemes and Phoneme-Blends
3 years	Vowels: ē, ĭ, ĕ, ă, ŏ, ŭ, ŏŏ, ōō, ō, ô, å, ûr Diphthongs: ū, ā, ī, ou, oi Consonants: m-, -m-, -m, n-, -n-, -n, -ng-, -ng, p-, -p-, -p, t-, -t-, -t, k-, -k-, b-, -b-, d-, -d-, g-, -g-, f-, -f-, -f, h-, -h-, w-, -w- Double-consonant blends: -ngk
3.5	Consonants: -s-, -z-, -r, y-, -y- Double-consonant blends: -rk, -ks, -mp, -pt, -rm, -mr, -nr, -pr, -kr, -br, -dr, -gr, -sm
4 years	Consonants: -k, -b, -d, -g, s-, sh-, -sh, -v-, j-, r-, -r-, l-, -l- Double-consonant blends: pl-, pr-, tr-, tw-, kl-, kr-, kw-, bl-, br-, dr-, gl-, sk-, sm-, sn-, sp-, st-, -lp, -rt, -ft, -lt, -fr Triple-consonant blends: -mpt, -mps
4.5	Consonants: -s, -sh-, ch-, -ch-, -ch Double-consonant blends: gr-, fr-, -lf
5 years	Consonants: -j- Double-consonant blends: fl-, -rp, -lb, -rd, -rf, -rn, -shr Triple-consonant blends: str-, -mbr
6 years	Consonants: -t-, th-, -th-, -th, v-, -v, -th-, -l Double-consonant blends: -lk, -rb, -rg, -rth, -nt, -nd, -thr, -pl, -kl, -bl, -gl, -fl, -sl Triple-consonant blends: skw-, -str, -rst, -ngkl, -nggl, -rj, -ntth, -rch
7 years	Consonants: -th-, -th, z-, -z, -zh-, -zh, -j Double-consonant blends: thr-, shr-, sl-, sw-, -lz, -zm, -lth, -sk, -st Triple-consonant blends: skr-, spl-, spr-, -skr, -kst, -jd
8 years	Double-consonant blends: -kt, -tr, -sp

SOURCE: *Certain language skills in children* by Mildred C. Templin, Child Welfare Monograph No. 26. University of Minnesota Press, Minneapolis,©Copyright 1957 by the University of Minnesota. P. 51.

The Baby Builds Lexical Elements * of Language

Early Vocabularies. The vocabulary that the very young baby uses in his oral expression has been variously described. Lewis presents

---

* *Lexical elements* are those elements that relate to words, word formatives, and vocabulary, as distinct from grammatical forms and construction.

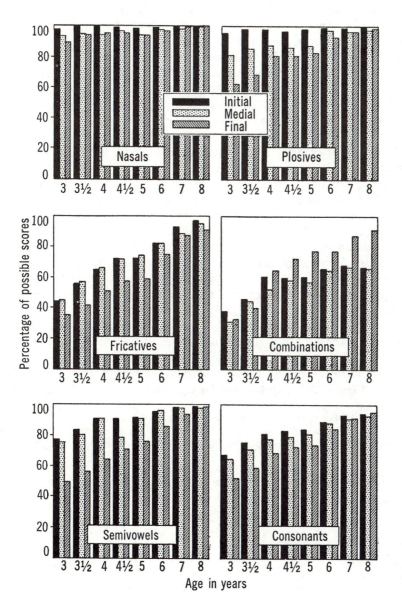

Figure 5-1. Development of phonemic classes. Mean percentages of possible scores on initial, medial, and final nasals, plosives, fricatives, combinations, semivowels, and consonant elements by age.

SOURCE: *Certain language skills in children,* by Mildred C. Templin, Child Welfare Monograph No. 26. University of Minnesota Press, Minneapolis, © Copyright 1957 by the University of Minnesota.

the typical early vocabularies of children of different nationalities which he calls the "international language of babies." In Table 5-2 only six fundamental words, or types of words occur in early baby-language: *mama, nana, papa, baba, tata,* and *dada.* They consist of *m, n* words and *p, b, t, d* words. Phonetic reduplications apparently are a significant part of the early vocabulary. *Da da, pa pa, ma ma, gog gie, tae-tou* (telephone), *tick tick, too-too* (toot-toot), and *shu-shu* make up the bulk of first words.[32] These words refer neither to a single figure nor a single object; rather they represent constellations of experiences, associated with figures or objects. The constellation generally is diffuse, sometimes impermanent.[33] In terms of perception, the word is the phrase, the sentence. Usually between the eighteenth and twentieth month when the child extends the use of the word *mama* to designate any smiling woman, or *dada,* any receptive man, he has by rudimentary reasoning and implicit speech entered upon the significant linguistic stage of extension of meaning. Like a traveler in a foreign land whose only speech resource is a strange phrase book, the child frequently employs bizarre extensions of the meaning of the words in his little vocabulary. Should his parents reinforce the extensions, they undoubtedly will remain for several years.

Second Words and Intelligible Speech. We use *second words* in a metonymic sense to indicate the true onset of speech. *Mama* frequently is the baby's first word and it may be separated by a considerable time interval from the simultaneous appearance of second, third, and fourth words. Figures 5-2 and 5-3 are derived from a study of 225 children

[32] M. M. Lewis, *How children learn to speak.* London: Harrap, 1957. Pp. 80–83.
[33] A. R. Luria and F. Ia. Yudovich, *Speech and the development of the mental processes of the child.* London: Staples, 1959. P. 40.

Table 5-2. Children's earliest words and their meanings.

Meanings	Forms					
	m	n	p	b	t	d
1. mother	mama					
2. nurse	amma	nana		baba	tete	deda
aunt	muhme				ta(n)te	deda
grandmother	amma			baba		
3. food	mum	nana	pap	bap		
4. bed, sleep		nana		bye-bye	tete	dodo
5. child himself				baby		
6. father			papa	baba	tata	dada
7. play: ball				ba		
clock					titta	didda
thanking					ta	da
good-bye					tata	ada

SOURCE: From *How children learn to speak,* by M. M. Lewis, Basic Books, Inc., Publishers, New York, 1959. Table VII, page 80.

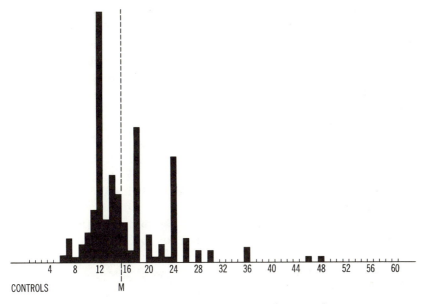

Figure 5-2. Onset of speech (in months).

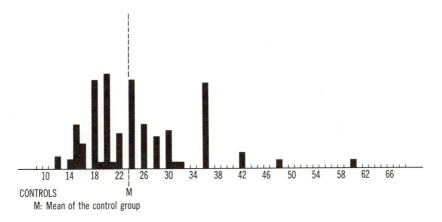

Figure 5-3. Development of intelligible speech (in months).

SOURCE: M. F. Berry, The developmental history of stuttering children. *J Pediat* (February 1938), 12: 215–216.

entered for routine pediatric care from four months through sixty months. The results are not based primarily on the report of the mother but on records of the child's speech made by pediatricians and speech clinicians. We present charts both on onset and development of intelligible speech, but, in our view, the latter is the more significant. It emphasizes the wide age range in this phase of development: the speech of one sizeable group is intelligible at 18 months but another group reaches this goal only at 3 years. The median in the use of intelligible speech is 2 years.

Vocabulary Development. A yardstick for measurement of vocabulary is difficult to find. What is a word in a child's speech? A 2-year-old youngster uses words only as a sequence in a phrase or a sentence, and he understands its meaning largely by its intonational pattern, not by its word composition. This step in language development, the use of intonational patterns for communication, has scarcely been studied. We know that some children use strings of sound with meaningful intonational contours as early as 11.9 months.

The vocabulary of comprehension apparently is somewhat ahead of the vocabulary of use. Interjectional speech normally is understood by the seventh month but not used before the eighth or ninth month. The baby understands such directional words as *no, bye-bye,* and *hot* by the ninth month but he may not use them before he is somewhat over 12 months old.[34] By this time the child follows simple instructions and understands many action words. At 15 months he is using many of these action or directional words: *out, go-go, baby bye-bye, no-no bed.*

Increments of Vocabulary Growth. At about 18 months, vocabulary development will begin its spiral of development, shooting up with tremendous rapidity at first and then slowing down to a 10 percent increase at 5 years. Between 2.6 and 3.0, for example, a child almost doubles the number of words he uses in speech. In this period his vocabulary may jump from 460 words to 910 words. By 4 years, however, he is increasing his vocabulary only by approximately 20 percent. His vocabulary of use then may total 1,500 words.[35] (For the complete table of vocabulary growth, see p. 373.)

Growth of vocabulary depends, not only upon intelligence and physical health, but also on so many environmental or socioeconomic factors that after the age of 4 years a child's standard vocabulary age can scarcely be set. Because children at all socioeconomic levels now are exposed to adult communication via radio and television, possibly vocabulary growth might be assessed more exactly than it was 25 years ago. On the other hand, we know that passive listening is scarcely conducive to language learning. If the child's social environment became *actively* linguistic because of television, of course we would have greater assurance of vocabulary growth.

[34] J. Cameron, N. Livson, and N. Bayley, Infant vocalizations and their relation to mature intelligence. *Science* (July 21, 1967), 157: 331–333.

[35] M. E. Smith, An investigation of the development of the sentence and the extent of vocabulary in young children. In *Univ Iowa Stud Child Welfare* (1926), 3 (5). Iowa City: The Department of Publications, State University of Iowa.

The Baby Experiments with Grammar: 2.0–3.0 Years

Two-Word Sentence. The one-word "sentence" usually prevails in the baby's speech until he approaches his second birthday. The word, as as we have noted, connotes sentence meaning and is the precursor of a primitive grammatical system. For a time imitation may play a role in learning syntactic form, although the baby has his own "innate system" for generating a basic grammar (p. 132). What he imitates actually are the *stressed segments* of speech because it is these peaks that he perceives and which usually carry the most information. Consequently his primitive sentences are made up of noun-phrases, so-called *pivot words,* combined with *operator words* that are used either preceding or following the pivot words. Operator words are particularly significant because they mark the emergence of a grammatical system. These high frequency words generally appear in a particular position in the sentence and define the meaning of the sentence as a whole. They may be either true function words or words that are used as substitutes for them. The baby hears, for example, *more milk?, more juice?,* until *more* becomes an operator word. Soon he says, *more car, more bye-bye, more bath,* "more everything." As a rule, he joins pivot words with operator words in order to command action, as in *shoe off, see Santa, Mummy car, Kim up.* Gradually he differentiates these words, employing them as possessive nouns and pronouns, articles, numbers, and adjectives. Miller and Ervin present in tabular form (1) classes employed in two-word sentences and, (2) the vocabulary employed in demonstrative sentences in a child's (Christy's) language. In these charts, the demonstrative pronouns do not appear before 2.0 years. In other studies, incorporation of this class of words in a child's language has occurred somewhat earlier, 1.9 years. In our study the child used *this* frequently before 2.0 years but did not employ *that* except in a single phrase, *Wha-za* (What's that?) at this age. At 2.6 he used *that* only in response to a question: *That boy no!* (Not that boy). *This a bear; this a doggie,* were favorite sentences in this period, 1.9–2.0, but one could not be sure that the child did not say [ə], meaning *This is bear,* rather than *This a bear.*

Classes in Christy's Two-Word Sentences (2.0–2.3)

I   this, thisa, that, that's, that's a, 'sa, thata

II   a, the

III   here, there

A   arm, baby, bus, cat, Christy's, dolly, dolly's, fish, horsie, truck, pretty, yellow, etc.

B   come, doed, flying, go, goes, got, hold, see, sit, sleep, sleeping, turn, want, walking

C   away, in, on, out, way
D   in, on, over, under [36]

Demonstrative Sentences for Christy (2.0–2.3)

that	*that's*	*this*	*thatsa*	*this a*	*thata*	*'sa*
blue					blue	
broken			broken			
chicken	chicken					
dolly	dolly					
eye	eye					
elephant			elephant			
go		go				
hat	hat					
Joe	Joe					
pants	pants					
pretty			pretty			
truck	truck		truck	truck		truck
yellow	yellow					
			cup		cup	
airplane	bus	one	car	A	doggy	arm
blocks	milk		coffee		horse	baby
bowl	quack-quack		girl			block
cat			owl			boy
Christy's			pig			ear
Daddy's			plane			lion
dolly's						rabbit
fish						Wick
horsie						
huke *						
kitty						
neck						
pin						
pink						
po *						
Sarah						
turn						
yellow [37]						

* *Po* and *huke* were the names of two nonsense shapes of play-doh.

[36] Adapted from W. Miller and S. Ervin, The development of grammar in child language. *The acquisition of language.* Monogr Soc Res Child Develop (1964), 29: 21.

[37] Adapted from W. Miller and S. Ervin, The development of grammar in child language. *The acquisition of language.* Monogr Soc Res Child Develop (1964), 29: 19.

Further Improvisation of Syntactic Forms. Once the child possesses a vocabulary of operator words, he no longer imitates adult speech but develops his own grammatical system. This period of freewheeling construction, appropriate for a child 2.6–3.0 years, is a critical stage of language development. The independent improvisations may be ingenious, often bizarre, but they indicate experimentation. If a youngster continues the use of single words into his third year and fails to make even a trial run of a single syntactic form, the prediction of normal language development is poor.

Expanded Noun-Phrase. Children who make up rudimentary sentences easily forge ahead in the expansion of their vocabulary of noun-phrases. Kim (2.6 years), for example, used pronouns and conjunctions in describing the circus to her grandmother: *Little dog and a big dog and a big-big* (bigger) *dog . . . and in a fire* (jumped through a fire hoop); *and all of 'em in fire.* A linguistically handicapped child may try to describe the event, but if his noun-phrases are only single words, the listener gains no knowledge of size or group action of the dogs.

Designative Constructions. By the age of 3 and sometimes earlier, the child begins to construct sentences, generally in question form, in order to verbalize names and actions in his environment. *What that thing go round?,* he asks; or *Where Daddy go, bye-bye car?;* or *Why Dolly head off, Ellie fix on?* Any mother cooped up with a 3- or 4-year-old can multiply these questions by a hundred in a single day. The failure of the linguistically handicapped child to reach this milestone may be interpreted, as Lee says, "as a personality manifestation, an undeveloped curiosity about the world . . . or it might just as easily emanate from a lack of linguistic skill." [38] In our experience it is precisely this lack of skill that tethers him. He cannot effect the transformation in syntax or expansion of noun-phrases to form the question.

Subject-Predicate Sentence. Another significant marker in linguistic development in the latter part of this period, 2.6–3.0 years, is the expansion of noun-phrases and verb-phrases into full blown subject-predicate sentences. By the use of the verb *is,* or more frequently *'s,* a child normally will expand such a construction as *Dolly head off* to *Dolly's head's off* or to *My dolly's head's off.* This represents a tremendous gain in comprehension of syntactic construction, for as Lee says, it now is a "simple-active-declarative kernel sentence, compatible with adult standards." [39] The *linguistically different* child frequently fails to reach this level without intensive training. If he still is without the chief tool of making expanded predicative sentences, i.e., the use of auxiliaries *is,*

[38] L. L. Lee, Developmental sentence types: A method for comparing normal and deviant syntactic development. *J Speech Hearing Dis* (November 1966), 31: 327.
[39] *Ibid.,* p. 321.

have, and *can,* when he reaches his fourth birthday, he probably is seriously handicapped in language.

Advancing Sentence Construction. The young child still must jump several hurdles in language making before he is able to express himself verbally so that others understand him. *Number, verb tense,* and *suffixes* are three hurdles of language that he may stumble over for several years. Although children at 3 years may comprehend the meaning of the number *two (two boys, dolls, balls),* they rarely attempt to count in series 1–2–3 at that age. Instead they will repeat *one,* as in counting lights while riding in a car at night: *One light and one light and one light.* Note, however, that the noun remains singular. They will pluralize it in all other combinations *except* when it is preceded by a numeral.

Another step in sentence-making is the development of verb tense. It is not an easy conquest and apparently is not an imitative process but another example of independent improvisation. The *perception* of the past tense, for example, precedes by six to eight months its proper use. At 3 the child understands the necessity of past tense and attempts to form it by the addition of *ed* to the present form. So he says, *I tell-ed Terry to stop, I stand up-ed, I catch-ed it, I breaked my airplane, I cutted my finger.* Parents are as nonplussed as we are in explaining this rather persistent practice in the speech of their 3-year-old children. The most resistant of all verbs in tense shifts is *have* when it is used as a main verb. *I had it* is a rare expression in the speech of 3-year-olds.

Another marker in the child's development is the use of suffixes in nouns and verbs. At 2.6 these suffixes generally are established for nouns but the child does not recognize changes in form before 3.0. In other words he is consciously imitating his models in major morphological sequences but overlooks changes in form both in verbs and nouns. The errors in our group of children at 2.6 followed the pattern observed by other students of children's speech, and fall into the following categories. (1) Omissions: *I* (am) *going* (to) *draw a house.* (2) Overgeneralization of morphophonemics: *My foots are cold; I breaked it all-up; The nice mans catch-ted the bad man.* (3) Doubly marked forms: *That's mine's; this's yoursez.* (4) Verbal transformations: *I didded it yesterday, I tell you!* In this last category we reach a critical point in the development of language since comprehension depends heavily upon the ability to use verbal transformations and verb restrictions in discourse agreement. The child's use may be unstable for many months but if he is able to "pass the test," he is on his way to responsive discourse.

Objective Assessment of Early Development of Language

The majority of the aspects of linguistic growth which occur before the age of 3 years has not been measured. Perhaps they are not measurable

or more probably children at this early age are not available for laboratory observation. At any rate, comprehensive studies of intonational
contours, the development of the two-word sentence, noun-phrases,
designative constructions, predication, and speech quantity are scarce.
Has anyone assessed, for instance, the *volume* of talk in the homes of the
language handicapped? Or do we know whether volume of early talk
bears any relation to later retardation? If a young child talks freely
and much, the gains from such practice should be reflected in all measurable skills. Feedback alone must accelerate language development. The
language deficits of some cleft palate children may be attributed, in part,
to the small amount of language they use. Vocabulary is meager, sentence
structure is unstable, phonemic production is seriously disturbed. All
too often we have observed 3-year-old youngsters, handicapped by facial
clefts, who are entirely silent. They behave as if they had not talked
because they were not expected to talk, because their speech attracted
unfavorable attention, or because they knew they would not be understood. Perhaps their greatest gains in speech skill were in sheer volume
of talk.

Quantitative indices of some aspects of language development have
been computed for children 3 years or younger in age. They concern
vocabulary size, grammatical forms, sentence length, and structural complexity. McCarthy's analysis of the use of grammatical forms of the same
age group is presented in Table 5-3.

Notable in this table is the very great increase in the use of adjectives and the decrease in nouns and interjections from 18 months to
36 months (particularly among the boys). In several respects, McCarthy's

Table 5-3. Mean percent of each part of speech by age and sex.
(based on total number of words used)

Age in Months	Sex	Nouns	Verbs	Adjec.	Adv.	Pro-nouns	Con-junc.	Prep.	Interj.	Misc.
18	B	43.6	16.7	5.1	5.1	12.8	.0	.0	16.7	.0
	G	51.5	13.1	10.7	8.5	9.8	.6	.0	5.5	.3
	All	50.0	13.9	9.6	7.9	10.3	.5	.0	7.6	.3
24	B	49.3	15.3	5.8	3.7	15.0	.0	2.0	3.4	5.4
	G	35.5	22.6	11.6	8.0	14.5	.7	4.1	2.2	.8
	All	38.6	21.0	10.3	7.1	14.6	.5	3.6	2.4	1.8
30	B	25.4	24.9	14.4	6.3	21.0	.5	4.3	1.5	1.8
	G	26.0	22.3	14.3	6.9	17.6	2.5	4.9	3.8	1.7
	All	25.8	23.4	14.3	6.7	19.0	1.7	4.6	2.8	1.8
36	B	23.6	23.5	15.4	7.8	21.3	1.1	5.4	1.5	.6
	G	23.2	22.5	16.7	6.3	17.3	3.7	8.4	1.5	.5
	All	23.4	23.0	16.1	7.0	19.2	2.4	6.9	1.5	.5

SOURCE: D. A. McCarthy, *The language development of the preschool child.* Child Welfare Monograph No. 4.
University of Minnesota Press, Minneapolis, © Copyright 1930 by the University of Minnesota. P. 114.

Table 5-4.   Percentage of scores of 8-year-old subsample
or 5-year-old subsample on the major language measures
attained by the subsample at age 3.

Total articulation	55.8
Ammons vocabulary*	62.4
Sound discrimination vocabulary*	79.0
Number of different words	55.5
Total words in response	54.1
Five longest responses	55.7
Complexity of response	44.1
No grammatical errors	63.0
Use of subordination	19.1

*5-year-old subsample

SOURCE: *Certain Language Skills in Children* by Mildred C. Templin, Child Welfare
Monograph No. 26. University of Minnesota Press, Minneapolis, © Copyright 1957 by the
University of Minnesota. P. 134.

study reflects the same slight superiority of the boys over the girls in the
development of linguistic form which Templin also found.

Templin's mode of analysis differs somewhat from that of Mc-
Carthy's. Templin takes the mean score at the oldest age tested (8 years)
as a measure of terminal status in all but two tests. The percentage of this
terminal score attained by the 3-year-old group then is calculated. In
two tests, Ammons Full-Range Picture Vocabulary and a sound discrimination test, the achievement of the 5-year-old subsamples is taken as
a measure of terminal status. Assuming that 8-year-old children receive
a score of 100 percent, Templin then calculates what percent of that
linguistic skill has been achieved by age 3.[40] Although the score for each
younger age group was calculated, we present the comparative tabulation
only for the age 3.0 group.

Table 5-4 presents items from Templin's comparative age study of
selected linguistic factors. Although we recognize that linguistic structure
is simple at age 3.0, we are impressed by the relative freedom from
grammatical errors in this sample. It is significant that this schedule is
predictive of relatively slow growth in sound discrimination vocabulary
between 3 and 5 years. It is interesting also to note that at the age of
3 years, the mean achievement of the boys is four percentage points higher
than that of the girls, but this acceleration for the boys does not hold
throughout the age range studied.

The stretch remaining for the child learning language is a long
one. Indeed it is never truly finished. By his second birthday he no
longer exclaims only about objects and persons present in his own immediate and limited environment. He now may be able to tell you where
the ball is which has rolled out of sight. He is aware of the form of

[40] M. Templin, *Certain language skills in children*. Minneapolis: University of
Minnesota Press, 1957. Pp. 122–123.

language and is demonstrating a generative system of grammar. By his third birthday his vocabulary is growing rapidly; he has made even greater strides in his sound discrimination vocabulary; and sentence structure is sufficiently complex to enable him to extend and abstract some experiences. Now the child may tell his grandmother over the telephone that he is going to the supermarket with his mother and that his daddy has gone to the office.

The Child Advances in Language Learning

Changing Purposes of Language. The child's purposes for speaking, which once served him well, no longer are adequate. The satisfaction of personal needs, the exploration of one's environment, and the proclamation of what one sees, hears, touches, and feels continue but their roles become less dominant as the world around the child becomes more complex. The transitional period from 3 to 5 years has been called the closed and prefatory open verbalization cycle. The child sometimes uses speech to develop his perceptual processes but is not communicating them (closed cycle), and on other occasions he may share his percepts and elaborate them by listening to the experiences of others (prefatory open cycle).[41] So he engages both in egocentric speech and in a kind of communication with others characterized by commands, requests, threats, and by questions and answers about his immediate environment. He verbalizes to himself about the behavior of others as well as his own, mainly in order to sharpen his perception. Yet occasionally he tries to communicate his ideas, using language both to elaborate and to modify them in accordance with the percepts of others.

Aspects of Language Maturation. We cannot identify all markers along the route of maturation of language and some that we present here may fade as research in psycholinguistics and communications is intensified. From 3 years of age the child's development seems to proceed along these lines: (1) growth and decline of egocentric speech; and (2) advances in implicit language and perception, in the form and substance of language (morphology, syntax, and vocabulary), and in articulatory and prosodic skills.

Egocentric Language: Its Growth and Decline. For several years linguists have engaged in dialogue over Piaget's theory that a child's language is highly egocentric and does not become adaptive before the sixth year. Piaget, however, defines egocentrism as

the initial inability to decenter, to shift the given cognitive or mental perspec-

[41] E. D. Mysak, Organismic development of oral language. *J Speech Hearing Dis* November 1961), 26: 377–384.

tive . . . in social and other relationships (in which language plays a part). The unconscious egocentrism of thought is quite unrelated to the common meaning of the term, hypertrophy of the consciousness of self. Cognitive ego-centrism . . . stems from a lack of differentiation between one's own point of view and the other possible ones. . . .[42]

It is, as we have suggested, a closed cycle in which the child vocalizes his perceptual processes. He is using language as a tool by which he analyzes and synthesizes his perceptions, always, however, in terms of himself at this stage. If he must solve a puzzle or assemble a toy, he talks aloud to himself about it. By the use of language, he is obviously trying to stir up CNS pools previously formed and so to synthesize circuits bearing upon his task. Egocentric language then becomes an instrument of thought in the clarification of ideas and solution of problems.[43]

Because the young child's world is egocentric and small, he makes systematic errors of thought. He may ask, "Why?" again and again but actually he makes little effort to absorb, to understand the explanation. To him subordinate clauses become coordinate, independent statements. In his scheme of syncretistic comprehension, he grasps the whole but he cannot analyze the parts and so perceives no causal connection.

Egocentric expression declines but it rarely vanishes completely. Even adults return for short or long spells to egocentric speech. The beginning instructor in his lectures often is incomprehensible to his students because he is talking to himself. So the young child thinks and talks for himself and not until his sixth year does he begin to learn how to place himself at the point of view of others. He assumes, as does the young instructor, that he is talking to others but actually he is thinking and talking for himself, or more accurately, according to himself. As egocentrism declines his *why* questions suggest adaptation. Piaget notes three principal kinds of *why* questions. (1) Causal explanation: *Why is it dark now?*; (2) Motivation: *Why are you going away?* (3) Justification: *Why do we have . . .?* [44] In these types of questions the child attempts to intervene in and extend his environment, the better to understand its reality. The third type of question undoubtedly is particularly har-assing to the mother yet it is an indication of mental activity in the child. Indeed if he is not asking these kinds of questions by the fifth year, the parents should be concerned.

The shift from egocentric speech to communication is reflected in different attitudes and percepts. The child now exhibits a cooperative

[42] J. Piaget, Comments on Vygotsky's critical remarks concerning *The language and thought of the child.* Cambridge, Mass.: M. I. T., 1962. Pp. 2–4.

[43] L. S. Vygotsky, *Thought and language.* Cambridge, Mass.: M. I. T., 1962. Pp. 16–17.

[44] J. Piaget, *The language and thought of the child.* London: Routledge, 1959. Pp. 164–199.

give-and-take spirit, an elementary rational reciprocity. He begins to develop concepts of number, speed, of time and space, and of elementary physical phenomena which affect and interest him. He is beginning to comprehend more fully the world and his relation to it. From the sixth year the average child ceases to answer another's questions only with *because,* although he still cannot verbalize causal relationships. He talks freely and associates verbal labels with many specific signals. These signal-label links "thus become a tremendous factor which forms mental activity, perfecting the reflection of reality and creating new forms of attention, of memory and imagination, of thought and action." [45] Between the seventh and eighth year, egocentric thought and language represent but 25 percent of the total. When he achieves this stage in language learning, two processes emerge: (1) the accelerated development of inner language, and (2) perceptual growth resulting in adaptive thinking.

Acceleration of Inner Language. An increase in rate of development occurs when the young child of 4 years exhibits a great advance in sentence construction and saccadic increases in vocabulary and prosody. Inherent relationships and inner signs are subtly reflected in rhythmic patterns and vocabulary. Now the child relegates to *soundless inner speech* much of that which he has said aloud in his egocentric period. He begins to think words as he utters them. Internal speech is not disappearing; it is going underground. There it assumes a planning function serving both autistic and logical thought.

Growth in Perceptualization. The psychology of perception has been fully discussed in Chapter 4. We present only a summary here in order to correlate perceptual development with other processes of language maturation in this age period, 3 to 8 years. Decades of time have been devoted to vocabulary counts in the belief that they are the critical index of growth in language. Admittedly the *quality* of a child's vocabulary is important; the *number* of words he uses is relatively unimportant for the reason that they may be unimportant words. More significant than the words a child uses are the percepts they represent.

In the early stages of perceptual formation, children rarely understand each other—but they think they do. Children, 5 to 6 years of age, reply to *why* questions only by juxtaposition for they have meager concepts of temporal, causal, or logical relations. Sentences are linked by *and, and, and* to make up non-stop recitals. By the eighth year linguistic representation of percepts reflects a great change. Now the child is looking for explanations of things, of motives of action of his peers, of the reality of events (*Can this be true . . .?*). He must synthesize his

[45] A. R. Luria and F. Ia. Yudovich, *Speech and the development of mental processes in the child.* London: Staples, 1959. P. 12.

percepts so he engages in genuine arguments with others for the purpose of unifying, making consistent, and establishing his own beliefs.

This explanation, however, goes a very short way to an understanding of the *modus operandi,* the method by which percepts are constructed. The first phase of comprehension is marked by the acquisition of diffuse cues. Then slowly they emerge as figures upon ground. As they are refined, the figures defined, the child becomes aware of the need to learn cues.[46] He expects them; he watches for them, visually, auditorially, and tactile-kinesthetically. He begins to integrate sensory-motor cues. The second phase of the process entails categorization. Children use language to assist them in categorizing their percepts. A child smells, feels, and sees a bowl of artificial fruit, and then says of one item, "But that isn't a real orange; it just looks like one." At 5 years, he trusts his identification and does not attempt to taste it as he might have done at 2 years. So from sensory cues, linked with memory traces, and based on similarities and differences, he recognizes a strange object, person, or event, makes inferences about it and categorizes it. It is barely but rarely possible for categorization to take place without the aid of language tools. Certainly in the realm of perception of information and ideas, we make the categorization largely on the basis of its symbolic representation, language. *It's a table, a chair, a sofa*—so the child identifies and categorizes by means of language.

In developing percepts by the medium of language, verbal symbolization no longer is limited to the representation of the object or event of immediate experience. The youngster of 4½ years talks about other objects and events which he has experienced *or is likely to experience.* The object becomes symbolic by transference to other experiences of all percepts in that class. He places what he perceives in a class of percepts, thereby grasping or enriching the meaning. By language, too, the child is able to analyze and synthesize elements from a number of perceptions into new units. Just as with objects, so he selects and puts together those elements of experiences which seem to belong together. Sometimes he forms highly specific percepts from scattered bits of information. In other words, language is the instrument by which his ideas begin to grow.

In the sixth and seventh years, the growth of perceptualization is rapid. Events, objects, persons go through a whole series of transpositions before the final abstraction or generalization is made. In semantic terms he is abstracting from the members of the sequence those qualities which they have in common and thus placing all these experiences in the same class. So the child recodes the sequences and transforms them into a general statement. Language has become truly symbolic, for in no sense is

[46] R. L. Shelton, W. S. Arndt, and J. B. Miller, Learning principles and teaching of speech language. *J Speech Hearing Dis* (November 1961), 26: 368–376.

it limited to the representation of the sequence as it was experienced. By this process of differentiated perception, the child is able to analyze and synthesize elements from a number of perceptions into new wholes as perceptual units.[47]

Continued Development of Form and Meaning. Percepts are mediated by linguistic codes; they are the operative instruments of language. To construct the codes of language most easily and effectively, the child must follow the rules of language. Presumably he comprehends linguistic form earlier than he uses it in speech. He generally understands at 5 years the use of the auxiliary in such a question as, "Will you go out to play now?" although he would not ask this question. This difference is true, it seems, not only of linguistic functions but of any percept entailing action.[48] One can select, for example, the correct design among many faulty ones presented to him, but the perception is not sufficiently clear for him to *reproduce* the correct design. He perceives dimly what is wrong but he cannot *act* to set it right. The child who distorts the pronunciation of a word has a vague idea of the order in phonemic sequences and may even be able to select the correct pronunciation among several choices. Motor feedback from earlier trials, however, has not been sufficiently strong to insure proper execution of the movement patterns. The motokinesthetic aid to speech perception is weak.

Grammar and Syntax in Speech. By the time the child is 4 years old, he usually is advancing rapidly in the use of his self-made rules of grammar. Presumably he constructs sentences he has not learned from others (or he may blend two or more whole utterances which he has learned from others).[49] At the advanced age of 5 years, he is beginning to experiment seriously with several aspects of linguistic morphology. He experiments orally with various forms and grammatic inflections of words as they undergo modification for tense, number, case, or person. He learns the difference, for instance, between *was* and *is; am* and *are; sing, sang,* and *sung,* and uses them in his speech. He inflects nouns, both in the plural and the possessive. He makes distinctions between mass and particular nouns. His ability to utilize number and gender, however, matures more slowly than his accomplishment in other linguistic elements.[50] He employs negation freely in sentences, although, if he is an average child, he probably will not free himself entirely from the double-negative gremlins for a good many years. He makes errors particularly

[47] E. H. Lenneberg, *New directions in the study of language.* Cambridge, Mass.: M. I. T., 1964. Pp. 126–127. R. C. Johnson, Linguistic structure as related to concept formation and to concept content. *Psychol Bull* (November 1962), 59: 468–476.

[48] E. Maccoby, Developmental psychology. In P. R. Farnsworth, Ed., *Ann Rev Psychol.* Palo Alto, Calif.: Annual Reviews, 1964, 15: 208–225.

[49] C. F. Hockett, The origin of speech. *Sci Amer* (September 1960), 203: 94.

[50] E. Zigler, L. V. Jones, and P. Kafes, Acquisition of language habits in first, second and third grade boys. *Child Develop* (September 1964), 35: 725–736.

in the transformation of irregular verb forms. He sometimes makes
mistakes in pluralization (*I saw two deers*) and in the use of the reflexive
(*hisself* for *himself*). The inaccuracies may be present only in some
contexts. They change in character as the child works toward a more
mature form of expression.

In his sixth and seventh years the child is gaining the power to
generate an infinite variety of new linguistic combinations and to use
them in oral communication. He now is able to differentiate rules, to
generate, remember, and use different kinds of sentences. In Templin's
extensive study of children's speech, she found that only 3.3 percent
of the 3-year-old child's oral responses were made up of complex and
compound sentences whereas the speech of the child at 5 years comprised
8.7 percent; at 6 years 10.8 percent; and at 8 years 15.0 percent.[51] The
child, 7–8 years old, demonstrates skill both in subordination and coordination; he uses both complex and compound structures. Interjectional phrases are used very rarely, the imperative sentence has decreased in frequency, and the interrogative goes into a sharp decline.[52]
Now the declarative sentence comes to the fore, and with good reason. It
is an index of the child's significant growth in independence of perceptualization and expression.[53] At 8 years he has a fair command of syntactic tools which he uses both in the comprehension and expression of
language.

Sentence Length in Speech.   We have said very little about sentence
length, despite its wide acceptance as one measure of linguistic maturation. It is, as McCarthy has said, the most "easily determined, objective,
quantitative and easily understood measure";[54] but we wonder if it is
a very reliable index. Taped recordings of children's free conversations
leave the writer in greater doubt. How does one tell when a sentence
ends? By a pause? By the intonational and inflectional patterns?
Moreover, we find that sentence length changes with the situation. In
active play, the child ordinarily uses very short sentences. In a situation
where he feels unusually secure, he may use very long sentences, usually
of the add-on variety (*and-and-and*), with the result that we are unable
to determine the basic structure.[55] The length of a sentence is no indi-
cator of the child's ability in vocabulary or grammar.

Prosodic Patterns in Speech. We have discussed the comprehension-

[51] M. Templin, *Certain language skills in children.* Minneapolis: University of
Minnesota Press, 1957. P. 84.
[52] *Ibid.*, pp. 90–92.
[53] DeL. Lantz and V. Stefflre, Language and cognition revisited. *J Abnorm
Psychol* (November 1964), 69: 472–481.
[54] D. McCarthy, Language development in children. In L. Carmichael, Ed.,
Manual of child psychology. New York: Wiley, 1954. Pp. 550–551.
[55] S. Goda, Comment on "Temporal reliability of seven language measures."
J Speech Hearing Res (September 1964), 7: 298–299.

use of melodic qualities in language development in this and the preceding chapters. At 3 years rhythmic and intonational shifts become sharp markers of the child's knowledge of structure and meaning. At 5 years he is more adept and uses more subtle intonational and stress contrasts to denote specific word classes, phrases, and complexity in sentence structure. He has incorporated stress into his grammatical system.[56] When he is about 8 years old he will try out modulations in vocal quality and rhythm to express not only meaning and structure but also the emotional overtones of speech.

Morphemic Perception and Speech. The steady growth in intelligibility of a child's speech is evidence of a maturation of motor skill and also of the comprehension of sound sequences that make up morphemic units. He appreciates combinations and permutations essential for ordered expression, and muscle synergies learn how to perform as the nervous system directs. Until recently we have had few tests of the child's ability to order sequences of sounds but many tests of his ability to discriminate the isolated sound. We know that by the fifth year the child uses the /r/ phoneme in some positions, albeit inconsistently, and has stabilized /s/, /ʃ/, and /tʃ/ in some combinations. When he is 6 years old he is generally able to use /l/ in all positions and has improved his articulation of /j/ and /θ/. The phonemic hurdles of the seventh year are /z/, /ʒ/ and many sibilant blends. And having listed these phonemes, one must recognize at once that they do not test the child's ability to handle phonemic sequences in continuous speech. We have included charts of phonemic development in this chapter (p. 166) and tests of articulation in a later chapter (p. 273), but we do not believe that they are very significant measures of linguistic proficiency. What we should test is the number of linguistic units of expression the child has learned and still must learn; and that would entail notation of all the possible linguistic units in which these phonemes appear. Many a child is 9 years of age before he possesses mastery of this aspect of language use.[57]

Vocabulary Growth. We have alluded earlier to the close relation of syntactic form and vocabulary. A child, 6 to 7 years of age, does not perceive language by wandering through the total English vocabulary; he chooses only the appropriate lexical class—a noun-phrase, or verb-phrase. In short, he is restricted to the possible phrase structures about which he makes inferences. So in the sentence, "A skunk crossed the road," he must know that the noun-phrase (*a skunk*) is made up of an article and noun, and the verb-phrase (*crossed the road*) a verb and noun-phrase

[56] W. Miller and S. Ervin, The development of grammar in child language. *The acquisition of language.* Mongr Soc Res Child Develop (1964), 29: 28–29.

[57] A. G. Epstein maintains with considerable logic that "distortions are true speech defects but omissions and substitutions are defects in linguistic expression, an evidence of deficit in sequencing, a central linguistic ability."—A. G. Epstein, Phonemic testing. *J S Afr Logoped Soc* (December 1963), pp. 11–12.

(*the road*). It is this limitation of choice which the linguistically handicapped child does not have. In coding the incoming data he seems to range over a welter of words which have no sequential organization. They fit into no syntactic frame. Semantic rules, on the other hand, limit the *class of words* from which a listener makes his choice. Miller and Isard illustrate this point when they state that the child can find no meaning in such a sentence as "The boy spoke a triangle." [58] The normal child *expects* the noun-phrase to be in a certain semantic class. He is ready to hear *The boy spoke a long piece* or *spoke a short time* or *spoke a little while*.

In order to denote objects or experiences falling within one potential class or category, a child's vocabulary should reflect steady growth. If he does not possess these tools, he cannot form higher level percepts. For example, if one has no word for snow (the Lapps have no generic name for it), certainly his perception of snow is impaired. The child's ability to discriminate, to categorize, depends in some measure upon the vocabulary he possesses. If he has only a few words to denote a dimension of experience, his categorization will no doubt be unsatisfactory. The result is that he tends to disregard the dimension because he has few words to describe it. So shapes, directions, and qualities frequently are not recognized, are not interpreted. He cannot develop and verbalize the percept of a triangular shape, or of the southeasterly direction of the wind, or of the acridity of smoke, if he has no words to describe them. Furthermore these words must possess an exclusiveness in that they are the right words to denote essential elements of the concept. An automobile is a car but it is not a truck or a wagon. And the child of 7 years who defines car only as "a thing that moves" is categorizing unsatisfactorily, for *movement* certainly does not provide an adequate verbal base for the concept, *car*. The child's language equipment must enable him to make choices, to discriminate consistently among sizes and shapes without respect to the absolute size or shape or quality.

Assessments of the *number* of words that a child possesses at various stages in his language maturation appear in this chapter, "but more important than the number of words is the concepts they represent and the way in which they are used." [59] At present we have few reports of *qualitative* assessment of vocabulary. We know that the vocabulary of use lags behind the vocabulary of understanding, both in quantity and quality.[60] Both vocabularies increase substantially but not in equal

[58] G. A. Miller and S. Isard, Some perceptual consequences of linguistic rules. *J Verbal Learn Verbal Behav* (September 1963), 3: 217–228.

[59] M. Templin, Development of speech. *J Pediat* (January 1963), 62: 11–14.

[60] The child at 3.0 years reportedly has a *vocabulary of use* of 896 words; at 4.0, 1,540; at 5.0, 2,071; and at 6.0, 2,562 words.—M. E. Smith, An investigation of the development of the sentence and the extent of vocabulary in young children. *Univ Iowa Stud Child Welfare* (1926), 3 (5). At 6 years the *cognition vocabulary* is 16,900

increments from age to age. At 4.6, the referential meaning of words is enlarging rapidly. The child now abandons the one word-one meaning concept. He understands and uses discriminatively the several meanings of the word. He finds shades of meaning (*The sky is dark blue with some pink around the edge*). He also attempts to use quantitative words correctly (*some, any, several*), although he finds that they do not fit easily into his linguistic system. Between 6 and 8 years, the child engages in free associations (particularly of nouns and adjectives) that are grammatically similar to the stimulus word.[61] He also evinces an ability to handle new words grammatically. He tries new combinations of substantives and noun substitutions, some of which represent significant extensions of meaning.

Unfortunately, the phonological, syntactic, and semantic development of oral language is not complete and the rules of each dimension are not thoroughly learned by the ages of 7 or 8 years. The battle of language acquisition is not so easily won. At 7 years the child is still making errors in grammar. Verb and subject often disagree in number; the case of pronouns goes awry (*Him and her went*); the use of the prepositional phrase is uncertain and will continue to be, even among students of college age (*To you and I it seems right!*). The double negative persists at 8 years, and *ain't* cannot be washed out of American speech. Strange intonational and stress patterns often distort meaning. As for morphemic units, we know adults who cannot order the sound sequences in *supercalifragilisticexpialidocious*. As long as one talks, one must keep on learning how to talk.

---

words.—M. K. Smith, Measurement of the size of the general English vocabulary through the elementary grades and high school. *Monogr J Genet Psychol* (1941), 24: 311–345.

[61] W. Miller and S. Ervin, The development of grammar in child language. In U. Bellugi and R. Brown, Eds., *The acquisition of language.* Monogr Soc Res Child Develop (1964), 29: 28–29.

III

Evaluation of the Linguistically Handicapped Child

6

Longitudinal Study of Verbal and Nonverbal Behaviors

Procedure, Personnel, and Plan

Procedures employed in evaluation of language disorders necessarily must vary with the teaching situation. The speech correctionist in the public school generally engages in a screening survey of speech followed by the administration of tests of articulation and auditory acuity. Later he may request a report from the school psychologist of intelligence scores and occasional reports from the classroom teacher. In higher educational and medical centers the child is usually referred by school or medical authorities or by health and social agencies to a speech center. The center staff administers a battery of tests to the child generally in a single diagnostic session. On the same day a case history is taken by interviewing the parents. Results are tabulated and the case is presented in staff conference. Summary remarks ordinarily are followed by recommendation of admission and/or referral to other agencies.

Diagnostic Teaching. The procedures recommended in this chapter fit neither of these prevailing practices. They are adapted to the practice of certain educational and other institutions of habilitation which now admit children for study or diagnostic teaching. A few speech and language teachers in the public schools have turned recently to this plan of diagnostic teaching, but the great majority of them claim that it does not fit their needs because they work alone. They need not and should not work alone. If they have vision and energy, they can organize an excellent team. In their communities, if not in their schools, are psychologists, psychiatrists, audiologists, and pediatricians who can be

189

persuaded to assist them in this program of diagnostic teaching. Furthermore they have resources that one does not always find in a university center—classroom teachers, supervisors, and great numbers of children who seek their help in learning language. The period of diagnostic teaching may extend from eight to fifteen weeks or throughout the school year. In a public school setting, the children usually return to the regular classroom as they reach a minimum standard of competence in language.

Personnel. The team conducting the program is made up of special language teachers, classroom teachers, trainees, observers, and all those administrative, medical, psychological, and social service workers who may rightly be drawn into a program that encompasses both the child and his family. The leaders of the team are the special language teachers. Whenever possible we have avoided calling them clinicians, therapists, or pathologists, for this is an educational, not a clinical program. The terms *clinician, therapist,* and *pathologist* have unfortunate connotations and might best be completely omitted, but we have no apt, unambiguous title to propose for the special language teacher. In origin and practice, clinics, pathologies, and therapies are associated with hospitals and medical schools. Although speech and reading clinics now are more commonly known as *centers* with *center staffs,* we do not yet speak of *center teachers.* In the context of this book, the special language teacher is, or should be, an educator. He is a teacher in a class (perhaps a very small class), and his success will be determined in large part by his ability to coordinate his teaching with that of other classroom teachers and with all efforts of other members of the team.

Plan. Our educational plan is based upon group instruction, not individual tutoring. The team, in the course of its observation and teaching, will make a longitudinal study that will include the following evaluation procedures: (1) a case history; (2) the study of developmental factors contributing to the child's language behavior; (3) objective and exploratory measurements of the child's nonverbal and verbal behavior; and (4) periodic assessment of the child's gains in the comprehension and use of oral language. All these materials, synthesized and interpreted, will make up a cumulative record, the journal. An extensive anecdotal summary can be an exciting story of one child's conquest of language.

Guidelines to Longitudinal Study

Diagnostic study and teaching demand good record-keeping, whether the keeping is done by the computer or pen. To aid the staff in record-keeping, this and succeeding chapters present a series of outlines to follow: a case history form, exploratory materials, inventories, and tables of nonverbal and verbal behaviors, exploratory and objective measurement of the child's deficits and abilities in learning oral language, and tests of adaptive behaviors associated with language.

Areas of Study. This course of study and teaching is both intensive and extensive. As the program develops, the staff and assistants, under the leadership of special language teachers, will use the checklists and schedules of development as guides in observing and teaching. These materials include salient features of the total behavioral profile of the child. Depending upon the age of the child, some parts of this record will be historical and gained by conference with the parents and other members of the family. The exploratory materials, inventories, and tables provide both the means and the criteria for evaluating maturation of verbal and pertinent nonverbal behaviors, with the result that distinctive features of the deficit in language-learning should be identifiable.[1]

Some leaders of the team may protest that it is not necessary to record observations on so many facets of behavior; they are interested only in the child's *language behavior.* The crucial deficit in the child's language behavior, however, is often discovered by observing other facets of behavior. It may not *seem* important, for instance, to note evidences of motor awkwardness or bizarre movement patterns in avoidance of objects or in accommodation to space. It *is* important, however, because poor psychomotor coordination may be the first notable sign of a central neural deficit that also may have affected the child's language. A clutterer's disorientation in time and space, for example, may have a direct bearing on his "word-salad" speech. Or let us cite another child's problem. He is a nontalking child of 4 years, a faceless child, without identity. The questions one must raise will not be limited simply to his hearing or to his articulatory mechanism. Is his language delay part of a *general delay* in mental maturation? Is this child perceptually

[1] Although much of this information is the result of the writer's teaching experience, much has been borrowed, consciously or unconsciously, from the work of others. Acknowledgment should be made of the assistance of the following authors: J. Abercrombie, *Perceptual and visuomotor disorders in cerebral palsy;* T. Bangs, Evaluating children with language delay. *J Speech Hearing Dis* 26 (1): 16–18; N. Bayley, The development of motor abilities during the first three years, *Monogr Soc Res Child Develop* (1935), 1–25; R. Brown and U. Bellugi, Three processes in the child's acquisition of syntax, in *New directions in the study of language;* W. Daley, *Speech and language therapy with the brain-damaged child;* A. Gesell and C. Amatruda, *Developmental diagnosis;* E. Haeusserman, *Developmental potential of pre-school children;* M. M. Lewis, *Infant speech;* A. Luria and F. Yudovich, *Speech and the Development of mental processes in the child;* L. Scott, *The longitudinal study of individual development;* M. Shirley, The first two years, in *Inst Child Welfare Monogr* II (7); M. Templin, *Certain language skills in children;* and N. Wood, *Communication problems and their effect on the learning potential of the mentally retarded child.*

ready for speech? Does he have specific perceptual deficits? Why is he unable to imitate the simple rhythmic action of other children in the group? He watches them as they prance " 'round the mulberry bush so early on a Monday morning" or as they make up jingles to match their costumes: "Wiggle-waggle-woggle; we dance a pretty joggle." The silent youngster retreats to the opposite corner of the room. A staff member asks, "Is this an emotional problem?", and suggests that you investigate and appraise his socioemotional adjustment. One will need to know much about his cultural and social environment, about the size, economic status, and basic attitudes of the family. One will need non-linguistic criteria by which to make this evaluation.

In connection with this question of socioemotional adjustment, our observation of two little boys, 4 years of age, both handicapped by unrepaired palatal clefts, comes to mind. Jimmie, a child with poor but devoted parents, talked nonstop and was easily the most popular youngster in the summer resident Center. Dale came from a home in the upper middle economic group. In an initial conference, Dale's parents re-ferred frequently to their misfortune, to the tragedy which they must bear. Dale covered his mouth when he was called upon to speak. He ran screaming to his dormitory when he saw the photographer. A social maturity scale was completed for both boys. According to their parents' rating, Dale, who exhibited maladjustment at every turn, outranked Jimmie in social maturity. Formal tests have their place but they cannot replace judgment based upon continuous observation of behavior. You may need to apply all the neurophysiological and psychological knowl-edge you have acquired in the course of your evaluative study. You will be aided by inventories and tables of the normal development of verbal and nonverbal behavior; they will act as pegs for your comparisons. You will appreciate the fact that a language disorder may be a manifestation of major or subtle disturbances in the general behavior of the child. Longitudinal studies must be both extensive and intensive.

Objective Measures. Language diagnosticians who object to the time required for longitudinal studies are inclined to rely solely on ob-jective tests. We agree that objective measures are valuable and we in-clude them, but they are valuable only insofar as they become an integral part of the longitudinal study. Despite the skill of test makers in cate-gorizing symptoms, causes, and disabilities, we find few definitive con-clusions except as they are supported by longitudinal studies of the indi-vidual's total behavior. In foreign countries leaders in the field of lan-guage disorders are not so impressed as are our American colleagues with quantifying methods resulting in analyses of variance and covariance. As Teuber says, "Much analysis in current neuropsychology in the United States (though much less in England and France) makes large-scale use of standard tests . . . often at the expense of more versatile, qualitative tasks. . . ." [2] We do not decry the use of tests; both standardized and exploratory tests are presented in succeeding chapters. We believe, however, in a field where the bases of language have not been agreed upon, longitudinal studies are more productive. We think we can learn more about the child's language disorder by observing him when he is actively engaged in language learning than by his answers to questions or non-verbal performance in a formal test situation. Although a standardized test of motor skills is included, in our experience we have learned more by watching the child skip or bump along the corridor, run or awkwardly negotiate the stairs, regularly tip the drinking glass, or turn right when the rest of the group is turning left, than from such tests. We have watched him *with his peers;* we have appraised his motor maturation in relation to a control group.

Basic Relationships. Success or failure in a longitudinal study and teaching program will depend to a significant degree on the relationships that the team establishes with the family and the child. In interviewing parents for a case history or in counseling, basic attitudes may be established which can either break or make the learning situation. Fortunate is the family who finds in the team understanding and wise friends. Even more fortunate is the child if all the persons who teach him are motivated to enter a young life, to make an investment in a child, and to bring to him and his family a sense of worth and belief that they are an integral and valuable part of the program. Some children who have entered special classes, already defeated although they were only 4 years old, have almost perceptibly developed a sense of identity. One day when three 4-year-olds were creating hubbub outside the preschool room, the director happened along and admonished them. One turned and said, "Who are you?" Uncertain of her role at the moment, she mumbled, "I'm the boss." John scoffed that one off with: "Huh, we *belong* here." It behooves those teachers who conduct the interviews for a case history, the evaluative studies, and the tests and measurements to make an investment. If they do not do so, why should the child and his parents reciprocate? "Getting to know you" means more than *vis-à-vis* confrontation. It is the communication of fellows in a joint enterprise.

Meeting the Child's Special Behavioral Problem. The language teacher must understand and be prepared for all kinds of unpredictable behavior. Sometimes the problem is how to keep the youngster in the room or, if he is in the room, off the window sills or the desk. In other cases one must persuade him to leave his hideaway under the table. If the

---

[2] H-L. Teuber, Preface. In A. R. Luria, Ed., *Higher cortical functions in man.* New York: Basic Books Inc., Publishers, 1966.

child is hyperactive and somewhat destructive, the best injunction is to give him opportunities to move in specified activities and to engage him in a job which he must tackle with the language teacher. He must help in locating toys or putting a wheel on a wagon, and finally he will be drawn into a structured activity. Generally these children welcome structure and a firm hand. If the child seems to be autistic and completely removed from the environment, it is best for the teacher to become occupied with something at his table, neither ignoring nor attempting to make contact with the child for a time. He adopts what might be called conscious coexistence. He discovers a toy that he has learned the child likes. He plays the music box or talks to the doll as he puts on its coat and cap, finally leaving the doll close to the child. Sometimes the language handicap itself presents a problem. Not only must the teacher use nonverbal communication with many of these children but he also must learn the child's substitute for communication. Language-impaired children are prone to multiple sensory-motor handicaps, and these also pose particular problems for the staff. If the child is cerebral-palsied, for example, the examiner may not be able to follow the customary procedures in evaluation of his language deficits.

Use of Results of Study. Carefully documented, dated, and interpreted longitudinal studies should result in clear decisions at the end of the period of diagnostic teaching. These documents, contained in a journal, trace the rate of development of specific facets of language, the stops and starts, plateaus and heights. Correlation of problems of language learning with other kinds of learning and with behavioral factors, internal and external, must be made. The resulting composite picture of *this child,* the subject and substance of the anecdotal summary, should reveal how *this child* differs from every other child who seems to have a similar language disorder and also how he may best be taught. Well done, the longitudinal study becomes the touchstone of all future teaching.

Organization of Longitudinal Studies

Before the student begins his study of a linguistically impaired child, he should review the chapters on the normal development of oral language and its neurophysiological and psychological parameters. If he is to use the materials in this and succeeding chapters he must understand thoroughly the underlying matrix, of which language behavior is a part, and the rationale for the inclusion of the information and criteria he is to use.

Longitudinal Study I is devoted to the case history. Longitudinal Study II encompasses exploratory materials, schedules of normal development of verbal and nonverbal behaviors, and inventories identifying atypical behavior patterns associated directly or indirectly with language learning. In succeeding chapters (Longitudinal Studies III and IV), objective and exploratory assessment of linguistic function and tests of other functions associated with language learning will be described.

Longitudinal Study I: Case History

The skeleton outline of the case history may well seem uninteresting. It is lifeless until it is filled with information pertinent to the child's linguistic problem; then it becomes a lively and valuable document. The preparation of a case history is important and difficult; it should demand the most expert members of the staff. One must know not only how to establish the kind of relationship to which we have alluded in the preceding paragraphs; he also must know what questions to ask, how to ask them, and how to record them.

The interviewer must appraise what he is told. Parents' memories with respect to the early development of their child often are not accurate. (A baby book is a good resource for factual data.) Parents are proud, often defensive, and often have guilt feelings about the child. The interviewer must be sensitive to these responses. Not in the first interview, perhaps, but after a time the parents' report may be more accurate. Then the interviewer must go back and modify earlier entries in the case history.

The interviewer must feel free to digress from the printed form of the outline. One question leads to another. The child began to talk at about 1 year, the parent says, but you know that most parents make this statement, so you go on with other questions. When did second words appear (p. 168)? Was there a long plateau after second words? Did he stop talking altogether for a time? How does the parent account for this silent period? Was the child ill? Was there extraordinary emotional stress in the environment? If there was stress you suspect that one parent may talk more freely about it if the other parent is not present. The skillful interviewer detects this situation and finds an occasion to continue the interview when only one parent is present.

How can one interviewer record all information as rapidly as it is given? He must learn to be selective in asking only pertinent questions and in recording only pertinent information. He may record notes in a free shorthand, notes that he will later expand. Hopefully he may have the advantage of a tape recorder operating without the awareness of the parents. In this event he can give undivided attention to the parents. Moreover a recording permits him to evaluate the consistency of the parents' information after the interview is over.

Physical environment contributes much to the success of the interview. The writer has observed interviews conducted behind burners of a home economics laboratory in a public school or amid the coming and going in a teachers' lounge. She has observed parents sitting in a clinic room on children's chairs while the speech correctionist looks down on them from her perch behind a desk. Often one or two children of the family may be present with the parents. The implications are clear. The interviewer often protests, "These are factors beyond my control." He would be wise if he intervened in his environment in order to change it.

Techniques of interviewing are not learned by rote. Sometimes we say "we will play it by ear." If we do, it must be by an ear perceptive to all the nuances of the situation. Successful interviewing will depend upon knowledge of language disorders, upon friendly rapport and understanding, upon time and the physical environment, and all these will hinge finally upon the perceptive and personal qualities of the interviewer.

Case History

Name of Child _____ Date _____

Age _____ Birth Date _____ Sex _____ Race _____

Address _____ Telephone _____

City _____ Zip Code _____ State _____

Description of child's appearance _____

_____

Entered for _____

Name of Parents or Guardian _____

Address _____ Telephone _____

Siblings _____ Ages _____

Source of referral _____

Doctor's name and address _____

Names of persons filling in questionnaire _____

Relation to child _____

Nature and onset of problem: _____

Etiology suggested by referring agent: Mental retardation _____; Emotional

disturbance _____; CNS deficit or injury _____;

Environmental deprivation _____.

I. Family History

   Father: Name _____ Address _____

   Age _____ Height _____ Weight _____ Birthplace _____ National descent _____

   Living with family _____ dead _____ divorced _____ remarried _____

   Present occupation _____ Previous occupation _____

   Present state of health _____ How far did he go in school _____

   Which hand does he prefer _____ Was preference ever changed _____

   Mother: Name _____ Address _____

   Age _____ Height _____ Weight _____ Birthplace _____ National descent _____

   Living with family _____ dead _____ divorced _____ remarried _____

   Present occupation _____ Previous occupation _____

   Present state of health _____ How far did she go in school _____

   Which hand does she prefer _____ Was preference ever changed _____

   Siblings:

Name	Age	Hand Preferred	Age Started to Speak	Health	School Progress	Normal	Retarded
_____	___	_____	_____	_____	_____	_____	_____

II. Language and speech problems in immediate family. (Note relation of individual
    to propositus, severity of disorder, exogenous/endogenous.)
    Delayed development of language _____

    _____

    Retarded speech _____

    Language and/or speech disturbances resulting from CNS deficits or injuries
    (aphasia, mental retardation, cerebral palsy) _____

    _____

    _____

    Cluttering (tachyphemia) _____

    Stuttering _____

    Defective articulation (preadolescence to adulthood) _____

Hearing loss _____
Speech defects resulting from structural anomalies (cleft palate, palatal insuffic-
iency, macroglossia, dental malformations, micrognathia) _____
_____
Voice problems _____
Dyslexia (reading problems) _____

III. Medical history of immediate family.
Is there or has there been in the immediate family any of the following: diabetes;
convulsive disorders; congenital disorders of heart, eyes, ears, lungs; allergies; Rh-
negative blood; nervous disorders; mongolism; structural anomalies. (Identify
person; note severity, duration, treatment of disorder.) _____
_____
_____
_____

IV. Parents' family.
Mother's: Siblings: number and mother's position among sibs; health status;
    chronic diseases; language and/or speech retardation in sibs and offspring of
    sibs; education of sibs. _____
    _____
    _____

Father's: Siblings: number and father's position among sibs; health status;
    chronic diseases; language and/or speech retardation in sibs and offspring of
    sibs; education of sibs. _____
    _____
    _____

V. Pregnancy data.
How many pregnancies has mother had _____; Which was this child _____
Miscarriages _____; How many _____; Which pregnancy _____
Babies born dead _____; How many _____; Which pregnancy _____
Premature babies _____; How many _____; Which pregnancy _____
State of mother's health before this pregnancy _____;
during _____; after _____
Infectious diseases during pregnancy (rubella, scarlet fever, kidney infection)
_____
Other illnesses (anemia, hormonal deficiencies or excesses) _____
Rh incompatibility _____
Exposure to radiation during or shortly before pregnancy _____
Medication (contraceptive or other) before or during first trimester pregnancy
_____

VI. Perinatal history.
Child born in _____ Hospital; Address _____
Physician in attendance _____; Address _____
Was child full term _____; Premature _____
Delivery: Normal _____; Forceps _____; Cesarean _____
Duration of labor _____; Anesthetics _____
Presentation: Breech _____; Vertex _____
Birth condition of child:
    Anoxia (length of time) _____; Kernicterus _____; Jaundice _____
    Child cried, breathed, nursed normally _____

Incubation: _____ ; Oxygen _____

Signs of injury (scars, bruises, deformations) _____

Convulsions _____ ; Other _____

Child's health in first 10 days of life _____

Feeding _____; Left hospital with mother _____

VII. Developmental data.

Weight at birth _____ ; 6 months _____ ; 1 year _____ ; present _____

Age in weeks or months at which following first occurred:

Showed response to mother _____ ; raised head _____ ;

Tooth erupted _____ ; sat without support _____ ; crawled _____ ;

grasped objects readily _____ ; responded to environment _____ ;

stood with support _____ ; took first steps _____ ;

walked without aid _____ ; fell frequently _____ ;

gait normal _____ ; walked upstairs with alternating tread _____ ;

ate with spoon _____ ; drank from glass (cup) _____; coordinated

in fine and large movements _____ ; chewed and swallowed

normally _____ ; voluntary control of bowels _____ ,

bladder _____ ; asks to go to toilet _____ ;

cared for toilet completely _____.

Child sucked fingers _____; which hand _____; how long _____ ;

Age at which child showed preference for one hand _____ ; now definitely

right handed _____ ; left handed _____ ; ambilateral _____ ;

handedness influenced _____.

VIII. Health-medical data.

Present state of health: _____

Under medical treatment for _____

Physician's name and address: _____

Food habits: Appetite good _____ ; eats regularly _____ ;

snacks _____. Chews normally _____; swallows normally _____ ;

drools _____; enjoys eating _____.

Sleep habits: Regular _____ ; time of retiring _____ ; arising_____;

Does child share room_____; bed _____; _____.

Respiration: Breathing regular _____; noisy _____; mouth breather_____.

Systemic defects: Ocular: fixation, version, and vergence _____ ;

Aural (peripheral) _____ ; watches television at very close range _____ ;

Television volume excessive _____.

Childhood diseases: (Specify the age at which child had any of the following
illnesses. Specific information, such as degrees of temperature, medical treatment, coma, rigidity, and seizures should be included.)

Measles _____	Diphtheria _____
Whooping cough _____	Mumps _____
Scarlet fever _____	Chicken pox _____
Pneumonia _____	

Diseases of Central Nervous System:

Etiology	Evidence	Symptoms
A. Unknown	Neurological examina-	Convulsions
1. Abnormal pre-	tion	Ataxia
natal conditions	Air study	Gait disturbance
2. Prematurity	Increased intracranial	Lateral nystagmus
3. Neonatal apnea	pressure	
4. Birth injury	(hydrocephalous, etc.)	
5. Possible encephalitis		

B. Cerebral cyst or tumor — Increased intracranial pressure — Hemiparesis / Ataxia / Febrile convulsion

C. Encephalopathy caused by
1. Mechanical trauma — Neurological examination / Abnormal EEG / CNS involvement following accident — Hemiparesis / Convulsions—grand mal / Convulsions—focal

2. Inflammation
Meningitis, bacterial
Meningitis, viral
Encephalitis, viral — Neurological examination / Abnormal EEG / CNS involvement during illness / Associated generalized infection (fever, convulsions, etc.) / Agent bacterial / Agent viral — Hemiplegia / Convulsions / Questionable eye movements / Positive Babinski

3. Metabolic
Hypoglycemia caused by metabolic defect; pancreatic adenoma — Neurological examination and blood glucose levels / Abnormal EEG — Convulsions—grand mal / Variable dysfunction of CNS

Diseases Affecting Middle Ear:
Tonsillitis _____ Sinusitis _____
Otitis media_____: suppurative _____; high temperature _____
URI _____ ; chronic cough _____
Atopic diseases: Allergies
Eczema _____; Asthma _____; Hay Fever _____
Vasomotor rhinitis _____ ; Hives _____
Surgery:
Tonsillectomy and adenoidectomy _____; Other _____
Severe shock or injuries _____; when _____
Structural defects: mouth _____; nose _____; palate _____;
mandible _____; teeth _____.
Immunizations for: small pox _____; diphtheria _____;
tetanus _____; whooping cough _____; poliomyelitis _____;
others _____.

IX. Socioemotional Development.
Primarily responsive to objects _____
Especially alert to movements _____
Sensitive to vibrating sensations _____
Normal activity (behaviorally consistent) _____
Usually happy _____; sympathetic _____;
demonstrative in feeling _____.
Enjoys company of others _____ ; avoids company _____
Shows concern when separated from parents _____
Unaware of environment _____
Plays mostly by himself _____; with other members of family _____;
with children outside family _____; younger _____; older _____

Likes to play alone under table or in closet _____
Cooperates best with: mother _____ ; father _____ ; sibs _____
Shares toys or turns _____ ; willing to try new things _____
Initiates new play schemes, etc. _____ ; afraid of strange things _____
Lives in talking environment _____ ; bilingual environment _____
Answers ringing telephone _____ ; uses dial for telephoning _____
Sensitive to discipline _____ ; resistant _____ methods used _____
Angers easily when frustrated _____ ; temper tantrums _____ ;
   cries frequently (sheds tears) _____ .
Hyperactive _____ ; phlegmatic _____ ; rocks while sitting _____ ;
   bangs head (crib, chair, floor) _____ ; stares at lights, objects,
   people, into space _____ .
Adults beside father and mother living in home _____

X. Language and Speech Development.
   At what age was child sensitive to sounds in his environment _____ ;
      did he respond to loud sounds only _____ ; seem to ignore sounds _____
   Did child coo and babble as a normal baby _____ ;
      use gestures meaningfully _____ ; communicate by crying, smiling _____
   At what age did child comprehend speech of others (go bye-bye; Daddy's home,
   yum-yum—food, and so forth) with concrete stimuli present _____
   _____
   At what age did child comprehend speech when supporting, concrete stimuli were
      not present _____
   At what age did child show enjoyment of television _____ ;
      what programs does he watch now _____
   At what age did he attend quickly and purposefully to speech of others _____
   At what age did child use words or phrases _____ ;
      to communicate meaning _____
   What were the second phrases (after baby bye) _____
   At what age did child communicate meaning about stimuli which were not imme-
      diately present_____
   Was language meager in amount _____ ; in quality _____ ;
   Was there steady development of: vocabulary _____ ; sentence
      structure _____ ; syntax _____
   Are prosodic qualities of child's speech appropriate for age and sex _____
   What other means of communication has child used _____ ;
      does he use them now _____ .
   Is articulation appropriate to age? Phoneme order confused _____ ;
   phonemes omitted _____ ; substituted _____ ; distorted _____
   Are there known defects of tongue, palate, nose, throat, ears which may be re-
      lated to child's communication problems _____
   _____
   _____
   Are there injuries or illnesses, pre- or post-natal, which may have had adverse ef-
      fect on language/speech development _____
   _____
   What is child's present attitude toward oral communication:
   Attends readily to speech of others _____
   Ready to initiate speech as a means of communication _____
   Verbal output is excessive _____
   Pantomimes much of time _____
   Makes no attempt to communicate _____

What is parental attitude at present toward oral communication:
Mother's view of importance of communication _____
Father's view of importance of communication _____
Permissive attitude toward noisy, talking environment _____
Restriction on speech in home _____
Expectations of parents with respect to child's progress in communication
_____
_____

Parents' description of present status of child's communicative disorder:
_____
_____
_____

Recorder's description of child's language _____
_____
_____
_____

XI.   Educational record.
Does child attend preschool _____; kindergarten _____ ;
   elementary school _____; junior high school _____
Has child followed his age group in school _____ ; special difficulties
   in learning _____; in social adjustment _____
What subject or activity does he enjoy most in school _____
_____

XII. Special education in language/speech prior to or continuing at this time:
Clinical examinations and diagnosis at _____
_____
Teaching at _____
   for period _____
   by _____

XIII. Summary of Reports from Other Agencies:
A. Medical
   1. Pediatrician or general physician:
      a. General health index
      b. Appraisal of physical mechanism of speech
   2. Neurologist
   3. Psychiatrist
B. Psychological (from private or community agencies)
C. Educational
   1. Classroom teacher
   2. Teachers in special education (private or public school)
   3. School psychologist
   4. School nurse
   5. Social service staff
   6. Physiotherapy, occupational therapy staffs

Longitudinal Study II: Significant Developmental Factors in the Child's Verbal and Nonverbal Behavior

We cannot adequately consider all factors of behavior which undoubtedly have some bearing on the onset and growth of oral language. Many physical, psychosocial, motivational, and other environmental factors discussed in preceding chapters are referred to only indirectly in this chapter. Rather, only those data that are most significant milestones in the sequence of linguistic development have been chosen. Perceptual development in the child is one of these significant milestones in determining language learning. The child's early and meaningful interpretation, both of verbal and nonverbal stimuli bodes well for the later appearance of motor speech. And motor speech, the use of oral language, of course, must be charted in sequence. It is intimately bound up with the general processes of motor maturation, and hence much of the data on general adaptive behavior is concerned with motor development. Beginning with the motor theory of speech perception, we have emphasized throughout the book the importance of bodily coordination in the development of oral language. Bayley and colleagues have reinforced this view in recent reports of their longitudinal studies of development (p. 151).[3] Our data are concerned first with early motor activity and coordination of the extremities, postural shifts and locomotion, balance, and special sensory-motor behavior, and secondly with the later development of motor skills. The final section of normative data is devoted to socioemotional development and learning attitudes. This section is by no means complete, probably because this type of material cannot be easily sequenced or tabulated according to the chronological age of the child.

Longitudinal Study II is divided into two age periods. The materials in the first division concern the age group from early infancy to 3 years, the second division, 3 years to 8 years. The three aids to appraisal—exploratory materials, inventories, and tables—serve different purposes. Exploratory materials provide for the student or staff member the means of observing and extrapolating his observations of verbal behavior. Inventories are useful in the quick overview and identification of atypical behavior patterns; tables must be referred to in the detailed day-by-day

[3] J. Cameron, N. Livson, and N. Bayley, Infant vocalizations and their relationship to mature intelligence. *Science* (July 21, 1967), 157: 331–333.

study of all phases of verbal and nonverbal behavior associated with language development. They appear in the following order:

Longitudinal Study II-A: 1 Week–36 Months

    Table 6-1. Development of Nonverbal Adaptive Behavior, 1 Week–36 Months. Motor activity and coordination of the extremities; postural shifts and locomotion; balance; and special sensory-motor behavior.

    Table 6-2. Comprehension and Use of Oral Language, 1–36 Months. Comprehension of verbal and expressive signals; vocabulary; length of response; use of oral language.

        Materials. Exploring Use of Oral Language in Play Sessions, 11–36 Months.

        Inventory 1. Comprehension of Nonverbal and Verbal Stimuli, 1–36 Months.

        Inventory 2. Use of Oral Language, 11–36 Months.

Longitudinal Study II-B: 3–8 Years

    Table 6-3. Nonverbal Adaptive Behavior, 3–8 Years.

        Inventory 3. General Motor Development: 4–8 Years.

        Inventory 4. Socioemotional Behavior: 4–8 Years.

        Inventory 5. Attitudes in Learning: 4–8 Years.

    Table 6-4. Development of Some Aspects of Oral Language, 3–8 Years.

        Materials. Exploring Comprehension of Oral Language, 3–8 Years.

        Inventory 6. Comprehension of Nonverbal Stimuli, 3–8 Years.

        Inventory 7. Comprehension of Verbal Information, 3–8 Years.

        Materials. Exploring Use of Oral Language, 3–8 Years.

        Inventory 8. Use of Oral Language, 3–8 Years.

        Rating Form. Some Phonological Aspects of Oral Expression, 5–8 Years.

Longitudinal Study II-C: The Summing Up

Longitudinal Study II-A

Table 6-1. Development of nonverbal adaptive behavior, 1 week–36 months.

Age	Motor Activity and Coordination of Extremities	Postural Shifts and Locomotion	Balance Antigravity Behavior	Special Sensory-Motor Behavior
1–4 weeks	Nonpurposive arm and leg thrusts. Activity diminishes with attentional focus.	Lateral head movements. Crawling movements.	Lifts head at shoulders.	Visual localization.
8 weeks	Leg thrusts in play.	Much body movement, especially in anticipatory excitement.	Head erect in vertical position.	Turns eyes to light. Eyes follow pencil or moving person.
12 weeks	Watches play with hands. Pulls at clothing. Directs movement toward object. Holds toy actively. Crude palming movement. Puts object to mouth.	Reaches for ring. First gross shift in bodily position. Lifts head and chest (when on stomach); weight on elbows.	Balances head steadily. Dorsal suspension.	True visual fixation. Blinks at visual stimulus. Follows vanishing stimulus with eyes. Aware of strange situation. Markedly less crying. Smiles when talked to.
16 weeks	Plays with hands and fingers. Closure reflex disappearing. Beginning thumb apposition. Contact generally unilateral. Reaches for cube. Pulls dress over face.	Tonic neck reflex subsiding. Prone: Elevates self by arms.	Sits with support, 10–15 min. Holds self erect when pulled to sitting position.	Turns head to sound. Eye cooperation in reaching. Stares at rattle in his hand. Responds to human sounds more definitely.
20 weeks	Beginning to shift to bilaterality. Clutches in play. Grasps 1 cube. Recovers rattle; puts it in mouth. Partial thumb apposition. Pats bottle at feeding time.	Turns from back to side. Rolls over easily, automatically to retrieve toy. Supports some of his weight when held in standing position.	Sits with slight support. Head erect; steady for moment. Bounces up and down.	Grasps cube as he looks at second one. Smiles at mirror image. Discriminates strangers.
24 weeks	Shift to bilaterality. Grasps foot. Grasps and holds 2 objects. Simultaneous flexion and thumb apposition.	Cannot yet stand with holding on. Turns to observe fallen spoon. Tries to creep or roll toward object.	Sits alone 30 secs. or longer. Holds head and trunk erect. Leans forward from sitting position. Sits up easily when attention is purposive.	Discriminates between people.

Table 6-1. (continued)

	Motor Activity and Coordination of Extremities	Postural Shifts and Locomotion	Balance Antigravity Behavior	Special Sensory-Motor Behavior
28 weeks	Bilateral reaching but with some spatial error. Likes physical play. Puts foot in mouth. Holds foot in hands. Lifts cup with handle.	Stepping movements. Moves himself one foot by creeping.	Stands and bounces actively.	Smiles. Reaches and pats mirror image.
32 weeks	Reaches unilaterally and persistently for toys. Complete thumb apposition. Holds 2 cubes.	Steady posture. Maintains standing position briefly (hands held). Creeps rapidly from room to room.	Sits alone.	Bites and chews toys.
36 weeks	Shift to unilaterality; left hand open. Rotates wrist. Picks up pellet with thumb and finger tips. Retains ball; tries to throw it. Radial digital grasp of cube. Hits, pushes cube with cube. Bilateral reaching discontinuous, then continuous with little spatial error.	Leans forward as he sits. Movements in straight line.	Pushes from stomach to sitting position. Re-erects body while sitting.	Feeds self cracker.
40 weeks	Plays pat-a-cake. Attempts to scribble imitatively. Rotates wrist.	Creeps well. Early stepping movements. Takes side-steps, holding on.	Pulls self to standing position.	Plays peek-a-boo. Rings bell purposively. Laughs and covers face. Playful response to mirror.
44 weeks	Holds crayon adaptively. Removes cube from cup. Extends toy but will not release it.	Stands up. Takes first independent step.	Standing by rail, lifts, replaces foot.	Beginning to drink from cup.
12 months	Reaching: smooth, continuous; little error. Release of hand poorly timed in throwing.	Sits down. Walks alone or with 2 hands held. Walks on feet and hands, knees off floor.	Pivots while sitting. Broad base when trying to pick up toy.	Plays with noisemakers. Responds to music. Expresses fear, anxiety, affection.

206

Age					
18 months	Strikes doll in imitation. Repeats performances that bring attention. Eats with spoon.	Grasp, prehension, release fully developed. Hurls ball. Turns 2-3 pages of book together. Builds tower: 3 cubes with difficulty. Feeds self; often spills. Puts cover on box on command. Plays with pull-toy. Carries doll. Helps dress self. Manipulates objects.	Walks; seldom falls. Walks backward. Walks upstairs, downstairs with help. Climbs into adult chair.	Squats in play. Seats self on small chair with only fair aim. Crawls downstairs backward.	Places square or triangle in form board. Vigorous imitative scribble in drawing.
24 months		Shift from unilaterality to confused laterality. Bilateral use of nondominant hand. Kicks ball; throws ball into box. Pulls on simple garments in dressing. Turns pages of book one at a time. Inserts key in lock. Can string large beads. Feeds self without turning spoon upside down.	Walks; runs; little falling. Walks up and down stairs alone but does not alternate steps.	Can quickly alternate between sitting and standing. Can stand with heels together. Drinks from cup without spilling.	Mouthing of objects almost stopped. Some mimicry. Pays attention to other children. Beginning to match two like objects. Imitates circular motion with crayon.
30-36 months		Good hand and finger coordination. Can move digits independently. Holds crayon securely with fingers while drawing. Builds tower: 6 cubes. Pushes toy with good steering. Carries household objects. Pulls off socks. Assists with washing hands.	Walks on tiptoe. Walks in line.	Jumps from chair. Jumps off floor with both feet. Reaches with one hand without using other to balance. Rises from prone to standing position without turning.	Tries to remove wraps when removal is initiated by parents. Makes vertical strokes with crayon.

Table 6-2. Development of comprehension and use of oral language, 1-36 months.

Age in Months	Comprehension of Verbal and Expressive Signals	Vocabulary (Mean No. of Words)	Mean Length of Response	Use of Oral Language
1	Responds to sound. Reflex smiling to tactile and kinesthetic stimulation and mother's voice.			*Precursory stage:* Crying sounds that change in pitch; sign of bodily discomfort. Most frequent sound [n]; other vowel-like sounds: [ɛ] [æ] [ʌ]
2	Attends readily to speaking voice. Aware of his own sounds.			*Precursory stage:* Babbling begins. Reflex activities associated with breathing, swallowing, hiccoughing produce sounds resembling nasalized front and middle vowels (not true speech sounds). Coos and gurgles in vocal play.
3	Aware of many visual and auditory stimuli in environment.		2 syllables (non-speech).	*Precursory stage:* Vocalizes feelings of pleasure in response to social stimuli. Makes many vocal noises resembling speech sounds.
4	Motor response to outstretched arms: raises arms to be picked up. Responds to noise and voice by turning. Vocalizes social stimulus.		*Precursory:* repetitive sound chains (4-5 syllables): *ba-ba-ba,* etc. (comfort sign).	*Precursory stage:* Continued babbling. Cry changes with bodily state. Sound vocabulary changes with bodily position: [m], [n], [p], [b]. Vocalizes in self-initiated sound play.
5	In absence of visual contact responds to voice by head turning. Responds to angry tone by crying. Responds to pleasant speech by smiling and laughing.			*Precursory stage:* Continued babbling: (a) vocalizes emotional satisfaction; (b) tuning up speech organs, an integrative process. Imitates his own noises: *oohs, ahs, bas, das.*
6	Distinguishes between friendly and angry talk. Listens to his own voice.		Several syllables (prespeech).	*Precursory stage:* Lalling begins. Vocalizes [ma] or [mu]. Pleasurable repetition of sounds and syllables. Tries to repeat heard sound-sequences. Uses intonational pattern with jargon speech in "talking to person." Directs sounds and gestures to objects.

7	*Precursory stage:* Enjoys imitating sound sequences. Vocalizes emotional satisfaction or dissatisfaction.			Pays attention to speech of family. Pays attention to many sights and sounds in environment. Smiles at onlookers. Listens to his own private vocalizations.
8	Lallation continues; back vowels now more like speech sounds. Vocalizes syllables: *da, ba, ka.* Vocalizes interjections and recognition. Copies inaccurately intonational contours.			Listens to greetings and other familiar phrases. Eyes and ears alert to all stimuli in immediate environment.
9	*Precursory stage:* Echolalia (*da-da*), etc. Copies melody pattern of familiar phrases: greetings, interjections, etc. Enjoys making lip noises. Tries out variety of pitches. Facial and arm gestures accompany vocalizations.	3–4 syllables in chain response but varies syllables (*ba-ba-da-da,* etc.).		Rudimentary comprehension of symbolic gestures and intonation patterns. Action response to verbal request (opens mouth when asked). Comprehends *no-no, hot,* his name.
10	*Annunciatory stage:* Tries to name familiar object upon seeing it again, *viz.,* bottle (*babo*). Many speech and nonspeech sounds used in random vocalization. Imitates melody of phrase pattern but phonemes inaccurate.	Says word-like syllables *ma-ma-ma; da-da-da.*		Pays attention to face of speaker. Comprehends *bye-bye;* waves *bye.* Action response to verbal request: "Where's Baby's shoe?"; shakes head *yes, no* to some questions.
11	*Rudimentary language,* largely annunciatory; proclaims biological needs and psychological satisfactions. "Talks" to himself in mirror.	Median age of *first word.*		Differentiates family and strangers. Understands many action words.
12	*Communicative speech* begins. Copies melodic patterns more accurately but in jargon speech.	1-word sentences.	5–6 words: *mama, dada, babo* (bottle), *bye-bye, baw* (ball)	Understands phrase-wholes, simple grammatical patterns. Responds in action to commands. Enjoys rhymes and simple songs. Understands arrival and departure signals.

Table 6-2. (continued)

Age in Months	Comprehension of Verbal and Expressive Signals	Vocabulary (Mean No. of Words)	Mean Length of Response	Use of Oral Language
18-24	Understands most linguistic units but does not separate sequences into word units. Recognizes names of many familiar objects, persons, pets. Heeds to *here, now.*	50-75 words. Nouns: 50% of vocabulary. Many words made by phonetic reduplication: *da-da; pa-pa; ma-ma; gog-gie; tato* (telephone); *tick-tock; too-too* (toot-toot).	1.5 word-sentence.	Interjectional speech prevails. Begins extension of meaning (*mama* designates any smiling woman). Perceives and imitates stressed segments of speech, pivot words *with modifiers: more car; more milk; more bye-bye;* etc. Particles *off, on* used with nouns. Uses one word for many unrelated things. Repeats syllables or word-sequences in easy manner. Much vocal overflow with little or no phonetic value (laugh, sigh, whisper). Vocal inflection fair; pitch uncontrolled; tends to rise. Communicates by pulling person to show him object, person, situation.
24-30	Does not understand many specific words but develops "functional equivalents of comprehension." Action response to verbal request (*close door*); sometimes repeats request. Distinguishes prepositions *in* and *under.* Listens to simple stories, especially liking those he has heard before.	272 Of total response: nouns: 38.6% verbs: 21.0% adverbs: 7.1% pronouns: 14.6% unclassified: 18.7%	1.8 word-sentences	*Egocentric speech* prevails but some socialized speech (adapted information and emotional expression) also used. Extension of meaning develops. Asks simple questions about own concerns: "Where ball?" "Go bye-bye?" Expresses emotions massively; attended by clapping, dancing, etc. Names or describes object in environment; names one color. Uses "language of reference": accompanies speech with pointing. *Grammar:* Development of generative grammar begins. Some improvisations: *doed, goded* (went).

30–36

446

3.1 word-sentences.

Comprehension of sentence structure, syllable-sequences, and prosody develops rapidly.
Understands: *yes-no; come-go; run-stop; give-take; grasp-release; push-pull.*
Comprehends time words.
Understands three prepositions.
Enjoys rhythmical repetitions of others.
Identifies action in pictures.
Listens to longer and more varied stories.
Understands semantic difference in subject-object by position of noun (*Show us the car pushing the truck. Now show us the truck pushing the car.*)

Uses demonstrative pronoun, *this*, accompanied by gesture.
Adjectives and adverbs gaining steadily at expense of interjections.
Phonology: All vowels, labial and labio-alveolar consonants in sequences, but they are not stabilized.
Telescopes phrases.
Pitch control improved.
Copies speech rhythms.
Final and medial consonants slighted or omitted.

Continues *egocentric speech;* talks about himself to himself.
Gives full name.
Repetition of heard phrases more marked than at 24 months; first repetitions to himself.
Names 5 pictures on card.
Recites 1–2 nursery rhymes.
Relays telescoped message to another person.
Grammar: Begins to use question-making sentences.
Independent improvisations of syntactic forms: *Look me no* (don't look at me); *stove bite yes* (stove will burn me).
Uses demonstrative pronouns *this, that.*
Uses two or three prepositions.
Shifts between *me* and *I* in referring to himself.
Phonology: Much telescoping of words in primitive sentences with medial consonant still slighted.
Pronunciation is unstable.
Wide variability of pitch but has established firm base.

Materials for Exploring Use of Oral Language in Play Sessions:
11–36 Months

The language of the very young is not amenable to formal measures
of testing yet it is in this early period of development that the "slow to
talk" are most frequently referred for evaluation. The play-study situations described in this section are conducted only under conditions of
stimulated and imitative play of the child with the mother and the
teacher. No single session will suffice for the assessment of a baby's oral
expression. Indeed as many as six to eight play sessions probably will be
necessary for a satisfactory appraisal. All sessions are taped for subsequent
study. In play situations, the attempt is made to establish the baby's
language development in three principal areas: (1) vocabulary; (2) linguistic structure; and (3) articulation. The equipment for the series
of tests is simple: toys, objects, and such picture books as the following:
Baby's First Book,[4] *My World,*[5] *Play Time,*[6] *Animal Friends for Baby,*[7]
Where's the Bunny?[8] and *The Country Noisy Book.*[9]

Appraisal of Vocabulary and Linguistic Structure

Use of Single-word Phrases, Accompanied by Gesture: 11–18 Months.
The baby uses the single-word phrase purposively, usually in order to
elicit verbal or actional responses from others. Employing proper motivation, the teacher should be able to elicit the following word-phrases in
four or five play sessions.

1. baby	9. kitty
2. truck	10. doggie (bow-wow)
3. dolly	11. duck (quack-quack)
4. bye-bye	12. apple (apu)
5. car	13. clock (titta or dedda)
6. bottle (babo)	14. food (mmmm-)
7. Daddy (da-da)	15. thank you (ta-da)
8. Mommy	16. ball (baw)

Use of Two-word Sentences: 15–24 Months. The task is to elicit
equivalents for each of these expressions of *semantic content:*

1. Push car	4. Baby fall
2. Ronnie bye (Baby bye)	5. Hurt baby
3. Water duck	

[4] ———, New York: Platt, 1950.
[5] M. W. Brown, New York: Harper, 1942.
[6] ———, Chicago: Hampton Publishing Co., 1961.
[7] ———, Chicago: Hampton Publishing Co., 1954.
[8] R. Carroll, New York: Henry Z. Walck, 1950.
[9] M. W. Brown, New York: Harper, 1940.

Generation of Noun-phrases Using Mass Nouns: 19–24 Months. Equivalents for each of the following expressions should be found:

1. Two tinker-toy	6. A Nancy
2. More milk	7. A Daddy-car
3. That Bobbie	8. Two sock
4. Two water	9. More light
5. A coat	10. No night-night

Development of Syntax, First Level: 18–30 Months. The objective in this play situation is to observe imitative or echoic speech in which the number of morphemes will be reduced. The teacher may note equivalents for each of these expressions:

1. Model: There goes one (truck)
   Baby: There go one
2. Model: He's going bye-bye
   Baby: He go bye-bye
3. Model: It's not the same dog as Heidi
   Baby: Doggie Heidi no
4. Model: Throw it to Mommy
   Baby: Throw Mommy
5. Model: He sat on a wall
   Baby: Sat wall

Development of Syntax, Second Level: 30–36 Months. In this play situation we are watching for another phase of syntactic development: the imitation of speech but with expansion, not reduction, of morphemes. The teacher may note equivalents for each of these expressions:

1. Model: Dolly says Hi
   Baby: Dolly say Hi-there Baby
2. Model: Kitty's lost
   Baby: Kitty lost now no more
3. Model: Here comes Daddy
   Baby: Here come Daddy car beep-beep!
4. Model: Eat your cereal please
   Baby: Eat-ed cereal all up, p(l)ease
5. Model: Clock goes tick-tock
   Baby: Clock go titta-titta-titta

Development of Syntax, Third Level: 33–36 Months. At this level of syntactical development, the child begins his independent development of sentence structure through a process of induction of the latent structure. Hopefully the teacher will find equivalents for each of these expressions:

1. Model: Throw the ball to Mommy.
   Baby: Me no throw ball Mommy; throw (to) Bobby.

2. Model: What do you have in your mouth?
   Baby: Look me no; no candy.
3. Model: Did you bring your dolly today?
   Baby: Dolly sick; me no bringded it.
4. Model: Look, it's raining now.
   Baby: Raining; Mommy can't go out; (but) me go out play.
5. Model: Come along; let's go in Mommy's car.
   Baby: O.K. I (me) go home now; bye-bye.

Appraisal of Articulation: 11–36 Months

As Templin and others have pointed out, the pattern of articulation in this age range is so inconsistent as to preclude the establishment of definite norms.[10] Although the check list employed here is called a test, its author agrees that it is a gross measure. It is nonetheless a valuable tool in appraising the articulatory development of the child within a broad age range.

The Houston Articulatory Test [11] for children, *1 to 3 years of age,*

measures consonants that are produced according to certain specificity of muscular development. . . . Labials are articulated by the average child at 24 months, dentals at 30 months and velars at 36 months. Any method of eliciting a response can be used (pictures with auditory stimulation, pictures alone, auditory stimulation alone). The method that seems to fit the individual case may be used. The examiner should say, 'Let me hear you say . . .' (using the words in the test list) as this is the fastest way to test. If the child fails to respond, the word is elicited by use of a picture dictionary.[12]

The test words will be found on the record sheet for this test, Figure 6-1.

[10] M. Templin, *Certain language skills in children.* Minneapolis: University of Minnesota Press, 1957. Pp. 11–13, 23–25.
[11] M. Crabtree, *The Houston test for language development.* Houston: The Houston Test Co., 1958.
[12] *Ibid.,* p. 8.

Figure 6-1. Record sheet for Houston articulatory test.

SOURCE: M. Crabtree, *The Houston test for language development.* Houston: The Houston Test Co., 1958. P. 8,

Name:			
Articulation Group I (Labials)	Initial	Medial	Final
Baby, Bob			
Puppy, Top			
Mamma, Come			
Watch			
House			
Group II (Dentals)			
Top, kitty, hat			
Daddy, good			
Nose, pony, down			
Group III (Velars)			
Cat, monkey, book			
Gun, bigger, dog			
Bang			
Group IV			
For, elephant, knife			
Very, oven, five			
Sun, horses, bus			
Zebra, fuzzy, buzz			
Group V			
Shoe, washing, fish			
Treasure (zh sound)			
That, Mother, bathe			
Thank, birthday, bath			
Look, balloon, Bill			
Rabbit, carrot, car			

Symbols: (x) if missed, (–) if omitted. Record substitution.

Inventory 1.   Comprehension of Nonverbal and Verbal Stimuli,
1–36 Months

Name _____ Recorder _____

Age (C A) _____ Date of this record _____

Original enrollment date _____

First six months:
1. Does he return a smile from the mother? _____
2. Does he cry on hearing intense noises? _____
3. Does he turn toward you when you call his name? _____
4. (Intraverbal gesture) Does he smile and make comfort sounds on hearing mother's voice? _____
5. Does he like toys that make a noise: (squeaky rubber animal, music box, xylophone, bell)? If he cannot hold the toy by himself, does he show you that he wants you to produce the sound for him? _____
6. Does he like to have you sing to him? _____
7. Does he change the volume of his voice as his needs are met? _____
8. Does he coo _____; laugh out loud _____; squeal _____?
9. Does he show pleasure with pleasant, friendly speech; discomfort on hearing unfriendly speech? _____
10. Does he hold out arms to be taken? _____

Six months to one year:
1. Does he play pat-a-cake? _____
2. Does he point to indicate desires? _____
3. Does it frighten him when a dog barks? _____
4. Does he recognize his parent's step even before parent enters the room?
   _____
5. Does he discriminate faces in environment? _____
6. Does he recognize the voices of some of his favorite people outside the immediate environment (grandmother, aunt)? _____
7. Does he cry when the volume of television or radio is excessive? _____
8. (Echoic gesture) Does he wave bye-bye in response to mother's gesture, bye-bye? _____
9. Does he understand inhibitions (No)? _____
10. Does he turn toward you when you call his name? _____

One year to two years:
1. In answer to: Where's baby? (in mirror) does he point to reflection of self.
   _____
2. On seeing picture of smiling woman, does he say mama? _____

3. Is he easily frightened when people speak in a loud voice or when he hears a door slam? _____

4. Does he want you to read to him? _____

5. Does he imitate a familiar phrase or request (bye-bye, etc.)? _____

6. In response to Smell the pretty flower, does he bend over, smell flower? _____

7. Looks at blossom, says fa-fa ? _____

8. Does he name a familiar person or object upon seeing it again, almost in manner of greeting or recognition (babo for bottle)? _____

9. Does he look to mother when something goes wrong (bursting of balloon)? _____

10. Does he want you to tell stories to him? _____

11. Does he lift his foot when shoe is offered? _____

12. Does he like horns and drums to play with? _____

13. What does he do when you open a familiar box (crackers) in such a way that he has not seen what you are doing? _____

14. Does he respond to question, "What do you want?" _____

15. Does he try to pick up objects dropped on the floor? _____

16. Does he point (eye or hand) to indicate his wants or call attention to events? _____

17. Does he change volume of voice as needs are about to be met? _____

Two years to three years:

1. What is his favorite song? _____

2. Does he open mouth in action response to verbal request _____; stick out tongue _____ ; close eyes _____

3. Does he like to listen to story records on his record player? _____

4. Does he watch cartoons on television? _____

5. How long can he sit and listen to stories, songs, etc.? _____

6. What does he do when he hears: telephone bell _____ ; vacuum cleaner _____ ; airplane _____

7. Does he understand some spelled words (candy, bye-bye, etc.)? _____

8. Does he understand semantic difference in subject-object by position of noun? (Show us the car pushing the truck. Now show us the truck pushing the car.) _____

9. Does he parrot verbal request after he has complied (shut door)? _____

10. Is there action response to verbal request, Bring me baby's shoe, with his oral reinforcement Baby shoe? _____

11. Does he respond to simple questions about immediate concerns, Where is ball? Where did Daddy go? _____

12. Does he recognize sounds of: coughing _____; humming _____ ; hand clapping _____ ?

Inventory 2. Use of Oral Language, 11-36 Months*

Name _____ Recorder _____

Age (C A) _____ Date of this record _____

Original enrollment date _____

1. Talks to his toys using tonal modulation _____

2. Uses lalling sounds much of time _____

3. Imitates vocal sounds of others in his immediate environment _____

4. When he plays with cars or dolls, mimics representative noises _____

5. Uses reflexive jargon imitating melody, rhythm, etc. of mother _____

6. When he plays by himself hums _____; does it sound like a tune? _____

7. Duplicates syllables: da-da-da, etc. _____

8. Combines syllables _____; has single word phrases _____

9. Generates noun-phrases (more milk; two water, etc.) _____

10. Generates noun-phrases to express emotion (Mommy home; go bye-bye)_____

11. Use of noun-verb (in present tense); holophrases (two words as single utterance: baby fall; push car) _____

12. Names (with simultaneous pointing) objects and pictures _____

13. Imitates speech of others with reduction (reduces imitation to 2–4 morphemes with semantic content as in He bye-bye; There go one) _____

14. Imitates speech of others with expansion _____

15. Begins to induce latent structure, freewheeling forms _____

16. Pluralizes nouns _____

17. Substitutes pronouns for noun-phrases (uses it) _____

18. Includes low information words _____
    a. Possessive inflections ('s) _____
    b. Progressive inflections (ing) _____
    c. Modal auxiliary verbs (will, can) _____
    d. Contraction of auxiliary verbs (is, are)_____
    e. Inflection of third person in verb (goes) _____
    f. Inflection of little words (articles, prepositions, conjunctions) _____

19. Unstressed syllables still weak or omitted (raff for giraffe) _____

20. Has vocabulary of 10-20 words _____

21. Has vocabulary of 20-100 words _____

22. Repeats four-line nursery rhymes (may not know meaning) _____

23. Sings simple nursery songs (Rock-a-bye-baby) _____

24. Answers in automatic speech these questions:
    a. What is your name? _____
    b. Are you a little girl (boy) ? _____

*Check list of progressive development from item 1 at 11 months to item 24 at 36 months.

Longitudinal Study II-B

Table 6-3. Nonverbal adaptive behavior, 3–8 years.

Age	General Motor and Manual Coordination	Locomotion	Balance	Special Sensory-Motor Behavior
3.0	Rides tricycle using pedals. Can put on shoes himself. Can unzip clothing. Handles kitchen utensils, such as small pitcher in pouring milk.	Alternates forward foot going up stairs. Jumps from bottom steps (30 cm.) Walks in line. Runs but stumbles occasionally.	Walking board; alternates part way. Can maintain balance in tiptoeing, 3 meters. Rises from prone to standing position without turning.	Draws; names own drawing. Copies circle. Completes simple puzzles. Plays with toys; then shifts. Enjoys children's records. Watches cartoons on television.
3.6	Marked shift to bilaterality. Washes hands on request. Builds bridge from model.	Walks up 3 steps with alternating steps. Runs smoothly with acceleration and deceleration.	Skillful in balancing on toes. Stands on 1 foot, 2 secs. Jumps over rope, 20 cm. high. Distance jump: 30–60 cm. Can erect self from squatting position.	Removes wraps without assistance. Plays happily alone, but will play with peers. Frequently shows dependence; ("Watch what I do.")
4.0	Catches ball in arms. Touches point of nose with eyes closed. Puts 20 coins in box. Clasps hand: right, left, both. Still lacks poise in reaching.	Descends stairway with alternating steps (some help). Rides bike with guard wheels.	Hops on right foot less than 2 meters. Distance jump: 61–80 cm. Hops in same place, feet together, 7 times.	Uses crayons; enjoys color books. Follows cartoon stories on television. Completes 8-piece form-board puzzle. Draws square after model.
4.6	Unilateral right hand dominance in most activities. Grasps with thumb and medial finger. Describes circles with index fingers, arms extended at sides. Washes face and hands when told to do so. Dresses self except for tying shoes.	Does simple dances, rhythms, jigs. Skips but not with alternating step.	Hops on left foot less than 2 meters.	Makes little response to minor injuries. Has imaginary companions who assume blame for mishaps.

219

Table 6-3. (continued)

Age	General Motor and Manual Coordination	Locomotion	Balance	Special Sensory-Motor Behavior
5.0	Draws circles. Makes ball with thin silk paper. Prints simple words with pencil. Dresses without assistance.	Uses roller skates, sled. Rides junior bike. Descends stairway with alternating step.	Hops on 1 foot, 5 meters.	Plays simple card games. Reads first books by pictures. Dials telephone numbers correctly. Learns songs from television.
5.6	Reaching and grasping becomes one continuous movement. Unilateral right hand dominance in most activities. Rolls 2 meters of thread on spool. Catches ball with hands. Draws lines in small area; holds paper with other hand.	Boys wrestle; friendly fist fights. Girls skip and dance. Follow simple rhythmic tunes with action.	Balances, standing on one leg. Skips rope in rhythmic sequence.	Enjoys group play (small group). Behavior is noisy. Watches and listens to children's stories on television. New expressions: clenches and bares teeth. Begins to appreciate humorous stories.
6.0-7.0	Knows right and left. Throws ball at target (1.5 meters distant). Can tie bow knot. Uses table knife for spreading. Combs or brushes hair. Prints with pencil.	Movement is facile, easy, economical.	Jumps over rope 20 cms. high.	Makes simple drawings, angles fairly correct. Reads aloud simple stories.
7.0-8.0	Taps floor alternately with feet. Kicks box distance of 5 meters. Touches thumb to all fingers of same hand. Uses simple tools. Uses table knife for cutting.	Runs swiftly, surely; weight on ball of foot.	Crouches on tiptoe.	Knits eyebrows. Wrinkles forehead. Copies diamond.

Inventory 3. General Motor Development, 4–8 Years

Name _____

Age (C A) _____

Original enrollment date _____

Recorder _____

Key

A   Yes, or very good
B   Better than average
C   Average
D   Below average
E   No, or poor
√   Inconsistent
O   No opportunity to
     observe

Date of Record

Has a characteristic gait						
Arms move in cross pattern in walking						
Clumsy in hopping, skipping, running (A or E)						
Keeps step with others in marching						
Changes rhythm of march with shift in musical rhythm						
Facial muscles reflect subtle shifts in feeling (nonverbal communication)						
Dominant hand in unimanual activities (LRM)						
Follows directions: in-out; up-down; right-left						
Executes sequential movement accompanying song, Looby-Lou						
Conceives properly the sequential pattern of movements which is required						
Knows left to right (pictures)						
Knows left to right (writing)						

Inventory 3 (continued)

Exhibits useless, extraneous movements (A or E)						
Works jaw and tongue when using hands (A or E)						
Exhibits uncontrollable responses (rocking) (A or E)						
Draws differentiated form and names (A or E)						
Draws undifferentiated form and names (A or E)						
Draws with brush pen: 1. straight lines 2. curved lines 3. diagonal lines 4. stick figure of man						
Cuts with scissors 1 inch or more						
Outlines with scissors						
Holds scissors so they will cut						
Follows detail with scissors (eye-hand coordination)						
In coloring scribbles within design						
In coloring follows details						
Writes within framework						
Makes reversals in writing (A or E)						
Posture in writing properly oriented						
Holds pencil and paper in proper position						
Catches ball (thrown from 3 yards) with one hand						
Makes circles with forefingers (arms extended 10 seconds)						

For the format and some items in these scales we are indebted to T. C. Bangs, Evaluating children with language delay. *J Speech Hearing Dis* (February 1961), 26: 16–18.

Inventory 4. Socioemotional Behavior, 4–8 Years

Name _____

Age (C A) _____

Original enrollment date _____

Recorder _____

Key

A Yes, or very good
B Better than average
C Average
D Below average
E No, or poor
√ Inconsistent
O No opportunity to observe

Date of Record

Plays mostly by self (A or E)						
Peer play, parallel						
Peer play, cooperative						
Teacher-child relationship						
Adult-child relationship: Withdrawn (hides in closet or under table)						
Eye contact most of time (A or E)						
Personal hygiene						
Contributing member of group						
Socially acceptable behavior at school						
Avoids catastrophic reactions						
Demonstrates compulsive behavior (A or E)						
Shows feeling, pity (A or E)						
Shares toys or turns						
Plays group games						
Generally hyperactive in play (A or E)						
Dependable						
Parent cooperation, mother						
Parent cooperation, father						

Comments: (Number item on which you wish to comment. Record comment, with date, in space below chart.)

Inventory 5.   Attitudes in Learning, 4–8 Years

Name _____

Age (C A) _____

Original enrollment date _____

Recorder _____

Key

A   Yes, or very good
B   Better than average
C   Average
D   Below average
E   No, or poor
√   Inconsistent
O   No opportunity to
    observe

Date of Record

Approaches test or learning situation with motivation							
Attention span							
Distractible (A or E)							
Pervasive hostility toward learning situation (A or E)							
Awareness of error							
Corrects own errors							
Works purposively							
Hyperactive (A or E)							
Ability to shift							
Completes assignment on time							
Completes assignments, but not on time (A or E)							
Has power of self-criticism							
Withness							
Meticulosity							
Neatness of work							

Comments: (Number items on which you wish to comment. Record comment, with
date, in space below chart.)

Table 6-4. Development of some aspects of oral language, 3-8 years.

Age: Years, Months	Phonological Development	Syntactic Development	Semantic Development
3.0	*Fairly intelligible speech.* Substitution, omission and distortion of many phonemes inconsistent, varying with position in word and context. Final consonants appear more regularly than at 30 months. *Speech melody* develops rapidly although easy repetitions are present. Voice usually well controlled.	Generative grammar develops (development by his own rules). Experiments with *many syntactic forms.* *Two-word phrases* most frequent form: *That boy (is) naughty; Mommy car stop* (Mommy's car stopped; wouldn't run). *Designative constructions* coming into use: Phrases expanded into subject-predicte sentence.(*What that thing go round?*) *Mean length of response:* 3.4 words.	Egocentric speech prevails. Dramatizes, combining words and actions for his own pleasure. Asks questions about persons, things, processes. Names two colors. Tells sex; full name. Verbalizes toilet needs. *Vocabulary.* Mean number of words: 896.
3.6	*Phonemic gains.* All English vowels and following consonants are used: /m-/, /-m-/, /-m/; /n-/, /-n-/, /-n/; /-ŋ-/, /-ŋ/; /t-/; /k-/; /p-/, /-p-/; /b-/, /-b-/; /f-/, /-f-/; /h-/; /w-/, /-w-/. Articulation still characterized by omission of many medial consonantal phonemes and syllables; does not remember unstressed bits. *Speech melody.* Blocking on initial syllables frequently interrupts rhythm. Rate of speech increased. Many responses in loud voice or yell.	*Grammatical categories.* Speech is made up of: nouns 17% conjunctions 2.2% verbs 22.8% prepositions 6.7% adjectives 6.5% interjections 1.7% adverbs 10.1% articles 6.9% pronouns 19.8% unclassified 6.3% Uses new adjectives: *strong, new, different.* Uses new adverbs: *maybe, too.* Uses auxiliaries: *might, could.* Gains skill in *permutations:* Makes questions from declarative statements. *Mean length of response:* 4.3 words.	*Closed-cycle linguistic development.* Egocentric speech, perception, and inner language reciprocally augmented. *Communicative speech* developing. Directive speech: Commands, requests, threats. Question asking, "why" stage. Relates experiences with fair understanding of sequence and closure. Says nursery rhymes. Names primary colors. Repetitive use of one in counting: *one light and one light,* etc. *Vocabulary.* Mean number of words: 1222. Misuses many words; imperfect understanding.

Table 6-4. (continued)

Age: Years, Months	Phonological Development	Syntactic Development	Semantic Development
4.0	*Phonemic Development.* 98% of speech intelligible. Articulatory omissions and substitutions sharply reduced. *Speech melody (prosody).* Vocal pitch controlled. Uses some adult patterns of rhythm. Repetition reduced, thus improving rhythm. Some blocking and associated overt mannerisms may continue.	Skill increasing in *transformations* (modification in sentence which transforms kernel). *Sentence structure* advances rapidly: Beginning to use complex and compound sentences, 6–8 words in length. Mean sentence length: 4.2 words. *Grammatical categories.* Speech is made up of: nouns 16.3% verbs 23.1% adjectives 6.7% adverbs 10.4% pronouns 20.3% conjunctions 2.8% prepositions 7.5% interjections 1.3% articles 7.5% unclassified 4.1%	*Verbal syncretism* still dominates understanding, but he is beginning to show interest in isolated word meanings. In general still deals with whole sentences without analysis of words. Uses many *how* and *why* questions in response to speech of others. *Perception still is realistic, first person.* Ideation, however, becoming less concrete: alludes to objects, persons, events not in immediate environment. Engages in collective monologues with other children but there is little cooperative thinking. Tells tales; talks much; threatens playmates. Counts 3 objects. *Vocabulary.* Mean number of words: 1540. Uses slang.
4.6	*Phonemic gains.* Appearance or stabilization of phonemes: /s-/, /-s-/; /ʃ-/, /-ʃ-/, /-ʃ/; /tr-/; /kr-/; /-tʃ-/, /-tʃ/. Phonemes /l/, /r/, /s/, /θ/ not stabilized in any position. Reverses order of sounds within word occasionally: reflects lack of memory for bits. *Speech melody.* Frequently disturbs basic melody by beginning sentence with (ʌm) or (ʌ). Voice well modulated and usually takes on intonational and rhythmic patterns of mother.	Use of complex and compound sentences increasing. Reverses syllabic and word order occasionally in sentence. Elaborates sentence by use of conjunction; makes spontaneous corrections in grammar. Mean length of response: 4.7 words.	*Egocentric speech declining;* uses more adaptive language (social communication). *Verbal syncretism* still dominates understanding. Employs extension of meaning in interpreting speech of others. *Discrimination.* Perceives differences in concrete events. *Recall.* Links past and present events. *Vocabulary.* Mean number of words: 1870. Vocabulary now reflects his linguistic culture; uses many colloquial expressions. Defines simple words. Tries to use new words, not always correctly.

5.0

Phonemic gains. Articulation generally intelligible but phonemes /f/, /v/, /l/, and /s/ are not stabilized in all positions or in all contexts.

Grammar. Reasonably accurate; Makes many spontaneous corrections. Sentence structure expanding rapidly in accuracy and complexity. *Embedding* more common. Develops relative clause. Mean length of response: 4.8 words.

Engages in *responsive discourse.* Gives and receives information; change from egocentric speech to rational reciprocity. *Develops percepts* of number, speed, time, space. *Shows inner logic* in recounting plots of children's plays (television and theatre). *Names and describes objects* in composite pictures. Names penny, nickel, dime. Employs some *imaginative thinking,* but is mainly realistic. *Abstraction* still is meager. *Categorizes* concrete events on basis of likeness and difference. *Vocabulary.* Mean number of words: 2072. Percentage increase in *vocabulary of use* slight; *comprehension of vocabulary* increasing markedly. Defines simple words.

5.6

Intelligibility of speech: 89%–100%.

Permutations. Great gains in sentence making of all types. Uses all basic structures. Mean length of response: 4.9 words. *Grammar.* Makes some errors but corrects them spontaneously.

Language is becoming symbolic. Significant gains in relating present and past events. *Conversation is socialized* in sense that listener is associated with speaker; little true collaboration of thought. Child still speaks chiefly of himself, his actions, and thoughts. *Primitive argument* develops: clash of unmotivated assertions. Advances in *categorization and synthesis* of percepts. *Vocabulary.* Mean number of words: 2289.

Table 6-4. (continued)

Age: Years, Months	Phonological Development	Syntactic Development	Semantic Development
6.0–7.0	*Phonemic proficiency* established in /l-/, /-l/, (-l-); /-t-/; (-θ-/, /-τ/, /-r-/, /ʃ-/. *Sentence melody* imitative of adults in environment. Child experiments with rhythmic patterns. Facial expression accompanying speech changes with rhythm; more varied patterns of expression.	*Grammatical categories.* Speech is made up of: nouns 17.1% verbs 25% adjectives 7.6% adverbs 10% pronouns 19.2% conjunctions 2.6% prepositions 7.6% interjections 1% articles 8.3% unclassified 1.6% Sentence length and complexity develops sharply; has command of every form of sentence structure. Mean sentence length: 6.5 words.	*Comprehension of morphemic sequences* develops sharply. Anticipates closure in speech of others. Perception and inner language make great gains; asks for explanations, motives of action, etc. Understands roughly differences between time intervals. Understands seasons of year. Generally distinguishes left from right in himself. Attempts to verbalize causal relationship. Counts three objects without error. *Vocabulary.* Comprehends meaning of 4000 words; uses (mean number of words): 2562 (7 years).
7.0–8.0	*Phonemic proficiency* established in /-z-/; /ð-/, /-ʒ-/; /-st/; /-lz/; /-lθ/; /-tr/; /-kt/. *Speech melody.* Subtle rhythms and intonational contours present. Facial and hand gestures underscore speech rhythms.	*Grammar.* Chief errors now are common to his cultural environment. Mean length of response: 7.2 words.	*Egocentric speech* has gone underground, and inner language shows marked development. *True communication* develops. Ideas shared; speech reflects understanding of causal or logical relations. *Vocabulary.* Comprehension of words races far ahead of vocabulary of use. Understands 6000–8000 words. Vocabulary of use: 2562 to 2818 words (7-8 years).

Materials. Exploring Comprehension of Oral Language: 3–8 Years

During the diagnostic teaching period the language teacher will have the opportunity to observe carefully the child's responses to visual, tactile-kinesthetic, auditory—to all kinds of sensory-motor stimuli. Visuomotor responses may be as important as auditory responses in the evaluative data with which he must deal. Perception of language is multimodal; it does not depend on a single avenue of input.

Several structured situations are presented as starters for the study. Inventory 1, which follows these examples, will suggest other ideas for exploratory techniques.

Auditory Perception. The language teacher is familiar with tests of *auditory acuity* but he is not concerned at this point with the child's *peripheral hearing.* Others presumably have ascertained that the conductive mechanism of the ear is intact and that sound waves reach the cochlea. His interest now is in knowing what happens to sound in the cochlea and the CNS. He will observe carefully the child's discrimination of the ordinary sounds in his environment. Does the child interpret correctly the sounds of the toy animals or other noisemakers when they are not visible? Upon hearing the sound can he select the picture of the toy animal or noisemaker from among several in a picture book? When the examiner speaks to him does he comprehend more easily if one speaks slowly? If one presents a three-beat rhythm (e.g., da-dit-dit), is he able to imitate the tapped pattern? Does he understand one better if there is a pleasant controlled background of sound? Does he respond at all if noise is uncontrolled? Can he identify the speech of other children when he does not see them? Can he interpret familiar sounds in a strange setting? A child with normal acuity did not heed his teacher's warning at a circus although she stood directly beside him. Apparently there were too many strange sounds battering his auditory coding mechanism; he could not select the proper ones to which to respond. The questions suggest the type of appraisal of perception that can be made in one area.

Visuo-motokinesthetic Perception: Pretended Action Technique, 4–5 Years. The average young child responds quickly to facial expression, but here is a child whose bodily response, like his speech, is faceless. The language teacher tries pretended actions with him. After a few trial demonstrations, the teacher says, "Now I am going to pretend to do something. Can you guess what I am doing?" The examiner pretends to (1) drink through a straw; (2) spread butter on bread; (3) bite into and chew food (bread, piece of candy, apple). If the child does not interpret the action correctly, repeat the pantomime and then explain the action. Then say, "Now I want you to pretend. First pretend you are drinking from a glass. Now pretend you are combing your hair. Pretend you are eating ice cream with a spoon. We brush our teeth after eating, so pretend you are brushing your teeth. Finally you must wash your hands. Pretend you are washing your hands."

Perceptual Capacity: Identification, Discrimination, Memory. Furnishing the Dollhouse, 3–5 Years. In this exploratory technique one is not asking the child to respond orally but to comprehend oral sequences which increase steadily in complexity. After a warm-up period, the teacher places the empty dollhouse before the child with the furniture in proper orientation but in random order to the child's right. He says, "Let's look at this dollhouse. Here, you see, is the large room; we call it the living room, don't we? Next to it is the dining room, and here is the kitchen where Mommy cooks. The counters already are in place. Upstairs you see the bedroom and the bathroom. The tub and toilet have been put in by the plumber. Now let's furnish the doll house. Let me tell you where to put the furniture the first time, and then when we have finished, you may change it around if you like. 'Turn up the dial' on all your 'listeners' so you will know where to put each piece. Are you ready?

1. Put the bed in the bedroom.
2. Put the sofa (couch) in the living room.
3. Put the biggest chair of all in the living room.
4. Put the stove in the kitchen.
5. Put the towels and the soap-dish in the bathroom.
6. Find a chest of drawers (dresser) and put it inside the bedroom but near the door.
7. Put the big table and three little chairs in the dining room.
8. Place two little tables on each side of the sofa in the living room.
9. Here is the kitchen sink. Take it and the refrigerator. Put them close together in the kitchen.
10. Put the large rug in the living room and the small rug in the bedroom.
11. The two big red lamps should go on the tables in the living room and the little green lamp on the chest in the bedroom.
12. Count four plates, four cups, and four glasses. Put them on the table in the dining room.

Now if you would like to change some pieces, move them to other rooms; go ahead." The average child, 3–4 years of age, will follow the first six commands to successful completion. Commands 7–12 normally will be executed successfully by the average child, 4–5 years of age.

Comprehension of Syntactic Structure. Scrambled Sequences: I, 6–8 Years. Here we are exploring a more advanced comprehension of word order or sentence structure. Just as in the perception of nonverbal symbols, in which the significance of figures is confused by background, so in this "game" the meaning of the sentences is disturbed by the word order, irregular syntax, and faulty use of function-words (*on, in, under*).

Presented in the form of a game, many children enjoy working out the puzzle, particularly if other children are involved. The language teacher has two lists of sentences: the first is made up of sentences confused in structure; in the second list the structure and word order have been corrected. First he will ask the child to repeat the scrambled sentence (after he has said it himself) and then the sentence in correct form. What we wish to know is which type of sentence the child repeats more readily. Does he have as much difficulty repeating the sentence with correct order as with the misplaced elements? If he does, it is possible that his perception of syntactic structure is so atypical as to deter him in comprehending language. Here is a list of scrambled sentences from the speech of a 6-year-old boy with serious language retardation:

1. Look me no.
2. Lost mittens me.
3. Me go buy candy more.
4. He school no go Saturday.
5. Me untry do it.
6. No stand table please.
7. Boat how much want.
8. Drink milk bottle yes, cup no.

Discrimination and Immediate Recall of Sound Sequences. Scrambled Sequences: II, 6–8 Years. In this speech game the child is asked to listen to phonologically distorted or scrambled sequences, uttered, however, with appropriate stress and rhythm. If the child does as well in repeating these scrambled sequences as he does after hearing the phonologically accurate units, we may assume that his ability to discriminate and remember sound sequences probably is impaired. The directions to the child are: "I am going to say a little rhyme and I want you to repeat what I say line by line. You may not understand what I say. All you have to do is to repeat just what you hear. I will wait after each line for you to repeat what I have said." Before the second recital the child is told: "Now I am going to say it again but in a different way. After each line I will wait for you to repeat what I have said." The teacher repeats the verse using conventional pronunciation, stress, and rhythm.

1. Remi tat a ritle bam (Mary has a little lamb)
   Sa sleef saw taigh a woe (Whose fleece was white as snow)
   Du yerviyou ta remi ten (And everywhere that Mary went)
   Ta bam so oosh ta go. (The lamb was sure to go.)
2. Said the molice pan to the piddle-um
   (Said the police man to the little bum)
   Gimme um. Ont!
   (Give me gum); (I won't)
   Gol I sot, said the piddle-um.
   (All I've got, said the little bum)

Inventory 6.   Comprehension of Nonverbal Stimuli, 3–8 Years

Name_____

Age (C A)_____

Original enrollment date _____

Recorder _____

Key

A   Yes, or very good
B   Better than average
C   Average
D   Below average
E   No, or poor
√   Inconsistent
O   No opportunity to
      observe

Date of Record

Matches color						
Matches objects by use						
Matches pictures in cartoon sequence						
Matches objects to pictures						
Matches form						
Does easy puzzles						
Recognizes change in size						
Finds things that go together (form, use, color)						
Furnishes doll house						
Selects clothes belonging to father, mother						
Knows right and left						
Points accurately to object						

Retrieves toy without bumping (A or E)							
Does not turn around to see chair he wants to sit on							
Steps easily over board (A or E)							
Usually catches the ball (A or E)							
Moves hand to wrong position to catch ball.							
Handles spoon (fork) skillfully (A or E)							
Tries to tie shoe (A or E)							
Unzips coat when in house (A or E)							
Walks down stairs without clinging to bannister (A or E)							
Often underreaches or overreaches							
Steps too high or not high enough							
Drops crayon frequently while drawing or coloring							
Finger frequently loses contact with dial notch in telephoning							
Is spatially oriented with reference to room or familiar street							
Counts objects in space accurately (A or E)							
Perceives position of his body in space (A or E)							

Inventory 6 (continued)

Copies bead design (A or E)							
Can draw square surveying the results as he draws *							
Copies rhythm by tapping (A or E)							
Hops rhythmically (A or E)							
Skips rhythmically (A or E)							
Maintains rhythm in marching							
Is sensitive to sticky foods on tongue (A or E)							
Is sensitive to food about lips (A or E)							
Tongue responds by resistance to pusher (A or E)							
Exhibits extraneous bodily movements when attending (A or E)							
Exhibits tremor in facial and articulatory muscles in response to stimuli (A or E)							
Attends selectively to stimuli							
Attends only to fringe areas of auditory, visual, haptic perception							
Sees "what others see" in picture							
Identifies geometric forms (square, circle, triangle) by haptic means							

* When laterality is disturbed, child often cannot draw the square if he looks at the strokes he is making. Visual perception thus is connected with laterality.

Inventory 7. Comprehension of Verbal Information, 3–8 Years

Name _____

Age (C A) _____

Original enrollment date _____

Recorder _____

	Date of Record					
Responds only to gestures (A or E)						
Makes appropriate gestural response in speech reading to: That's all I have; No more, etc. (A or E)						
Responds better to speech with gestures than to speech alone (A or E)						
Responds to words and phrases (A or E)						
Responds to speech continuum (A or E)						
Responds to speech when he is not looking at speaker (A or E)						
Responds to speech in background of noise (A or E)						
Comprehends morphemic sequences only at slow rate (A or E)						
Comprehends morphemic sequences at normal rate (A or E)						
Responds better to speech with gestures than to speech alone (A or E)						
Mimics facial and articulatory movements of speaker when attending (A or E)						
Taps rhythm of jingle or nursery rhyme						
Anticipates meaning of phrase or sentence						
Attends quickly, purposively to verbal stimuli (A or E)						
Attends only to fringe areas of speech, not to central cues (A or E)						
Exhibits tension or anxiety when attending to speech (A or E)						
Comprehends single linguistic structure (word order); syntax						
Comprehends vocabulary appropriate to age						
Reflects insight into problems (inner logic) (What must you do when: hungry, sleepy, cold, etc.)						
Tells what happens (comprehension of current events)						
Announces future action (comprehension of future events)						

Materials: Exploring Use of Oral Language, 3–8 Years

The roads to evaluation are limitless, as we have suggested in the introduction to this chapter. An ingenious and knowledgeable staff will devise many ways to study the child's use of speech in and out of the classroom. In the first weeks of evaluative teaching we have used both free and controlled activities that orient young children and stimulate them to engage in social talk. We suggest only a few that may assist the inexperienced staff member. In these activity sessions we concentrate on appraising the child's syntactic development since this dimension of language seems to be fundamental to the development of other aspects of language. Games and exercises which follow these activities are designed primarily to evaluate phonological and semantic aspects. The final picture story encompasses all three dimensions: phonological, syntactic, and semantic. (See Table 6-4.)

Free and Controlled Activities: Syntactic Development, 3–5 Years. The walls of the classroom are not the boundaries of teaching. Visiting the park, zoo, supermarket, Kiddieland, or watching a parade, circus, or ball game often has loosened the tongue of even the smallest and most silent youngster in our Center. In the classroom free play with toys, puzzles, and picture books may provide stimuli for talking in the initial period of evaluative teaching. Soon, however, speech should center around an activity. The activity is not an accident; it is planned carefully with consideration of its timeliness, interest, and reinforcement value. Making paper puppets, a house, a plane, or marching in a rhythm band has stimulated many a child in our Center to talk. Telephone "round robins," dramatization of nursery rhymes, holiday stories, and songs, or an activity so simple as pouring lemonade at a birthday party have given impetus to some silent youngsters to attempt to speak. Taped records of these activity sessions will afford the staff materials for analysis of the child's speech—his vocabulary, sentence formation, and melodic patterns. An outline, inventory, rating form, and table (6-4) are provided to assist you in analysis. In the outline you will note that elements of sentence form, grammar, and syntax are enumerated and/or illustrated by expressions from the speech of children in this age range. These examples from our journals are typical of the kinds of equivalent expressions one may expect. They are pegs of comparison.

Linguistic Form: Syntax, 3–5 Years

(Note use of equivalent expressions in each category.)

1. Form of verb tense:
   a. Larry didded it; I (me) didn't.
   b. He buyed two of (th) em.
   c. We (will) go Gramma's 'morrow?
   d. Dolly awful sick; I (will) call dokkor (doctor).
   e. You (*u*) take candy, p(l)ease.
2. Inflection of third person in verb: *goes*
   a. Heidi goes Bow-Wow.
   b. He goes fast, huh?
3. Progressive inflection: *-ing*
   a. Mommy washing dishes.
   b. Hello, what doing, Gramma? (on telephone)
4. Modal auxiliary verbs: e.g., *will, can*
   a. Bobby can jump over the fence.
   b. Cookie'll bring it 'morrow, O. K.?
5. Contraction of auxiliary verbs: *is, are, does* not.
   a. He's funny, isn't he, Mommy?
   b. She doesn't know that song.
   c. I'll sing it for you.
   d. They're silly; I don't like silly boys.
   e. We're going to buy a birthday present for Ellen.
6. Pluralization of nouns:
   a. Now I put on two sockses.
   b. One car and one car: two cars, see!
   c. My Mommy made free (three) pancakes an' I ate 'em all up.
   d. Tommy caught two fishes.
   e. This scissors isn't sharp.
   f. Two mans tried to start Mommy's car.
7. Substitution of pronouns for noun-phrases:
   a. He rides every day wif (with) Daddy.
   b. You ('re) bad boy; no candy.
   c. Me's pretty dress (I have a pretty dress).
   d. We go fast—huh?
   e. They (ten children) are coming to my party.
8. Introduction of functional words: articles, prepositions, conjunctions
   a. He ran and hit a fence—but it didn't hurt him.
   b. I'm playing wif (with) it; you can't have it.
   c. He likes to ride on a bike.
   d. I want two pieces of gum.
   e. Pin it on me, please.
9. Possessive inflection: *'s*
   a. Nancy's doll; more big (than mine).
   b. I want to ride in Daddy's car.

10. Sentence forms: declarative, interrogative, imperative.
   a. Can you count five pennies?
   b. Our cat caught two mice.
   c. Run fast; it's raining.
   d. Who's afraid?
   e. Wow! Not again!
11. Prosodic qualities in speech continuum:
   a. That's mine!
   b. Quick! Hide it! Daddy's coming.
   c. Mmmm—; I'm so hungry.
   d. Do I *have* to, Mom?

Word-Fun: Semantic Development. Many children enjoy playing with words, and it affords the language teacher many opportunities in the diagnostic period to study the child's knowledge and use of vocabulary. It also is an excellent index of the ability of the child to categorize on the basis of similarities and differences.[13] One often will find that many handicapped children respond in word games with acoustically similar but not semantically related words.

Game I: Semantic Development, 4–8 Years. The first game follows this procedure: After a demonstration, (preferably to a group of children), the teacher says, "Now can you give me the name of something that is like a (1) cat, (2) penny, (3) nail?" The teacher will accept any real likeness. Here is a list of suggestions to use in the game:

1. a knife (scissors, sword, saw, razor, stiletto)
2. a bed (sofa, couch, crib, cradle, hammock)
3. a pencil (pen, chalk, crayon)
4. an orange (grapefruit, lemon, tangerine)
5. a bicycle (motorcycle, scooter, trike)
6. an airplane (helicopter, kite, bird)
7. a letter (postcard, newspaper, telegram, postal package)
8. a boy's shoe (boot, slipper, sandal, clogs)
9. a girl's cap (hat, hood, bonnet, lid, headgear, scarf, beret)
10. a lady's dress (gown, robe, suit, formal, togs, get-up, frock, glad rags)

Game II: Semantic Development, 6–8 Years. Success in motivating the children in this game depends again on careful explanation and demonstration of the nature of the task. A possible procedure is the

[13] The goal is described by de Hirsch: Appraisal of the child's "ability to group verbally an array of objects or events in terms of features they have in common. Skill in this area . . . is a measure of the child's verbal integrative capacity." Three groups of items (in random order) were presented to the child to which he must assign class names. "Responses were scored in terms of the number of times the subject failed to assign an item to the correct category."—K. de Hirsch, J. Jansky, and W. Langford, The oral language performance of premature children and controls. *J Speech Hearing Dis* (February 1964), 29: 60–69.

following: The teacher says, "I am going to say something, and then I want you to say something that *means* the same thing or *means nearly the same thing* as what I said. Let's practice a bit first. If I say, 'The baby cried', what could you say that would mean about the same thing? Begin 'The baby _____.' " If the response is not immediate another child or the teacher helps by saying, "I know one word that means almost the same as *cried;* I will say, 'The baby bawled.' " The child then usually continues with such verbs as *howled, screamed, squealed, squalled,* or *sobbed.* The child may be able to give two analogues for each of the following phrases:

1. The little girl *ran.* (skipped, hopped, jumped, stumbled, flew)
2. Mamma is *angry.* (mad, cross, burned up, huffy, steamed up, annoyed, riled, furious)
3. Baby brother *smiles.* (grins, laughs, gurgles, chuckles, is happy)
4. Dan *walks.* (marches, hikes, tramps, jaunts, strolls, hobbles)

Game III: Semantic Development, 7–9 Years. This is not an easy game. It may require several sessions before the children in the group understand how to play by the rules. In this game the stimulus word is held constant but the child now is asked to find *two different uses* of the words in addition to the identification of the word as a part of the body of a person or animal. Again a practice game precedes the actual task. The examiner says, "In this game, I'm going to say one word and then I want you to use the word in many different ways. All the words will be parts of the body but I want you to show me how you may also use the word in other ways. For example, when I say *eye* you probably would say right off *my eyes* or *my dog's eyes,* but I want you also to think of other ways in which you use the word *eye.* You might say, *eye of a needle,* the *camera eye, bulls-eye, eye of a tornado, hook and eye,* or *to eye some one* (stare at). Do you understand how to play the game?" If the child is not sure that he understands, the teacher continues with "Now try the word *leg.* First you would say, *my leg,* or *leg of lamb,* or *frog's legs*—but then I want you to go on to use it in different ways. You might say _____ " (*chair leg; daddy longlegs; leg of a trip or race; dog-leg; bowlegged; legs of triangle; legged it over to his house*). The words and possible responses are:

1. mouth (mouth of a hole; of a river; mouthpiece; mouthful; loud-mouthed; to make a mouth [wry face])
2. head (head of cabbage; head of a pin; head of the class; head teacher; headpiece; headline; headstone)
3. tongue (tongue of a shoe; tongue of flame; French tongue (speech); wagon tongue; tongue of land)
4. foot (foot of the class; foot-long hot dog; foot the bill; footlights; footprint; footboard)

New Words in Context: Syntactic and Semantic Development, 5–8 Years. The child who enjoys talking and pursues it purposively likes and puts new words into his speech readily. These illustrative stories will give the teacher an opportunity to evaluate the child's ability to bring entirely strange words into his vocabulary, to integrate them in his contextual patterns of language, to retrieve, and to express them on demand. The words in the three stories that follow are set in a context with which the child has had no previous experience. The first story is geared to children 5–6 years; Story II, 6–7; and Story III, 7–8.

Story I: How to Prepare Pumme–yutut

Put on all your listening aids because I want to tell you how a little Eskimo girl in Alaska told her teacher about something she liked very much for supper. After I have given you the recipe, I want you to tell me how to get this dish ready for supper. This dish is called *pumme-yutut.* Can you remember how to say that word? Let's say it together three times. Remember, after I have finished telling you about *pumme-yutut,* you are going to tell me exactly how the children like to eat this food. This is the way the little Eskimo girl told it to her teacher. "*Pumme-yutut* is a little plant that grows on the ground a little way from the seashore. The leaves of the *pumme-yutut* are green and reddish-green. We pick the stem and leaves, take them home, put seal-oil on them (like butter), and eat them." Now you tell me about *pumme-yutut.*[14]

Story II: Recipe for Oogruk

Here is a recipe for fresh *oogruk* from Stewart, Morris, and Bert, three Eskimo boys in Shishmaref, Alaska. I'm going to tell it to you, and then I want you to tell me how the Eskimo boys prepared this dish. Remember the dish is called *oogruk* (seal). Are you ready to listen? Here is the recipe. "Cook the *oogruk meat,* adding salt. Boil it just a few minutes. Don't boil it too much. After the *oogruk* is boiled, remove it from the cooking pot. Next you cool it and then you put it with *blubber* and dried *oogruk* in layers in a *poke.*" (Poke is made by cutting out the inside of the seal, together with the head, through the head part of the sealskin. The skin is then turned, cleaned, and blown up for drying. It is used for storage.)[15]

Story III: Recipe for Ah-Zee'-Ach

(The third recipe makes use of four or five new words.) Here is a recipe from Peter Tocktoo, an Eskimo boy in Shishmaref, Alaska. I'm going to read it to you and then ask you to tell me exactly how to prepare this Eskimo dish. Remember all the directions just as if you were the cook. Don't forget a single one, or the dish may not turn out well. This is a recipe for *Ah-zee'-ach* (black-

---

[14] *Eskimo cook book.* Anchorage: Alaska Crippled Children's Ass., Inc., 1952. P. 3.

[15] *Ibid.,* p. 26.

berries) and *Ah-lowe'-kuk* (wild chard). Let's say the name of the dish together three times. First you put some *seal blubber* and a little water in the pot. Then you put in the *ah-lowe'-kuk* and cook it until it is very soft. Next you put it aside to let it cool. When it has cooled for a time, take out the pieces of blubber. Then you mash the *ah-lowe'-kuk* with the *tuh-gooh* (seal meal). When it is cold, put it into the *poke*. Now you must wait until the *ah-zee'-ach* are ripe and then you gather the berries. When you have gathered the berries, take the *ah-lowe'-kuk* from the poke and mix the two together, *ah-lowe'-kuk* and *ah-zee'-ach*. Yum, yum, it's good! [16]

Patterning the Speech Melody: Phonological Development, 4–8 Years. A very important key to a child's comprehension of language is the prosodic quality, the melody of his speech. It involves the perception of linguistic structure, closure, and fusion and the use of intonational contours, stress, and rhythm. These instruments of prosody, in turn, are dependent on visual, auditory, and tactile-kinesthetic feedback.

We suggest three types of materials by which one can gain insight into the child's ability to copy the teacher's melodic patterns or the speech melodies of other children. Undoubtedly one can think of other methods and materials. The teacher's speech should be accompanied by facial and bodily gestures since patterns of speech melody emerge from the matrix of general motor coordination.

I. *Rhymes*

4–5 years: One-two; buckle your shoe
Three-four; close the door
Five-six; pick up sticks
Seven-eight; open the gate
Nine-ten; begin again.

5–6 years: Hickory-Dickory-Dock
The mouse ran up the clock
The clock—struck—ONE
The mouse ran down
Hickory-Dickory-Dock.

6–7 years: Kitty-kitty-kitty-cat
Where are you—in the house?
Kitty-kitty-kitty-cat
Now I know; you've seen a mouse!

7–8 years: Who am I? Just ME!
Capital M and E for ME!
Sometime I'd like to be a Cat-ME
And climb high up in the maple tree;
There I would be for all to see,
A fine-fine-EVER-SO-FINE-CAT-ME!

[16] *Ibid.*, p. 14.

II. *Emphatic Command Utterance,* 4–6 Years
   (Stress italicized words)
   1. Wait for *me!*
   2. *Is* she *crying* again?
   3. *Wait* a minute; I'm *first,* Daddy.
   4. Hide in *here; quick!*
   5. What is the *matter* with *Mary Jane?*
   6. I didn't want *two apples,* just *one* apple.
   7. Tell him to *stop* it *right this minute!*
   8. Give it to *him; I* don't want it.
   9. Will you *please* be *quiet?* I want to *talk.*
III. *Conversational Melody Patterns,* 6–8 Years
   1. I *don't* know; he's coming—I guess.
   2. What's *he* doing?
   3. *All* of them are *gone.*
   4. What's *your* name?
   5. Did you *eat?*
   6. I know why he said *that!*
   7. *That's* O.K., *isn't* it?
   8. Can't you *really* fix it?
   9. Here I *go: hippety*-hop; *hippety*-hop.
   10. He did it, I'm *sure*—or *almost* sure.
   11. Would you like a piece of candy? It's *marvelous!*
   12. I'm *too tired* to yawn, *too tired* to sleep.
   13. I'll tell you a *big secret*—but come over here—*quick!*
   14. May I go to Jerry's house? *Just* for a *little* while, *please*—Mom?

Controlled Conversational Speech: Picture-Story, 5–8 Years. As the teacher progresses in his evaluative study, he will need larger samplings of the child's conversational speech in a controlled situation. Tests of factors of language have been constructed (to be discussed in chapter 8), but at this point we want to appraise the child's developing competence in an *organized continuum* of expression. One way is *via* the *picture-story* technique. In the hands of the skillful teacher, this technique gives an opportunity to explore phonological, syntactic, and semantic dimensions of language. The outline of the critique that follows the story includes the following subordinate dimensions: (1) its substance or ideational level, (2) lexical elements, (3) functional elements, (4) linguistic form, (5) prosody, and (6) articulation and resistance to articulatory disintegration.

We present one *picture-story* in detail, which through use may become a standardized measure. The materials consist of a series of eleven 4×6 line drawings (Figure A-1, pp. 374–379) that present the part of the story which the child is to reconstruct. The pictures are placed in order before the child. The teacher says:

You've been watching television, haven't you? Do you remember the last flight of our astronauts, _____ into space? Well, you and I together are going to make up a story about a boy, Scott, who also watched that last space flight. I said, *we* would do it together because I'm going to begin the story. I will tell it up to the point where the picture-part begins. Then with the help of these pictures you go on and make up all the rest of the story. The pictures are only a help. You probably will think of many more things to put in the story than the pictures suggest. I want you to make up your own story. Are your "listeners" ready? I'll begin.

Let's call the story *Mission Scottie-O*. Scott is a boy 6 years old. One night he had a dream which was not like his other dreams. Maybe he'd eaten too many ice cream bars or lollipops—or hot dogs. He had been watching television that day, a Friday, and it was the most exciting thing he had ever seen. Two men, one with his own name, Scott, had gone up into the air in something that looked like a swordfish. He had seen a swordfish at the aquarium last Saturday. There was so much smoke around this swordfish thing that he couldn't see it start off exactly but when it got up a way, there it was as plain as a sky rocket or a great hawk flying straight up into space. It was hurtling along so fast that very soon—poof!—it was gone. Where had it gone, he wondered. When he asked his father that question after supper, Daddy said, "to the moon, I guess," but Daddy was reading his paper, and that's no time for a boy to ask questions. Then his Daddy added, as if to stop Scottie, "Someday you'll probably be going up in one of those things, all right." So Scott went to bed and dreamed about it all night—or so he thought—about going up in a space ship.

When morning came—it was Saturday—Scott was up so early that his mother thought he must be sick. No, he wasn't, he said, but he wanted his breakfast early. Why? Well, he thought he had better get started because this was to be his big day! He really wanted a spaceman's breakfast, steak and potatoes, but if he'd asked for it, his mother would come up right off to take his temperature and put him to bed. And that he didn't want—at least not before he got into his gear that Uncle Charley had given him for Christmas last year. Everyone except Scott had thought it was such a funny present from Uncle Charley, but it really wasn't. Maybe he should eat breakfast before he tried on that gear. Then no one would ask questions. So what does Scottie do, (child's name)? Here he is in the bathroom. You go on making up the story. Make up a good one about Scottie and Mission Scottie-O. Here are the pictures to help you (pp. 374–379).

Motivation of Ideas. If the child remains silent after he has been urged to go on with the story, the teacher may say, "See! Here is Scott in the bathroom. He's getting ready for his big day. What is he doing?" The teacher's questions should suggest a description in form of action but if the child is very young, he may respond only with enumeration. As Scott puts on his space suit, the teacher prods the child to the imaginative-descriptive or interpretive level of thinking with these questions: Why is Scott putting on that kind of a suit? Where do you suppose he is going? If, in response to picture 8, the child says, "He's landing on the moon," the teacher should ask him, "And what kind of a place is the moon? Are there real people or moonsters on the moon?", thus urging him on to the abstract-descriptive level.

If the child is under 6 years of age, he may need questions at every step of the way to spur him on. On the back of the cards the following questions appear which will prompt specific forms of answer.

Card   1. What is the boy doing?
          Has he forgotten to brush his _____?
Card   2. What do you suppose he had for breakfast?
          What do you eat for breakfast?
Card   3. What is the boy doing now?
          Won't he need longer socks?
          Could he wear his sister's leotards, do you think?
          Is he nearly dressed? How do you know?
Card   4. What is he putting on?
          Why is he putting on all these things?
Card   5. This boy has lost some of his _____.
          How many has he lost?
Card   6. What is he going to do?
          Will it get off the ground?
Card   7. Where do you suppose he is going?
          How long will it take him to get there?
          What do you call his space ship?
Card   8. Where is he now?
          What are those things around him? (moonsters)
Card   9. Oh! What does he see?
          Is he scared?
          Is his space ship all right?
          Can he get away?
Card 10. Where are the moonsters taking him?
          Who is the little man?
          What is he saying?
Card 11. Here he is fast asleep!
          How did the boy get to his own bed?

Projected Levels of Achievement. The child seriously retarded or disturbed in language simply may echo the examiner's remarks, "Scott in bathroom; what doing?" Judged by ideational planes, this child is on the echolalic or meaningless language level. The average child, 3–4 years of age, probably will go no further than the *enumerative level:* "I see a boy, soap, towel." The 4–5-year-old child enters into simple *description* of the picture: "Boy washes face. He eat(s) breakfast (supper). Put on socks, clothes, cap." The average child at this age probably would not proceed beyond picture 6. The average 6–7-year-old child will begin to interpret meaning with picture 3 and continue on the concrete-imaginative level of interpretation until he reaches picture 9. With picture 9 the child, 8–9 years, should enter upon the abstract-descriptive level of interpretation. Here, as Myklebust has pointed out,[17] the child would introduce concepts of time and sequence. We believe that he also may introduce emotional interpretations at this age. So to picture 9 he might well say, "I'll bet Scott was afraid of those moonsters." He may go on to narrate things which happen to him before he gets back from his moon-trip. Finally he may reach a high order of interpretation and insight, if to picture 10 he responds, "You know I think this whole thing was a dream!" In other words, he now has employed ideation which is beyond the observable. He has exercised his imagination at the abstract-imaginative level.

Evaluative Data. No score of language-age may be obtained by this *picture-story.* More valuable than a score is the complete profile of the child's language development. By repeated review of the taped record of the child's responses and the notes of observers, and with the help of inventories, tables, and the critique-outline that follows, the team should have the necessary materials for the task.

I. Substance of Language: Ideational Levels
  A. Enumeration
    1. Names people, objects, physical surround.
    2. Simply reproduces visual situations.
  B. Literal description
    1. Presents formless, disorganized bits of information.
    2. Describes only what he sees without attempting to establish relations or continuity.
    3. Groups information according to some plan.
  C. Imaginative description
    1. Introduces unseen figures and objects which are incorporated in the story.
    2. Employs deliberate invention of details: romancing.
    3. Reflects syncretistic understanding (whole is understood before parts are understood).
  D. Interpretation: Level I
    1. Interprets concrete details and relates them to the plot of the story.
    2. Reflects little egocentric thought.
    3. Attempts to explain events and motives of action.
  E. Interpretation: Level II
    1. Introduces forms of analysis; synthesis of ideas and events in perception.
    2. Introduces imaginative and abstract materials suggested by the picture sequence.
    3. Abstracts qualities or meanings from stimuli; forms constructs transferable from situation to situation, using materials that are tangible, abstract, or numerical.

[17] H. Myklebust, *Development and disorders of written language, vol. I.* New York: Grune & Stratton, 1965. P. 140.

  II. Language Behavior
- A. Enjoys verbalizing about exploits and behavior of the child adventurer.
- B. Develops percepts logically from sense impressions.
- C. Identifies with the child in the story in some respects.
- D. Uses speech to elaborate new connections.
- E. Uses gestures, mimicry, movement, demonstration to accompany language.
- F. Uses communicable logic (guided by memories of earlier reasoning and by expressed deduction).
- G. Uses loose referential lexical meanings (*He needs to* _____ instead of *He wants to* _____).
- H. Uses rigid language structure.
- I. Uses egocentric logic (no real connections).
- J. Shows anxiety, inability to tolerate visual or auditory stimuli (defense against anxiety).
- K. Uses autistic language: highly organistic; grotesquely imaginary.

  III. Use of Lexical Elements of Language. Content words: Nouns, Verbs, Adjectives.[18]
- A. Word use
  1. Total number of words used in each class.[19]
  2. Limits choice of words to semantic class.
  3. Uses quantitative words correctly (some, any, several).
  4. Uses noun substitutes.
- B. Word Substance: Qualitative assessment of perceptual value.

  IV. Use of Functional Elements of Language: Structure Words [20]
- A. Uses prepositions and conjunctions.
- B. Uses interrogatives.
- C. Uses noun determiners.
- D. Uses auxiliaries.

  V. Use of Linguistic Form
- A. Sentence type, complexity, and elaboration [21]
  1. Total number of complete sentences.
  2. Total number of complex sentences employing:
     a. modifying phrases
     b. subordinate clauses
  3. Total number of compound sentences.
  4. Preponderant sentence types: Interjectional? imperative? interrogative? declarative?

---

[18] See Table A-1, p. 373, for *Increase in Size of Vocabulary with Age.*

[19] See Appendix A for *Rules for Counting Number of Words.*

[20] These words of function have high frequency and few members in a class. See W. Miller and S. Ervin, The development of grammar in child language. *The acquisition of language.* Monogr Soc Res Child Develop (1964), 29 (1): 13.

[21] See Table A-2, p. 373, for *Classification of Sentence Structure* and for *Sentence Complexity Scores.*

    B. Grammar and syntax
       1. Uses atypical word order:
         a. inverts subject-verb-object order
         b. makes remote inversions
         c. makes attempt to fit words into syntactic frame
       2. Uses incomplete sentences:
         a. interrogative fragments
         b. interjectional phrase fragments
       3. Uses verbs not in agreement with subject.
       4. Omits auxiliary.
       5. Makes errors in formation of tense.
       6. Uses double negative.
       7. Misuses nouns and pronouns.
       8. Makes errors in formation of plural forms of nouns.
       9. Makes errors in gender.
 VI. Prosody: Melody of Speech
    A. Uses a rhythm that is:
       1. conversational
       2. measured
       3. staccato
       4. tachyphemic
    B. Employs intonation patterns that:
       1. are appropriate to meaning
       2. are stereotyped, meaningless, atypical
       3. follow morphemic sequences
    C. Stress is:
       1. placed on proper morphemic units
       2. expressed by changes in:
         a. pitch-stress
         b. duration
         c. intensity
VII. Articulation and Resistance to Articulatory Distintegration [22]
    A. Distorts, omits, or substitutes consonantal phonemes.
    B. Distorts, omits, or substitutes vowel phonemes.
    C. Confuses phoneme order.
    D. Maintains articulatory proficiency throughout story.
    E. Articulatory disintegration is notable:
       1. in long sentences
       2. at end of story
       3. with increase of excitement or anxiety

[22] Children at this period of language development may demonstrate excellent articulatory competence in the repetition or voluntary production of simple sentences in response to pictures or objects yet may exhibit singular articulatory disintegration when they must organize complex thought units into verbal form. The organizational load which involves the projection of the *gestalt* into movement patterns simply becomes too heavy. The synthesis of input-output breaks down and articulatory sequences disintegrate.

Inventory 8. Use of Oral Language, 3–8 Years

Name _____

Age (C A) _____

Original enrollment date _____

Recorder _____

Key

A Yes, or very good
B Better than average
C Average
D Below average
E No, or poor
√ Inconsistent
O No opportunity to observe

Date of Record

Has two-word sentences (A or E)							
Has more than two-word sentences (A or E)							
Imitates phrase sequences without distortion (A or E)							
Repeats sentences of 12–13 syllables (A or E)							
Uses only simple sentence structure (A or E)							
Uses complex sentence structure (A or E)							
Responds without lag to questions (A or E)							
Voluntarily asks for objects by name							
Uses plurals correctly							
Uses pronouns but in incorrect case (A or E)							
Uses pronouns correctly							
Uses past tense in proper form							
Uses subject-verb in agreement							
Articulates phonemic sequences but omits or distorts some phonemes (A or E)							

Articulates phonemic sequence accurately (Eg.: Rain goes pitter patter; My puppy plays with kitty.)						
Confuses phoneme or word order (A or E)						
Omits little words in sentence (A or E)						
Often has unintelligible speech (A or E)						
Uses single words and phrases (A or E)						
Has meager vocabulary (A or E)						
Has vocabulary appropriate to C.A.						
Demonstrates prosody in contextual expression						
Often has cluttered speech (A or E)						
Gives full name (A or E)						
Names his sex (A or E)						
Misnames objects, people (A or E)						
Names objects, people correctly (A or E)						
Voice abnormally loud (A or E)						
Voice abnormally soft (A or E)						
Pitch changes follow shifts in meaning						
Loudness changes follow shifts in meaning						
Voice is monotonous (A or E)						
Voice is harsh (A or E)						
Voice is nasal (A or E)						
Voice is breathy (A or E)						
Speech rhythm is measured (A or E)						

Inventory 8 (continued)							
Speech rhythm is irregular (explosive)							
Imitates speech rhythm of others							
Enjoys act of speaking							
Responds easily to salutation, etc.							
Verbalizes purposively							
Verbalizes rarely (A or E)							
Uses variety of sentence forms (declarative, interrogative, etc.)							
Uses grammar appropriate to C.A.							
Tells story demonstrating semantic relations							
Imitates melodic expression of others (pitch-stress, duration, etc.)							
Articulatory stability maintained throughout story							
Articulation patterns disintegrate before end of story (A or E)							
Reflects intent to remember and replicate story exactly as it is printed							
Tells essential features of story							
Puts together string of nonessential features (A or E)							
Recalls more nonessential than essential cues of story (A or E)							
Recalls essential cues of story							
Demonstrates immediate recall							

For the format and some items in these scales we are indebted to T. C. Bangs, Evaluating children with language delay. *J Speech Hearing Dis* (February 1961), 26: 16–18.

Rating Form. Some Phonological Aspects of Oral Expression, 5-8 Years

Name _____ Age _____ Sex _____
Date _____

PITCH: 1 2 3 4
___ Too high
___ Too low
___ Pitch pattern
___ Monotonous
___ Pitch breaks
___ Other

LOUDNESS: 1 2 3 4
___ Too loud
___ Too soft
___ Monotonous
___ Loudness pattern
___ Other

RATE: 1 2 3 4
___ Too rapid
___ Too slow
___ Rate pattern
___ Monotonous
___ Jerkiness
___ Others

PROSODY (Speech Melody): 1 2 3 4
___ Intonational patterns
___ Stress patterns

ARTICULATION: 1 2 3 4
___ General misarticulations
___ Plosives misarticulated
___ Fricatives misarticulated
___ Semivowels misarticulated
___ Nasals misarticulated

___ Glides misarticulated
___ Vowels misarticulated
___ Diphthongs misarticulated
___ Substitutions
___ Distortions
___ Omissions
___ Voicing errors
___ Other

VOICE QUALITY: 1 2 3 4
Laryngeal Function:
___ Breathiness
___ Harshness
___ Hoarseness
___ Glottal attack
___ Other

Resonance:
___ Hypernasality
___ Hyponasality

FLUENCY: 1 2 3 4
___ Interjection of sounds, syllables, words, or phrases
___ Part-word repetitions
___ Word repetitions
___ Phrase repetitions
___ Revisions
___ Incomplete phrases
___ Broken words
___ Prolonged sounds
___ Unvocalized intervals

Longitudinal Study II-C: The Summing Up

The final profile chart included in this section will provide one type of summary; much more important is your interpretive anecdotal account encompassing all case history and comparative data you have assembled from your observations of the linguistically handicapped child. This is the most difficult of all tasks prescribed in this chapter, yet if it is not well done, all previous study goes for naught. Here the student must coordinate all his findings, reconcile those that often are contradictory, and present a consistent, well-ordered, analytical and interpretive story of central and contributory causes of linguistic deficit, the present status and prognosis of language learning. If he has learned how to recognize, record, reason, research and write, he will find this the most challenging task of all.

Longitudinal Study II-C

Developmental Profile: General Rating Sheet

	Poor	Below Average	Better than Average	Very Good	Remarks
Name _____ Age (C A) _____ Original enrollment date _____ Length of evaluation period_____ Recorder _____					
I. Table 6-1. Development of Nonverbal Adaptive Behavior, 1 Week–36 Months					
II. Table 6-2. Comprehension and Use of Oral Language, 1–36 Months Inventory 1. Comprehension of Nonverbal and Verbal Stimuli, 1–36 Months					
Inventory 2. Use of Oral Language, 11–36 Months					
III. Table 6-3. Nonverbal Adaptive Behavior, 3–8 Years Inventory 3. General Motor Development, 3–8 Years					
Inventory 4. Socioemotional Behavior, 4–8 Years					
Inventory 5. Attitudes in Learning, 4–8 Years					
IV. Table 6-4. Phonological, Syntactic, and Semantic Aspects of Oral Language, 3–8 Years Inventory 6. Comprehension of Nonverbal Stimuli, 3–8 Years					
Inventory 7. Comprehension of Verbal Information, 3–8 Years					
Inventory 8. Use of Oral Language, 3–8 Years					
Rating Form. Some Phonological Aspects of Oral Expression, 5–8 Years					

7

Diagnostic Testing of Oral Language

Comprehensive Measures of Oral Language

Because coding embraces an unbroken continuum of language, the customary practice of dividing language into comprehension and use may be a convenience but it is not consistent with our knowledge that modification of comprehension goes on throughout the act of oral expression. From initial discrimination in analyzers outside the CNS to the oral utterance of the sentence, perception is being modified. The only possible rationale for such a division might be based on the assumption that measures differ in their value on the denominator of comprehension-use. No test measures exclusively comprehension or use, and no single test can be said to measure all aspects of comprehension and use. We shall consider first four experimental diagnostic tests designed to measure linguistic deficiencies in several dimensions of language learning, *viz.,* the *Illinois Test of Psycholinguistic Abilities (ITPA)*,[1] *Utah Test of Language Development (UTLD)*,[2] *The Houston Test for Language Development*,[3] and *The Michigan Picture Language Inventory*.[4] They will be followed by descriptions of tests that assess deficiencies in specific aspects of oral language.

[1] J. McCarthy and S. Kirk, *Illinois test of psycholinguistic abilities* (experimental edition). Urbana, Ill.: The University of Illinois, 1961.

[2] M. Mecham, J. Jex, and J. Jones, *Utah test of language development* (revised edition). Salt Lake City: Communication Research Associates, 1967.

[3] M. Crabtree, *The Houston test for language development.* Houston: Houston Test Co., 1958.

[4] W. Wolski, *The Michigan picture language inventory.* Ann Arbor, Mich.: The University of Michigan, 1962.

254

Illinois Test of Psycholinguistic Abilities (ITPA). Of the four tests to be described this is easily the most comprehensive and most highly standardized. The final test battery was standardized on 700 children between the ages of 2.6 and 9.0, and language age and standard score norms were calculated. Yet the authors of this test emphasize its experimental nature. The measure is based upon

three major dimensions . . . (that are) postulated to specify a given psycholinguistic ability; they are levels of organization, psycholinguistic processes, and channels of communication. . . . The representational level . . . is sufficiently organized to mediate activities requiring the meaning or significance of linguistic symbols. The automatic-sequential level . . . mediates activities requiring the retention of linguistic symbol sequences and the execution of automatic habit chains. (The second dimension, psycholinguistic processes, encompasses the acquisition and use of the habits required for normal language usage.) There are three main sets of habits to be considered: *Decoding,* or the sum total of those habits required to ultimately obtain meaning from either visual or auditory linguistic stimuli; *Encoding,* or the sum total of those habits required to ultimately express oneself in words or gestures; and *Association,* or the sum total of those habits required to manipulate linguistic symbols internally. Tests which demonstrate the presence of association ability include word association tests, analogies tests, similarities and differences tests, etc.[5]

ITPA is composed of nine subtests: (1) auditory decoding, (2) visual decoding, (3) auditory-vocal association, (4) visual-motor association, (5) vocal encoding, (6) motor encoding, (7) auditory-vocal automatic ability, (8) auditory-vocal sequential ability, and (9) visual-motor sequential ability. The kind of task required is exemplified in such measures as auditory decoding, auditory-vocal sequencing, and vocal encoding. In the auditory decoding subtest the examiner assesses understanding of the spoken word; it is, according to its authors, "a controlled vocabulary test." This measure consists of 36 three-word questions of this type: *Do airplanes fly? Do apples fly? Do dresses drive? Do goats eat? Do daughters marry? Do dentists drill? Do carpenters kneel? Do carbohydrates nourish? Do meteorites collide?* The auditory-vocal sequencing subtest presumably evaluates the child's "ability to correctly repeat a sequence of symbols previously heard. It is assessed by a modified digit repetition test." [6] The range extends from two to seven digits. In the vocal encoding subtest the subject is asked to describe the following objects: *ball, chalk, block,* and *celluloid.*

Criticisms of the test will undoubtedly be met in the revised edi-

[5] J. McCarthy and S. Kirk, *Examiners manual; Illinois test of psycholinguistic abilities* (experimental ed.). Urbana, Ill.: The University of Illinois Press, 1961. P. 3. A revised edition appeared as this book was going to press.
[6] *Ibid.,* p. 6.

tion. We believe that the experimental edition falls short of expectations for these reasons:

1. ITPA does not test certain parameters of language which we consider vital in locating disabilities of the language-handicapped child. There is little opportunity to appraise the child's comprehension or use of contextual language, yet this is one of the major problems of children with linguistic handicaps; they are unable to interpret or use "swaths of language."

2. We believe language must be assessed for its *substantive value*. There is almost no opportunity to make such an assessment in ITPA. We need to know the *quality* of understanding and use. In our view this is the most important inquiry that we can make relative to a child's acquisition of language. In preceeding chapters we have discussed the consequences of a breakdown in the mechanics of language, but we also have tried to make clear that failures in comprehension of the *substance of language* usually contribute to the breakdown. This is a reciprocal relationship: "You can't have one without the other." It is true that the auditory decoding test poses 36 questions of this type: "Do babies eat"? "Do bicycles drink?" These questions cannot be regarded as a measure of substantive comprehension. In another subtest, vocal encoding, the child is asked to "tell me all about" four objects: *ball, chalk, block,* and *celluloid.* In our experience with the test, we have found the objects to be inadequate as stimuli for provoking substantive expression.

3. We do not regard the automatic-sequential test of ITPA as automatic. The auditory-vocal automatic subtest is an example: *Here is an apple; here are two* ———— ; etc. This subtest appraises grammar and syntax. Such an ability implies that the child has acquired the rules of grammar. A child in the stage of learning the rules of grammar does not operate language codes automatically. Indeed, one wonders if grammar ever becomes an automatic process.

4. Another subtest is called the auditory-vocal association test. (*I sit on a chair; I sleep on a* ————.) If the example for the automatic-sequential measure, *Here is an apple; here are two* ———— , is automatic, then why is not the example from the auditory-vocal association subtest also automatic?

5. The relationship between digit repetition (auditory-vocal sequencing subtest) and the auditory-vocal sequencing of linguistic patterns has not been supported by the research of other psychologists.[7]

6. Another limitation applies to the theory of the design of ITPA. The tripartite concept of coding, *viz.,* input, association, and output, runs counter to prevailing neurological theories of the unitary nature of coding. The process of "internal manipulation" of symbols has no established neurological correlate.

7. The final limitation applies to the rationale of the test. It is well

[7] See E. Taylor, *Psychological appraisal of children with cerebral defects.* Cambridge: Harvard, 1961. P. 432.

expressed by Spradlin: "The rationale for the ITPA assumes that the test items are measuring implicit processes within the person and that the language responses are merely effects of these processes. Since the implicit processes are not observable independently of the language responses, the rationale involves problems of dualism and circularity. The authors often slip outside of their 'theoretical' system as when they say, 'Encoding is the sum of those abilities required to express *ideas* in words or gestures.' In this statement the term 'idea' is extraneous to the system. Moreover, while the authors claim to be operational in their definitions of constructs, such constructs as 'representational level' and 'association' cannot be reduced to operations." [8]

Utah Test of Language Development (UTLD). This is a very simple measure and may be most useful as a checklist of the normal development of language before one undertakes a thorough study of the child's linguistic deficiencies. Its authors claim that it "provides the clinician with an objective instrument for measurement of expressive and receptive verbal language skills in both normal and handicapped children." [9] The age range is 1 to 15 years. Since it has been designed for use with "aphasic and hyperactive brain-injured individuals," it is not a timed test and can be administered in more than one sitting. Ordinarily the test takes approximately 30–45 minutes to administer. The raw score may be translated into a language-age equivalent, but because of the small sampling (twenty children for each chronological age level from 1.6 to 12.5 years), standard scores and percentile equivalents could not be established. It is assumed by the authors that the 51 items of the scale have good face validity because they were chosen from other standardized sources. Their indebtedness to general classification scales is evident, for example, in the test items for the child of 2–3 years: (1) names common pictures; (2) repeats two digits; (3) responds to simple commands; (4) identifies action in pictures; (5) names one color; and (6) makes eight or more correct responses to pictures of (*a*) table, (*b*) bird, (*c*) ball, (*d*) sitting, (*e*) leaf, (*f*) catching, (*g*) hitting, (*h*) fly, (*i*) peeking. (The score sheet for years 1 to 8 and the classification of language items according to linguistic processes are included in Appendix B.)

The Houston Test for Language Development. [10] Part I of this test is a checklist for the teacher-observer team of the behavior of the very young child, 6 months to 3 years of age. They are to observe such specific categories of language as melody of speech, accent, gesture,

[8] J. E. Spradlin, Language and communication of mental defectives. In W. Ellis, Ed., *Handbook of mental deficiency.* New York: McGraw-Hill, 1963. P. 522.
[9] M. Mecham, J. Jex, and J. Jones, *Manual of instructions: Utah test of language development* (rev. ed.). Salt Lake: Communication Research Associates, 1967. P. 1.
[10] Margaret Crabtree, Ed. D., *The Houston test for language development.* A language-age score may be obtained by administration of the entire test. The complete kit, which includes manual, score sheets, and vocabulary cards may be secured from The Houston Test Co., P. O. Box 35152, Houston, Texas.

articulation, vocabulary, grammatical usage, and dynamic content. When time does not permit the full use of the evaluation scales, the teacher-observer team will find that this section of the Houston Test provides a quick check of age equivalents for certain behavioral responses pertaining to language. The score sheet for part I is reproduced in Appendix B. Part II, employed with children from 3 to 6 years of age, attempts to tap several levels, channels, and processes of their language abilities. Spontaneous speech is elicited by use of the doll family and other materials included in the kit. The comprehensive nature of the scale may be judged by the variety of test items. Among the eighteen items in part II are included subtests of self-identity, vocabulary, gesture, auditory judgments, communicative behavior, temporal content, syntactical complexity, and melody patterns. The normative scores of language age are based on data collected from the administration of the tests, parts I and II, to 215 children from the age of 6 months to 6 years.

The Michigan Picture Language Inventory.[11] A slightly different technique is employed in this test: First, expression is tested, followed by comprehension. The materials of the vocabulary subtest, for example, consist of 35 cards, each card containing a key item and two foil items. After the establishment of rapport, the examiner presents the card "to the child in sequence *pointing only to the key item picture on each card, . . .*" and if he wishes may say, "What is this a picture of?" In testing comprehension "the child is credited with comprehension of an item if he succeeds in the more difficult task of naming it, so now only those items are tested on which the child erred in the expression test." The child is directed to look at these pictures again, and this time the examiner names the picture and the child points to the one named. Each item has a point value of one. Total expression and comprehension scores are obtained by totaling the number of correct responses. The standardization sample is limited to children 4–6 years of age.

The Inventory also includes a test of language structure in which fifty picture cards are presented to children 4 to 6 years of age. They should elicit 69 responses of expression and a like number of comprehension responses.

The test is divided into nine principal sections, each testing a particular class of words. These word classes are: (1) singular and plural nouns, (2) personal pronouns, (3) possessives, (4) adjectives, (5) demonstratives, (6) articles, (7) adverbs, (8) prepositions, and (9) verbs and auxiliaries. . . . Each section is tested separately following a particular three-step procedure: (1) the examiner first describes every card within the section to provide the context of the responses which the child will later be required to give, (2) returning to the first card the

[11] W. Wolski, *The Michigan picture language inventory.* Ann Arbor, Mich.: The University of Michigan, 1962.

examiner tests the key items for expression, and (3) again returning to the first card the examiner presents the set of cards a third time to test for comprehension of the items.[12]

After describing the picture of a boy, a girl, and a rabbit out playing, for example, the examiner says,

"In this picture *he* ran to the tree. In this picture *she* ran to the tree, and in this picture *it* ran to the tree." In testing *expression* the examiner returns to this card and says, "In this picture *it* ran to the tree. In this picture *she* ran to the tree, and in this picture _____."

The child completes the sentence. This procedure is followed throughout the test.

Testing Specific Dimensions of Oral Language

The tests that we have just described attempt to measure all aspects of language. Several scales have been devised, however, which deal chiefly with one dimension of language: syntactic, semantic, or phonological. Since linguistic structure seems to be basic to the other dimensions, we are inclined to place greater weight on this parameter than on the others. Several purposes may be served by each of the tests to be described in this section. A test of oral discrimination of sound sequences, for example, may test both one's comprehension of meaningful elements (semological) and morphemic components that are frequently categorized both as phonological and syntactic in purpose. Language measures also vary in temporal reliability,[13] so we have included several tests in each category. Moreover, no one set of tasks in any category is likely to establish a reliable and specific pattern of deficit. The measures vary in yet another way. Some are standardized, possessing statistical validity; others are exploratory measures that indeed could be more valuable than standardized tests in terms of effective diagnostic evaluation of the child's linguistic abilities and deficits. In the remainder of the chapter specific factors to be explored are (1) linguistic structure, (2) auditory discrimination of morphemic units, (3) vocabulary, (4) special semantic elements (verbal patterning of sequential information, comprehension span, closure, memory), and (5) articulation.

[12] W. Wolski, *Language development of normal children 4, 5, and 6 years of age as measured by the Michigan picture language inventory*. Doctoral dissertation, University of Michigan, 1962. P. 5. Microfilm No. 63–479. Ann Arbor: University Microfilms, Inc.

[13] F. Minifie, F. Darley, and D. Sherman, Temporal reliability of seven language measures. *J Speech Hearing Res* (June 1967), 6: 139–148.

Tests of Linguistic Structure: Syntax and Grammar

Experimental Test of Comprehension of Linguistic Structure (3–7½ years).[14] Although this measure still is in experimental form, it represents a significant advance both in breadth and depth of assessment of language development. Each one of the set of plates comprising this test contains one or more black and white line-drawings that represent referential categories and contrasts which can be signaled by form classes and function words, morphological constructions, grammatical categories and syntactic structure.

The plates which test the structural contrasts provide two or three pictures, one of which represents the referent for the linguistic form being tested; the alternate picture(s) represents the referent(s) for the contrasting linguistic form(s). For example, to test comprehension of the linguistic signal for future tense as contrasted with present and past tenses, a plate was designed to illustrate an action in the temporal sequence of present, past and future. The stimulus in this case is in the future, i.e., 'will jump.'

The form classes and function words tested by the instrument are nouns, verbs, adjectives, adverbs, and prepositions. Morphological constructions tested are those formed by adding *er* and *ist* to free morphs such as nouns, verbs, and adjectives. Grammatical categories that are evaluated involve contrasts of case, number, gender, tense, status, voice, and mood. Syntactic structures of predication, complementation, modification, and coordination are also tested.[15]

No oral expression on the part of the child is required.

The results of testing 162 children in seven age groups, 2.10–7.9 years, are presented in tabular form in Appendix B, pp. 385–387. An examination of the tables shows that the test is more comprehensive than many in that it attempts to assess the child's implicit knowledge of the basic rules governing linguistic production. In other words, it encompasses general linguistic competence. The table presents the age groups at which 60 percent of the children comprehended "linguistic items" in the following categories: (1) form classes and function words, (2) morphological constructions, (3) grammatical categories, and (4) syntactic structures. In the discussion of results the author makes these significant observations:

1. Girls advanced more rapidly than boys in language development at every half-year level except at 3.0 years.
2. In comprehension of form classes, such as verbs, the children understood the verbs, *jump, run,* and *eat,* at 3.0 years but did not understand a verb such as *give* until they reached the 4.6 year level. All adjectives of color, another form class, were understood by 60 percent

---

[14] M. A. Carrow, The development of auditory comprehension of language structure in children. *J Speech Hearing Dis* (May 1968), 33: 99–111.

[15] *Ibid.,* p. 103.

of the children by the age of 3.6, but adjectives of number or relative quantity, except *two,* were understood from two to three years later.

3. Sixty percent at 4.6 years comprehended the morph, *er,* tested by contrasting nouns, as *farm/farmer.*

4. At age 4.0, the grammatical categories of gender and number in pronouns were comprehended by 60 percent of the children.

5. Verb tense was understood in the following order: present progressive, past, future, and present perfect.

6. Response to categories of syntactic structure varied with the length and complexity of the structures. Sixty percent at 3.0 years comprehended a noun-phrase with a single adjective modifier but six of ten children were 4.6 years old before they comprehended a noun-phrase with two adjective modifiers.

7. Comprehension seemed to depend on the particular linguistic structure used, on the referent for the linguistic structure, and possibly on the frequency with which that particular item is used in the language.

8. The children seemed to comprehend earlier those categories that are fundamentally unmarked and specified, such as present tense and singular number, and to have more difficulty with grammatical contrasts that are derived and marked, such as past and future tense, and plural number.

Exploratory Test: Development of Grammar, 5–8 Years.[16] An exploratory means of studying the ability of a young child to develop rules of grammar is a measure we have designed from research studies of Berko.[17] She found that children have morphological rules—rules of extension, learned consciously or unconsciously, which enable them to deal with new words and their forms. In Berko's study, the child made consistent and orderly answers, pronouncing many inflectional endings with exaggerated care. For example, he demonstrated, when asked to supply the correct plural ending to a noun which had been made up, that he had an "internalized working system of the plural allomorphs in English, and was able to generalize to new cases and select the right form."[18] The features of English morphology most commonly represented in the language of the first-grade child are: (1) the plural and the two possessives of the noun, (2) the third person singular of the verb, (3) the progressive and the past tense, and (4) the comparative and superlative of the adjective. The pronouns were avoided, both because of the difficulty involved in making up nonsense pronouns, and because of the limited number and irregularity of the pronouns. Indeed, one could hardly expect even adults to have any generalized rules for the handling of new pronouns. Moreover, one does not encounter new pronouns, whereas

---

[16] M. F. Berry and R. Talbott, *Exploratory test of grammar.* 4332 Pine Crest Rd., Rockford, Ill. 61107, 1966.

[17] J. Berko, The child's learning of English morphology. In S. Saporta, Ed., *Psycholinguistics.* New York: Holt, Rinehart and Winston, 1961. Pp. 359–376.

[18] *Ibid.,* p. 359.

new verbs, adjectives, and nouns constantly appear in vocabularies, so that the essential problem is not the same. A number of forms that might suggest irregular plurals and past tenses are included among the nouns and verbs.

In our design of the test 30 cardboard plates bear line-drawings of mythical figures which are called by mythical names and engage in mythical action. The invented nouns, verbs, and adjectives used in short passages appear below the figure. The child is asked to supply the appropriate inflection. Plates 1, 2, 3, 4, 21, 27, 29, and 30 and the record form of this test are reproduced in Appendix B.

Tests of Auditory Discrimination of Morphemic Units

Some tests described in this section have been designated by their authors as tests of phonemic discrimination but in reality they are tests of free morphemic discrimination.[19] In this and preceding chapters evidence has been advanced to show (1) that the phoneme of a language need not be discriminable before its symbolic significance *in the morpheme* can be appreciated [20] and (2) that the morpheme is the smallest discriminable acoustic unit.[21] These tests, then, do not measure phonemic discrimination, an ability the child does not possess, but are tests of morphemic discrimination. In common with all tests of language learning, age, socioeconomic, cultural, and ethnic factors must be weighed in the interpretation of their results.[22] Since the language-retarded child frequently is unable to relegate irrelevant signals to the background, tests of oral discrimination should be repeated in a controlled background of noise. If there is great disparity in results, figure-ground distortion may be one facet of the child's perceptual problem. Among the many available tests in this area, we describe one test of discrimination by Templin, Wepman's *Auditory Discrimination Test,* and Mecham's *Picture Discrimination Test.*

Sound Discrimination Tests by Templin. The test, designed for use with preschool children, 3 to 5 years of age,

[19] A *free morpheme* is the minimal unit of speech that is recurrent, meaningful, and can stand alone (see pp. 158–160).

[20] E. Gibson, Association and differentiation in perceptual learning. Unpublished paper, Cornell University, 1962. E. Gibson, Learning to read. *Science* (May 21, 1965), 148: 1066–1072.

[21] A. M. Liberman, Some results of research on speech perception. *J Acoust Soc Amer* (January 1957) 29 (1): 117–123. A. M. Liberman, *et al., A motor theory of speech perception.* Paper presented at the Speech Communication Seminar, Speech Transmission Laboratory, Royal Institute of Technology, Stockholm, September 1962.

[22] M. Byrne, *The Wepman auditory discrimination test as a clinical tool.* Paper presented to *Amer Speech Hearing Assn,* New York, 1962. Abstract in *Asha* (1962), 4: 383.

is based on the identification of similarity and difference in the acoustic value of familiar words which can be pictured. Pairs of pictures of familiar objects whose names are words similar in pronunciation except for single sound elements . . . were pasted on a single card and presented to the child. The child was asked to point to the picture of the thing denoted by the word the examiner said. Ninety-two words were used in fifty-nine pairs in the test. The child pointed out his choice of pictures in response to the stimulus word uttered by the examiner in at least two presentations of all the cards. . . . If the stimulus word was both correctly and incorrectly identified, a third presentation of the pair of pictures was made.[23]

Three different methods of scoring are suggested by Templin. The score is the number of items in which (1) *two out of three* responses are correct and no attention is given to correct identification of test words, or (2) *two out of two* responses are correct and no attention is given to knowledge of test words, or (3) *two out of either two or three* responses are correct and *both* discrimination words have been correctly identified.[24] The list of words is presented below, with the stimulus word in each pair italicized:

1. *keys*-peas	21. star-*car*	41. *lamp*-lamb
2. *chairs*-stairs	22. *bread*-bed	42. nose-*toes*
3. mouse-*mouth*	23. pen-*pin*	43. thread-*spread*
4. *dish*-fish	24. back-*bat*	44. *cone*-comb
5. bell-*ball*	25. *grass*-glass	45. *string*-ring
6. pin-*pig*	26. *clown*-cloud	46. hat-*cat*
7. clocks-*blocks*	27. pail-*nail*	47. pipe-*pie*
8. bat-*bath*	28. *cap*-cup	48. beets-*beads*
9. *sail*-pail	29. *rake*-lake	49. *horse*-house
10. *card*-car	30. *blocks*-socks	50. *cane*-can
11. bread-*red*	31. thread-*sled*	51. gum-*gun*
12. *peach*-peas	32. string-*spring*	52. train-*rain*
13. *seat*-feet	33. back-*black*	53. *bread*-thread
14. bag-*back*	34. sleep-*sweep*	54. *ring*-rim
15. horn-*corn*	35. *cat*-cap	55. tree-*three*
16. *stone*-stove	36. tie-*pie*	56. swing-*string*
17. gun-*drum*	37. *beads*-beans	57. *cone*-coat
18. *nail*-mail	38. *tail*-pail	58. *bread*-spread
19. *box*-blocks	39. *soup*-soap	59. hand-*sand* [25]
20. *coat*-goat	40. ship-*chip*	

For children 6 to 8 years old, Templin has constructed a sound discrimination test consisting of 50 pairs of nonsense syllables. Each pair is judged to be *same* or *different* by the child. Examples of the two types

[23] M. Templin, *Certain language skills in children.* Minneapolis: University of Minnesota Press, 1957. P. 14.
[24] *Ibid.*, p. 63.
[25] *Ibid.*, p. 159.

of pairs are *le-le* and *esh-ech*. The total possible score is 50, one for each correct response.

Auditory Discrimination Test by Wepman.[26] The child, with his back to the examiner, is asked to listen to 40 pairs of words presented orally by the examiner, after an initial trial period with five pairs. The child then indicates in some manner whether the word-pair is the same or different. Thirty of the 40 word-pairs, such as *vie-thy, led-lad,* are to be judged as *different* by the child, and ten, such as *bar-bar* and *wing-wing,* as the *same.* If the child of 6 years judges more than 5 of the *different pairs incorrectly,* his development of auditory discrimination is inadequate. Here is a sample of the word-pairs from Form II:

1. cad-cab
2. led-lad
3. ball-ball
4. rub-rug
5. gall-goal
6. cope-coke
7. zone-zone
8. fret-threat
9. lave-lathe
10. vie-thy
11. rich-rich
12. wedge-wedge
13. guile-dial
14. wreathe-reef
15. cuff-cuss

Picture Speech Discrimination Test by Mecham and Jex.[27] This is a particularly useful measure for young children because the line drawings are clear and the *words* that the pictures suggest are within the age range. They have been selected from the Thorndike list. The test requires a word-picture matching response on the part of the child who hears and identifies the picture correctly. Three pictures are mounted on each of 86 cards. While viewing the pictures on a card, the child hears a series of three words, spoken by the examiner. One of the words is the correct name of one of the pictures; the other two words are only *acoustically* similar to the names of the other two pictures. The child must point to the picture that was named accurately. For example, he may hear *seat, fun, money* and simultaneously see the pictures, *feet, sun, money.* The total error score is the total number of items missed on the test.

Need for Tests of Sentence Discrimination. A "similar sentence test" with which we have experimented [28] might more nearly approach the purpose of a discrimination test for young children (4–8 years) by assessing the child's ability to perceive words in contextual speech. As far as we know such a test is not available. We suggest that the special

[26] J. M. Wepman, *Auditory discrimination test, form I, II.* Copyright 1958, Chicago, by J. M. Wepman. Byrne found this test "too gross a measure of discrimination" of children 5–8 years of age.—M. Byrne, Abstract *Asha* (1962), 4: 383. Goetzinger, Dirks, and Baer found no relationship between test scores on the W-22 or Rush-Hughes tests and the Wepman test.—C. Goetzinger, *et al.,* Auditory discrimination and visual perception in good and poor readers. *Ann Otol* (March 1960), 69: 130.

[27] M. J. Mecham and J. L. Jex, *Picture speech discrimination test.* Provo, Utah: Brigham Young University Press, 1962.

[28] The writer is indebted to her student, Mary Scott, Texas Woman's University (Denton) for her collaboration in this test.

language teacher experiment with a technique following this general plan: A small picture (or object if possible) representing the object of the action in one sentence of a series of *morphemically and acoustically similar sentences* is placed before the child along with two pictures eliciting linguistically and acoustically similar expressions. These expressions, however, are not contained in the series of three sentences. The three sentences, uttered with the same prosodic pattern, have been taped. The teacher says to the child:

I want you to listen carefully to each of three sentences, and then I want you to take the picture (or object) named *in one sentence* and do with it what is asked. For example, if you hear, (1) Hand me the trees; (2) hand me the peas; (3) hand me the keys, you will pick up this picture of a basket of peas and hand them to me. Remember that there is a picture (or object) for only one of the sentences.

The *word* being tested in context in each series is italicized; it has been taken from Templin's lists.[29] As far as possible similar morphemes have been employed in each series in order to keep the contextual environment constant. Here are some examples from the series of 60 similar sentences, to be used in testing children's vocabulary of comprehension:

1. Hand me the trees. Hand me the *peas*. Hand me the keys.
2. Point to the bat. Point to the *bag*. Point to the back.
3. Show me the *blocks*. Show me the clocks. Show me the box.
4. Put the one in the box. Put the drum in the box. Put the *gun* in the box.
5. Show me the boat. Show me the *goat*. Show me the coat.
6. Point to the crocks. Point to the clocks. Point to the *blocks*.
7. Put the *string* in the box. Put the swing in the box. Put the spring in the box.
8. Show me the sail. Show me the *pail*. Show me the tail.
9. Show me *thread*. Show me bread. Show me spread.
10. Point to a guy. Point to a *tie*. Point to a pie.

Tests of Vocabulary

The comprehension of word meaning and the ability to name an isolated object or action is not an adequate index to the child's ability to use words in contextual speech. In all but two of the tests in this section only recognition and naming of the objects or pictures are required. They are vocabulary-comprehension tests but they do not assess the child's ability to understand words joined in language sequences or to use them in connected speech. We have included means of appraisal of

[29] M. Templin, *op. cit.*, p. 159.

the child's speaking vocabulary in contextual speech in exploratory studies of several dimensions of language (Chapter 6).

Among the several available measures of vocabulary we shall describe three: *Peabody Picture Vocabulary Test (PPVT); Ammons Full-range Picture Vocabulary Test, Form A;* and the *Vocabulary Definition Test.*

Peabody Picture Vocabulary Test (PPVT).[30] This widely used test of auditory comprehension of words is particularly well adapted to the needs of the teacher of language-handicapped children. It is an untimed test, and the pictures (four on each plate) are bold, simple line drawings. Further advantages are the high interest value of the pictures, speed of administration, objective scoring, and obviation of the need for specialized preparation. In the words of its designer, its purpose is "to provide an estimate of the subject's *verbal intelligence* through measuring his hearing vocabulary." [31] Verbal intelligence has so many aspects that we hesitate to equate its results with intelligence. It probably is neither an intelligence nor a language test, as it is called in some speech centers. It is a good measure of a child's comprehension of word meanings. Each plate is presented in order; the examiner says a word and the child (below 8 years) is directed, "Put your finger on the picture of the word I have just said." The key words to the first 25 plates reflect careful selection of the vocabulary: *car, cow, baby, girl, ball, block, clown, key, can, chicken, blowing, fan, digging, skirt, catching, drum, leaf, tying, fence, bat, bee, bush, pouring, sewing, wiener.* Although one is directed by the manual to begin the test at a level somewhat below the presumed mental age, it becomes a more satisfactory measure of the child's ability to comprehend spoken words if words are identified from the beginning of the scale.[32] The measure is most suitable for children 4.6 years and older but the sample for standardization included children of 2.3 years.

Ammons Full-range Picture Vocabulary Test, Form A. Another popular test, used both as an intelligence and vocabulary comprehension measure, is the Ammons test.[33] It consists of sixteen plates, each containing four cartoon-like drawings. There are 85 stimulus words of increasing difficulty. As the examiner speaks each word, the child indicates by pointing or other signal which of the drawings best fits the given word. Although two forms are available, Form A is better suited to the purpose of *word-identification.* Norms begin with a mental age of 2 years. A selected word list from Form A is contained in Appendix B.

[30] L. Dunn, *Peabody picture vocabulary test:* Minneapolis: American Guidance Service, 1965.

[31] *Ibid.*

[32] R. J. Love, Oral language behavior of cerebral palsied children. *J Speech Hearing Res* (December 1964), 7: 349–362.

[33] R. Ammons and H. Ammons, *Full-range picture vocabulary test, form A.* Missoula, Montana: Psychological Test Specialists, 1958.

Vocabulary Definition Test (Experimental Edition), 5–9 Years.[34] Essentially an extension of the *Peabody Picture Vocabulary Test, Form A,* this is an experimental attempt to appraise the vocabulary that cerebral-palsied children understand and use in connected speech. The child's task is to define 39 words selected from the Peabody test. The test list has been composed by selecting every third word from 1 to 100 and every tenth word from 100 to 150 from the *PPVT* list. The child's task is to define these words (39 in all). The author of the test employs the Terman-Merrill levels of measurement, *viz.,* (1) definition by usage; (2) definition by description; and (3) definition by categorization. The presumption is that if a child can talk about the meaning of a word, even at the lowest level, *viz.,* usage, he is employing the word in his daily speech. Definitions are scored quantitatively and then placed on a qualitative scale.

Appraising Certain Semantic Elements: Verbal Patterning, Comprehension Span, Closure, Retention and Recall

The appraisal of these semantic elements of language has been approached from several vantage points. Normally, contextual language is highly redundant, providing both main and supporting cues to the listener. The child must learn to use cues in several ways. First he must be able to select and relate main cues to supporting cues (verbal patterning of sequential information). Second he must hold cues in a sequence until he comprehends the meaning of the whole (comprehension span). Third he must be able to anticipate the sequence of cues (closure). Finally he must be able to retain the sequence of cues over a period of time (long-term retention). Although we call these cues semantic, we must recognize that insofar as phonological and syntactic learning is good, semantic cues will also be enhanced.

Almost all tests that we shall describe are experimental or exploratory. Their reliability and validity are yet to be established. If we would combine psychological methods and physiological techniques, as Luria suggests,[35] test reliability could be established more quickly. Luria and Vinogradova found by recording vascular reactions of children, for example, that they responded to *semantically similar* words but not to *acoustically similar* words. They hypothesize that this physiological technique can be used to assess the child's ability to make semantic connections. The administration of this test is comparatively simple: "The child has to press with his right hand every time he hears the

---

[34] R. Love, *op. cit.*
[35] A. R. Luria, Study of the abnormal child. *Amer J Orthopsychiat* (January 1961), 31: 1–16.

word, *cat,* and to ignore all different words (in the list of words said to him). . . . The vessel reactions to the test word (registered on the left hand) remain stable." [36] The second step is to record the vascular reactions when semantically related words to *cat* (*dog, mouse, kitten*), are uttered. The vessels respond with a vascular reaction similar to that of the specific test word.

Verbal Patterning of Sequential Information. Many general classification scales employ verbal patterning in testing intelligence of children (p. 278). Subtests in the *Illinois Test of Psycholinguistic Abilities (ITPA)*, to which we have made reference earlier in this chapter, also deal with this aspect of semantic development. *ITPA's Auditory-Vocal Association* subtest, for example, assesses "the ability to relate verbal symbols on a meaningful basis—in this case, by analogy (e.g., *I sit on a chair. I sleep on a _____*). To this end, a sentence completion technique is employed; *S* is required to supply the analogous term." [37]

The following measures must be considered purely exploratory; they represent experimental approaches to more extensive probing of the way a child develops verbal patterning. The task involves the selection and relation of cues in a story generally unfamiliar to children in this country. Both the examiner's and the child's renditions of the story are taped so that additional linguistic features which aid the retention of sequential information—for example, intonation patterns, stress—may be appraised. The essential sequences in this story have been italicized. The examiner notes the number of sequences the child puts into his rendition. He also records other pertinent information such as (1) omission of the setting; (2) illogical and irrelevant additions; (3) omission or distortion of the climax; (4) failure in listening to "suggest" expressive facial patterns; (5) failure to maintain articulatory mimesis of important sequences throughout the listening period; and (6) failure to copy intonational and stress patterns in telling the story.

Test-Story I, 5–7 Years. After gaining the child's rapport, the examiner says:

I want to tell you a story. In fact I am going to tell it to you *twice.* The first time I want you to listen only with your *ears.* The second time you are to listen with your *ears, eyes,* and with your *tongue* and *lips.* After I have told the story twice, I want you to tell it exactly as you remember it. Now hide your eyes and listen ever so hard with your ears. Are you ready? (The examiner tells the story below.) Now I want you to "listen" all *over*—with your ears, eyes, and mouth. Do you know how to listen with your eyes? You watch my face as I tell the story. When you listen with your tongue and lips, you do silently what I do out loud. When I say, for example, "Let's have a race," I want you

[36] *Ibid.,* p. 11.

[37] J. McCarthy and S. Kirk, *Examiners manual, Illinois test of psycholinguistic abilities* (Experimental ed.). Urbana, Ill.: The University of Illinois Press, 1961. P. 39.

to make a small copy of the way I say it *but* without voice. Let's practice the way you listen when I say, "Let's have a race." (The examiner should repeat the practice several times until the child understands what is meant by articulatory and facial mimesis.) Good, now you have the idea. Are you ready with all your listeners? After I have finished, I want you to tell the story exactly the way I have told it.

The Fox and the Crab

A fox and a crab were standing together and *talking. The fox said* to the crab: *"Let's have a race!"* The *crab said,* "Why not? *Let's!"* They began to race. As soon as the fox started, *the crab hung onto the fox's tail. The fox ran to the goal* and still the crab hung on. *The fox turned around to see where the crab was.* He shook his tail and *there was the crab on the ground.* "Well," said the crab, *"I've been waiting here* for *a long time."* [38]

Test-Story II, 7–9 Years. The second story, *The Stork in the Wheat,* is used in measuring comprehension of sequential information of older children. The procedure is the same as for Test I. The critical sequences are longer and more complex.

The Stork in the Wheat

On the other side of the ocean there is *a little country called Denmark.* In the spring the *storks move from their winter home* in Africa to this little country, *Denmark.* They make their nests on roofs of houses very close to the chimney. Well, *one summer when the wheat stood high* in the field, *a stork came to a little village* in Denmark called Mols. But the stork didn't stay near the houses. *Every day he flew off into the wheat field to look for frogs.* The people of Mols didn't like it a bit. They were sure that *the bird would trample down all their fine wheat.* Something must be done! *The men of the village* got together and *decided to ask the Mayor to go into the field and drive out the stork.*

But just as the Mayor was about to walk into the wheat field, one said, "Oh, look, *the Mayor has such big feet he is likely to trample down the wheat* even more than the stork." What to do? They couldn't let the Mayor walk in the wheat and yet he had been appointed to drive out the stork. *Then one of them had a good idea. They would carry the Mayor* and all would be well. His feet would not touch the ground. So *they took a field gate off its hinges, put the Mayor on it,* and *eight men carried him into the wheat field* to chase the stork. And *he did not trample down a single blade of wheat!*[39]

Comprehension Span Test. Rochford and Williams [40] maintain that one can measure the ability to comprehend a series of verbal pat-

---

[38] Adapted from a Russian fairy tale.

[39] Kaj Elle, *Old stories from Denmark.* Ebeltoft, Denmark: Kaj Elle, Ed. and Publ., 1953.

[40] G. Rochford and M. Williams, The measurement of language disorders. *Speech Path Ther,* (April 1964), 7: 5–8.

terns by responses of nonverbal performance. The test material, a series of eight pictures accompanied by verbal commands, is based on material in Gates' *Advanced Primary Reading Test*. The subject is told, "Look at this picture. I am going to tell you something about it. Listen and then do what I say." He is then given a simple command, preceded in the more difficult tests by one or two explanatory sentences. Every word spoken by the examiner has a high frequency of usage, but the commands themselves and the sentences preceding them gradually increase in length and complexity of construction. The memory span required to carry out the command itself remains fairly constant. Age norms for this test are not available. Note is made of the cards to which the subject can respond correctly and the stage at which he either makes no response or an incorrect response. The score equals the number of correct responses made. The test is reproduced on pp. 394–395.

Closure Tests. The average child learns early to predict the sequence of morphemic units. He anticipates, he "perceptualizes" ahead of the verbal flow. Closure reflects, in a sense, his ability to grasp phonological, structural, and semantic relations of language. In attempting to assess closure, test makers have turned frequently to subtests of the Wechsler (WISC) and Stanford-Binet scales. The *Auditory-Vocal Association Test* of *ITPA* (p. 268) also might be called a test of sentence closure. The *Intraverbal Test* of the *Parsons Language Sample* employs sentence completion.[41] Three practice phrases (*bread and butter; soap and water; right and left*) are followed by sentences of this type: (1) We wear shoes and socks on our _____; (2) We go to church on _____; (3) Our flag is red, white, and _____. The child's errors generally are of three types: he repeats the last noun; he makes a farfetched or irrelevant completion; or he uses an acoustically similar word to that which precedes the conclusion. At present we have no comprehensive, reliable test of linguistic closure. An exploratory measure of our own design, which we use with children 4 to 8 years, is composed of the oral presentation of 25 completion sentences (see p. 397).

Retention and Recall. Memory applies to all parameters of language but perhaps the greatest demand is placed on the retention and recall, both long- and short-term, of meaningful contextual speech. No tests are included in this section which make use of the recall of digits, nonsense syllables, or speech sounds in isolation. Certainly it is more useful, as Epstein points out, to "know to what extent (children) are able to repeat utterances of normal language." [42] Meaningful material is

    [41] R. L. Schiefelbusch, *et al.*, Studies of mentally retarded children. *J Speech Hearing Dis* (January 1963), Monogr Suppl, 10: 88.
    [42] A. G. Epstein, Auditory memory span for language. *Folia Phoniat* (1964), 16: 271–289.

easier to learn because it preserves short range associations. The ability to remember is determined by contextual dependencies extending at least over five or six words.[43] Much attention has been given to measures of auditory memory span but in reality any test that is presented orally measures not only auditory memory but several forms of sensory-motor memory. As we stated in Chapter 4, retention and recall depend for their development upon both auditory and tactile-kinesthetic modalities. Such factors as intonational and stress patterns, which are directly dependent upon tactile-kinesthetic perception and feedback, also are important hallmarks of memory. Although memory span continues to mature well beyond 7 years, it is manifested first in the average child between 2.6 and 3.0 years of age.

Of the two processes, retention and recall, the latter is the more important in language comprehension for it is the function of instant recall upon which language depends. The language-retarded child, like the adult aphasic, knows how it feels to be able to "say it too late." Probably because he did not comprehend clearly the sequences as he learned them, he now is unable to retrieve them in order. If retrieval order is confused, oral expression often breaks down. The resulting verbal confusion and dysfluency has been called *articulatory disintegration* by some scholars and *tachyphemia* (cluttering) by others.[44]

As is true of many tests in this chapter, tests of retention and recall bear the clear imprint of *WISC* (Wechsler Intelligence Scale for Children) and the Stanford-Binet Scale. The tests of memory of sentences and passages from these scales have been models for many adaptations.

Word Tests of Recall. Because we believe that memory, both short- and long-term, is largely contextual in nature, we do not place great reliance on the recall of isolated words, words out of context. If such tests have value, it must lie in the assumption that children probably do as well in the recall of contextual material as they do in a word test. In these circumstances it may be an instrument of some value in differential diagnosis.

Word Test I, 7–9 Years.[45] The object of the test is to determine how many words the child can recall from the reading of two lists. List A is read five times, List B but once.

List A: Drum, curtain, bell, coffee, school, parent, moon, garden, hat, farmer, nose, turkey, color, house, river.

[43] G. A. Miller and J. A. Selfridge, Verbal context and the recall of meaningful material. In S. Saporta, Ed., *Psycholinguistics*. New York: Holt, Rinehart and Winston, 1961. P. 204.

[44] G. E. Arnold, *Present concepts of etiologic factors; studies in tachyphemia*. New York: Speech Rehabilitation Institute, 1965. P. 15.

[45] E. Meyer and M. Simmel, The psychological appraisal of children with neurological defects. *J Abnorm Soc Psychol* (April 1947), 42: 193–205.

> *List B:* Desk, ranger, bird, shoe, stove, mountain, glasses, towel, cloud, boat, lamb, gun, pencil, church, fish.

In presenting List A the examiner says:

I am going to read a list of words to you. After I have finished, I want you to say them back to me. Try to listen carefully and to remember as many as you can. You do not need to say them in the order in which I read them. Here I go. Listen carefully.

Read List A clearly and slowly, with intervals of about one second between words. Then say, "Now you go ahead; tell me all the words you can remember." Record all the words the child quotes. If he says a word twice, record it but observe, "You said that one before." Make no comments to words he says that were not in the list. The list is repeated five times. According to Taylor:

norms established on a Swiss population with words equivalent to those listed here show that a normal seven to nine-year-old child may give four to six words after the first reading, eight to twelve words after the third reading, twelve to fourteen words after the fifth reading.[46]

Introducing List B, the examiner says:

Now I am going to read another list of words to you. But this one I am going to read only once; you are not going to learn it as well as you did the other one. Let us just see what words you remember if I read the list just once. You try to get as many as you can, but you know, of course, that you cannot get them all right in one try. Here we go.

Taylor poses other critical questions to the examiner in connection with this test: (1) Does the child begin by repeating the last words which he has heard? (2) Does he start with the first word or pick some words from the list at random? (3) Does he at first give a group of words in quick succession, and slow down later, as is common, or does he start almost immediately to grope for words to repeat? (4) Is he inclined to say them in the order in which they were read, or is any other specific order apparent, as for instance, the order of association (*farmer-turkey, school-bell*)? (5) Does he give only words from the list, or does he make substitutions or additions? (6) Does he say the same word twice, does he check such an impulse, or practice the necessary self-control only mentally?

Word Test II, 8–9 Years.[47] The *Word-pair subtests* 3 and 4 of the *Hunt-Minnesota Test* appraise recall and may be adapted for use with children. The examiner says:

[46] E. M. Taylor, *Psychological appraisal of children with cerebral defects.* Cambridge: Harvard, 1961. P. 426.
[47] H. F. Hunt, *The Hunt-Minnesota test for organic brain damage.* Beverly Hills, Calif.: Western Psychological Services, 1943.

I am going to read ten pairs of words, and I want you to do your best to learn and to remember which words you hear together. Then, later on when I say the *first word in each pair,* you are to tell me as quickly as you can the word that I read with it. For instance, if I say *cat-dog,* when I say *cat* later on you will say *dog.* We will go over the list *two times.* Listen carefully and do your best to learn and to remember which words you have heard together so that later on when I say the first word in each pair, you will be able to tell me the word I said with it.

The ten word-pairs are:

1. pin-key	6. house-cloud
2. hat-smile	7. tire-shoe
3. sun-rock	8. chair-food
4. watch-wheel	9. page-ink
5. door-brass	10. boy-tooth

After reading the list at a rate of five seconds per pair, the examiner says, "Now I want you to tell me the word I said with *pin.*" The examiner continues with the list, timing and recording the correct responses. Plurals and mispronunciations are considered correct. Subtest 4 is administered in the same way except that the stimulus order is changed. The tests are scored by multiplying the number of checks for correct responses by the time credits at the bottom of the column (on the record form) and adding the products.

This section is incomplete because objective measurement of the semantic dimension of language has just begun. In the preceding chapter, ways to evaluate informally such important dimensions of language learning as the decline of egocentric speech and the development of inner language, categorization and elaboration of percepts, and recall of contextual language have been described. It is regrettable that no report of reliable tests of these factors of language learning can be given.

Tests of Articulation

Assessment of the motor synergies producing voice—respiration, phonation, and resonation—are treated extensively in texts of voice science and need not concern us here. If there were a valid test of speech melody it would be included here. Articulatory competence is undoubtedly dependent both on syntactic form and prosody. Articulation is not an isolated bit of speech mechanics divorced from the total linguistic process. Indeed its determinants are mainly those which also shape language proficiency, *viz.,* (1) the accurate perception and recall of gestalten, (2) control and integration of feedback, and (3) adequate and sustained projections of fine movement patterns in the peripheral speech mechanism.

The market abounds in articulation tests. We describe only three: Hejna's *Developmental Test of Articulation*,[48] *The Templin-Darley Tests of Articulation*,[49] and *A Deep Test of Articulation* by McDonald.[50] Both Hejna's and Templin and Darley's measures elicit words and/or sentences either spontaneously in response to pictures or as replication of the model. McDonald also utilizes pictures and sentences but employs a unique method known as *deep testing*.

Hejna's *Developmental Test of Articulation, 3.6–7.6 Years.* This test consists of a series of 37 plates of pictures. Three stimulus pictures on each plate call for the production of the sound, in initial, medial, and final positions, respectively.[51] On the left margin of the score sheet appears the age at which each phoneme should be stabilized in the child's speech. The score sheet (Appendix B) suggests the order of presentation of the stimulus pictures. De Hirsch, *et al.*,[52] would supplement Hejna's test with the analysis by three "experts" of tape recordings of a story told by the child. The subsequent comparison between the child's articulation of single words and of connected speech probably provides a better appraisal of his resistance to articulatory disintegration in contextual speech.

The Templin-Darley Tests of Articulation, 3–8 Years. There are 176 items in the diagnostic picture test, 50 of which may be used as a screening test. The line drawings are clear but, as in all other tests of this type, the figures are not drawn to scale. In Plate 17, for example, the cat is somewhat bigger than a child's bed. The baby in Plate 26 is too large to fit into the adult bath tub. The problem may be insoluble but since visual perception of space frequently is distorted in language-retarded children, they may have unusual difficulty in accurately perceiving several pictured objects on a single plate which are unrelated in size. The test is carefully constructed and provides established age norms.

The sound elements tested include 25 different consonant sounds, 12 vowels, and 6 diphthongs. These elements are distributed among eight sound classifications as follows:

1. 12 vowels
2. 6 diphthongs

[48] R. Hejna, *Developmental articulation test.* Storrs, Conn.: R. Hejna, 1955.
[49] M. Templin and F. Darley, *The Templin-Darley tests of articulation.* Iowa City: Bureau of Educ. Res. State University of Iowa, 1960.
[50] E. McDonald, *A deep test of articulation* (picture and sentence forms). Pittsburgh: Stanwix House, 1964.
[51] Exceptions: [ʒ] and [ŋ] are presented only in the medial position; [ð] and [w] in initial and medial position; [h] in initial position only.
[52] K. de Hirsch, J. Jansky, and W. Langford, Oral language performance of two groups of immature children. *Folia Phoniat* (1964) 16: 109–122.

3. 68 single consonants in the initial, medial and final positions
4. 37 two-consonant blends
5. 23 combinations of a consonant with the syllabic or nonsyllabic vowel [ɚ]
6. 14 blends of a consonant with the syllabic or nonsyllabic vowel [l]
7. 7 blends of two consonants together with [ɝ], [ɚ] and the vowel [l]
8. 9 three-consonant blends [53]

The child is first induced to say a series of single words, each containing a test sound or group of sounds in a specified position. As the examiner shows the child each picture he has the choice of (1) attempting to elicit the desired test word spontaneously by asking him to name the object pictured or to complete a sentence requiring the use of the word, or (2) saying the test word and having the child repeat it after him. Subsequently for each sound. misarticulated, the child is given a clear auditory pattern of the sound in isolation, in a syllable, and in a word, and is asked to imitate this exercise. Finally an evaluation is made of the child's intelligibility in conversational speech.

Scoring. The table of norms, which represents the mean scores on 176 items, is included in Appendix B. The examiner counts the test sounds correctly produced. The total is then compared with the norm table in order to find the mean number of items produced by children of the age and sex of the subject. In this way the examiner may determine whether the articulation skill of a child is average, accelerated, or retarded in relation to that of his age peers.

A Deep Test of Articulation (Picture and Sentence Forms) by McDonald.[54] In an earlier chapter we discussed the sensory-motor approach to oral language and developed the concept of the syllable as a series of overlapping ballistic movements of the articulatory organs (p. 116). McDonald's test is predicated on this concept of the syllable as the basic unit in the coding process. The picture form that we describe here is used in testing children below third grade reading level. In order to evaluate a speech sound as an audible end product of these syllabic movement patterns, pairs of pictures are named as connected syllables. Having learned beforehand the most frequently misarticulated sounds in the child's speech, the language teacher proceeds to "deep test" these sounds. He demonstrates first how to name pairs of pictures in connected syllables as *tubvase, tubsheep, teethsheep*. After the child has practiced naming pictures in this way the teacher turns to the picture that ends with the sound he wants to deep test, for example /s/, and by linking pairs of pictures he assesses the child's ability to produce the s-sound in

[53] M. Templin and F. Darley, *The Templin-Darley tests of articulation*. Iowa City: Bureau of Educ. Res. State University of Iowa, 1960. P. 2.
[54] E. McDonald, *A deep test of articulation* (picture and sentence forms). Pittsburgh: Stanwix House, 1964.

fundamental phonetic contexts. During the test the teacher hopefully has identified correctly articulated phonetic contexts; if so, he will begin enforcement of the sound in these contexts. The method of determining the percent of correct articulations appears on the score sheet which is included in Appendix B.

8

Testing Abilities Associated With
Language Learning

By this time the student must appreciate the need to explore all behaviors linked, directly or indirectly, with verbal behavior. Some behaviors can be easily tested and judged in terms of normative developmental schedules. General mental ability is such a one; social maturity is another. Both can be assessed developmentally. In other areas our purpose is diagnostic, i.e., we are locating areas of deficit or dysfunction and attempting to assess the degree of deviation and its effect on specific parameters of language learning. So throughout the assessment we must keep in mind an either-or question: Does this child function at a generally lower level, or is the *patterning* of function different? Are the child's difficulties apparent in atypical melodic qualities of his speech, in his perception of sequential units of speech, or in his comprehension-use of syntactic structure? If the pattern deviates, we may find few reliable objective tests to help us. Exploratory measures must then be undertaken if we are to probe further into these problems. They may be very crude instruments but in the hands of a skillful clinical teacher who goes searching, they will give him productive clues, if not definite information. In some instances the teacher will use exploratory techniques in order to compare the progress of two groups that have been taught by different methods. If exploratory techniques unlock a door to the diagnosis or to an effective method of teaching, their value will have been demonstrated. Although exploratory testing techniques may run counter to prevailing practices in some institutions in the United

States, our foreign colleagues hold a divergent view. The use to which they put exploratory techniques is explained in their books.[1]

Some language clinicians or teachers are trained to administer all tests described in this chapter. Others may be equipped to give certain measures designed to locate special perceptual or motor or personality disturbances. Still others must rely entirely on the assistance of clinical psychologists. Projective techniques employed in evaluating personality problems, for example, are dangerous instruments in the hands of the un-skilled. Yet even if the special language teacher or clinician is not able to administer the test, he must have knowledge of these measures. He must understand standardized scales and projective techniques in order to in-terpret and use reports of the psychometrician and the clinical psy-chologist. He also needs to be able to communicate directly with the scientists upon whom he must call for help. If he cannot speak their language, communication shortly reaches a dead end. And certainly if he does not understand the purpose and scope of the tests, he will not be able to use their results. The psychologist's report then becomes a sifter of semantic quicksand. The task encompassed in this chapter is to evaluate facets of behavior that may bear, directly or indirectly, upon the child's language problem. In order to realize this goal, the special language teacher or clinician may become the Academy's best borrower, both for information and professional assistance of other personnel.

This chapter is concerned with tests of (1) general mental ability (general classification scales) both for infants and children 2–8 years of age; (2) perception of nonverbal stimuli (visuomotor, motokinesthetic, and auditory); (3) motor development and skills; and (4) socioemotional maturation and adjustment.

General Classification Scales (*Mental Ability*)

The tests of the development in infants of mental ability are less reliable, perhaps, than standardized scales for older children, but they may be even more important in assessing the language problems of the child. We shall describe two infant scales, the *California First-Year Mental Scale* and the *Cattell Infant Intelligence Scale;* and five widely accepted tests of general mental ability. They are the *Stanford-Binet Intelligence Scale (Form L-M), Arthur Adaptation of the Leiter Inter-*

---

[1] A. R. Luria and F. Ia. Yudovich, *Speech and the development of mental processes in the child.* London: Staples, 1959; A. R. Luria, *The role of speech in the regulation of normal and abnormal behavior.* New York: Liveright, 1961; A. R. Luria, *Higher cortical functions in man.* New York: Basic Books Inc., Publishers, 1966; J. Piaget, *The language and thought of the child.* London: Routledge, 1959; J. L. J. Abercrombie, *Perceptual and visuomotor disorders in cerebral palsy.* London: Heine-mann, 1964; R. Brain, *Speech disorders.* Washington: Butterworths, 1961.

national Performance Scale, Goodenough-Harris Drawing Test, Raven's Progressive Matrices Test, and the *Wechsler Intelligence Scale for Children (WISC).*

Infant Scales of Mental Development

The language clinician in a hospital center has frequent need of the psychologist's services in assessing the general mental abilities of very young children who have not begun to talk. Among the objective measures are the *California First-Year Mental Scale* (1–18 months)[2] and the *Cattell Infant Intelligence Scale* (2–30 months).[3] Both scales borrow heavily from the Yale developmental schedules but may be considered superior to them in that a mental age can be computed by finding the age equivalent of each item. A precise quotient cannot be found since the *SD* of mental ages does not increase proportionately with age.

Both tests are untimed and similar in composition. They both should be given serially by the psychologist over a period of weeks. They cover such things as postural and motor development, perception, attention to objects and to persons, vocalization, manipulation of objects, understanding simple language, naming objects, and solving simple form boards. In Appendix C may be found selected items of the California Scale.

Tests of General Mental Ability, 2.6–8 Years

Some of these tests extend in both directions beyond the age limits suggested here but we shall limit our description to the age range 2.6 to 8 years.

Stanford-Binet Intelligence Scale (Form L-M). Despite the fact that Cruickshank, *et al.,* adopted this test as the instrument for evaluating intelligence "in brain injured and hyperactive children," [4] we question its validity in evaluating general mental maturation in language-handicapped children. Success in this test is posited largely upon the comprehension and use of language, and hence this group of children enters the race with staggering, unposted handicaps. Moreover we need information from tests that assess more carefully than the Binet test purports to do the very young child's mental potential. Comprehension of verbal directions in the Binet test is a further handicap for children with delay or disturbance in language.

[2] N. Bayley, *The California first-year mental scale.* Berkeley: University of California Press, Syllabus Series, 1933, No. 243.

[3] P. Cattell, *The measurement of intelligence of infants and young children.* New York: The Psychological Corporation, 1947.

[4] W. M. Cruickshank, *et al., A teaching method for brain-injured and hyperactive children.* Syracuse, N. Y.: Syracuse University Press, 1961. Pp. 258–262.

Here are subtests that bear directly on specific dimensions of language learning:

Year II.   Visuomotor perception: Three-hole form board.
            Visuomotor perception; spatial relations: Block building (tower).
            Auditory perception; short-term memory of sequences: Repeating two digits.
Year III.   Visuomotor perception and motor skill: Stringing beads.
            Perception of spatial relations; motor skill (direction and form): Copying a circle.
            Visual discrimination of spatial relations: Patience pictures.
            Visual discrimination; motor skill: Sorting buttons.
Year IV.   Visual perception and memory storage: Pictorial identification.
            Visual discrimination of form: Discrimination of forms.
Year V.   Visual perception; closure; body image: Picture completion.
            Visuomotor perception; form; direction; spatial relationships: Copying a square, paper folding.
Year VI.   Visuomotor perception; motor skill, closure, body image: Mutilated pictures, maze tracing.
Year VII.   Visuomotor perception; spatial relations: Copying a diamond.[5]

The *Arthur Adaptation of the Leiter International Performance Scale*[6] is completely nonverbal and therefore commends itself as an instrument adapted to the language handicapped. It is also superior to many tests in that it covers a wide range of function, roughly analogous to those found in verbal scales. Because the test has no time limit and can be modified to meet the needs of many types of handicapped children the results are useful and reliable. The scale is scored in terms of mental age and an IQ ratio. Critics point out that there is no assurance that such an IQ retains the same meaning at different age levels. It remains, however, a truly cross-cultural test and a reliable tool of assessment of mental ability. Its administration is particularly adapted to the child handicapped in language because there is no need for instructions either spoken or pantomimic. Each test begins with a very easy task of the type to be encountered throughout the test. The initial task, once comprehended, obviates the need for instruction. The material consists of a wood frame into which is fitted the card containing pictures or designs which form the basis for matching. The subject chooses the blocks containing the proper response pictures and inserts them into the frame. The tests for the age levels in which we are interested are presented in order:

[5] *Stanford-Binet intelligence scale (form L-M)*. Boston: Houghton Mifflin, 1960.
[6] G. Arthur, *The Arthur adaptation of the Leiter international performance scale*. Washington: Psychological Service Center Press, 1952.

Year II (three months each)
1. Matching colors (present one block at a time).
2. Block design (present one block at a time).
3. Matching pictures (present one block at a time).
4. Matching circles and squares (present one block at a time).

Year III (three months each)
1. Four forms (present one block at a time).
2. Block design.
3. Picture completion (demonstrate first notch).
4. Number discrimination (one to three forms; a demonstration follows each failure).

Year IV (three months each)
1. Form and color.
2. Eight forms (present one block at a time).
3. Counts four (two of three forms).
4. Form, color, number.

Year V (three months each)
1. Genus.
2. Two color circles (colors only correct).
3. Clothing.
4. Block design (colors only).

Year VI (three months each)
1. Analogous progression.
2. Pattern completion test (demonstrate Form A; correlations allowed on marked notches in Form A).
3. Matching on a basis of use.
4. Block design.

Year VII (three months each)
1. Reconstruction (demonstrate signs).
2. Circle series.
3. Circumference series.
4. Recognition of age differences.

Year VIII (three months each)
1. Matching shades of gray.
2. Form discrimination.
3. Judging mass (two or three forms).
4. Series of radii.

Year IX (three months each)
1. Dot estimation.
2. Analogous designs.
3. Block design (angles $\angle$).
4. Line completion (demonstrate first notch).

Goodenough-Harris Drawing Test.[7]   This test assesses particular components of intelligence, notably accuracy of visuomotor perception and spatial aptitude. Its score, however, is not identical with the IQ derived from an individual intelligence test. Its value lies in the discovery of such specific aspects of visuomotor and spatial retardation as form, directional orientation, and body image. Three pictures are to be drawn: a man, woman, and a self-picture. The directions are simple:

I am going to ask you to make three pictures for me today. You will make them one at a time. On the first page, I want you to make a picture of a man. Make the very best picture that you can; take your time and work very carefully. Try very hard, and see what good pictures you can make. Be sure to make the whole man, not just his head and shoulders.

After drawing each picture, the child is praised and given a rest period. No suggestions or adverse criticisms are to be made. The test is followed by informal questions to determine the child's intentions and to clarify any ambiguous aspects of the drawings. The manual provides illustrative drawings and detailed descriptions of each item to be scored in each picture, but as Harris states, "While almost any adult can learn to score drawings with reasonable accuracy, psychological training is necessary to adequately understand the results."[8] *The Short Scoring Guide for the Woman Point Scale* is included in Appendix C. Tables converting raw scores to standard scores are included in the manual, both for the Point and Quality scales.

The reliability of the test on a test-retest basis has not been generally questioned although drawbacks have been found which seem to suggest possible reservations. It is neither a culture-free nor class-free test, and this limits its usefulness as a measure of intellectual maturity. In low socioeconomic groups in the Middle West, it was found that children in the Head Start programs had almost no previous experience in using either paper or crayons or in viewing picture books in which they might see simple line-drawings of people. Emotional attitudes in other children affected adversely their scores. Rapport and motivation assume unusual importance in this test. A shy, withdrawn child, uncomfortable in such a task, usually penalizes himself unduly. The test also has been used for special purposes. Bender, for example, believes that a low score on this test, two years or more below the Binet MA, is suggestive of CNS injury.[9]

Raven's Progressive Matrices Test.[10]   This measure, developed by J. C. Raven, director of psychological research at Crichton Royal Hospi-

[7] D. B. Harris, *Goodenough-Harris drawing test manual.* New York: Harcourt, Brace & World, 1963.
[8] *Ibid.,* p. 246.
[9] L. Bender, Psychological problems of children with organic brain disease. *Amer J Orthopsychiat* (July 1949), 19: 404–415.
[10] J. C. Raven, *Psychological principles appropriate to social and clinical problems.* London: H. K. Lewis, 1966. Pp. 55–57.

tal, London, was developed to assess these mental functions: (1) a person's capacity for orderly thinking, (2) his recall of information acquired as the result of past experience, and (3) the psychological significance of any discrepancies between his recall of information and his capacity for orderly thinking. In essence the test is designed to measure the individual's capacity for coherent perception and orderly judgment.

The *Standard Scale* consists of five sets of twelve problems, abstract designs, from each of which a part has been removed. The items are grouped into five series, each containing twelve matrices of increasing difficulty but similar in principle. The *Coloured Progressive Matrices Scale, Sets A, Ab, B* are adapted specifically to the assessment of the intellectual processes of normal young children and mentally retarded persons. Successful completion of *Set A* depends upon a person's ability to complete continuous patterns which, toward the end of the set, change first in one and later in two directions simultaneously. In *Set Ab* the child must be able to discriminate discrete figures as spatially related wholes, and to choose a figure which completes the missing part. *Set B* contains problems involving analogies and hence is concerned with the child's ability to think abstractly.

The *board form*, in color, of this test commends itself particularly to very young children. In contrast to the book form, the board form requires the subject to insert the right piece rather than choose the correct completion. Moreover, if the child is orthopedically handicapped, he may, when responding, use any form of signaling of which he is capable. There is no time limit. It becomes, therefore, a very useful and adaptable measure for children who have motoric as well as language handicaps.

In order to test the child's recall of information acquired as the result of intellectual activity, Raven would combine the use of the Matrices Scale with the *Mill Hill Vocabulary Scale*. Like other vocabulary tests it is constructed to span the range of verbal development from infancy to maturity.

The norms for the board form of the *Coloured Progressive Matrices Scale* are included in Appendix C, but Raven makes clear that:

the use of age norms for the quantitative assessment of general mental development and the calculation of IQs is always questionable. The most one can legitimately hope to do is to compare a child's behaviour with the behaviour of other children of the same age, and to assess his performance in terms of the frequency with which a similar performance is observed amongst other children of his age. Nevertheless all such quantitative comparisons rest ultimately upon the psychologist's ability to distinguish certain qualitative differences in the performance compared.[11]

[11] J. C. Raven, *Guide to using the coloured progressive matrices* (sets A, Ab, B). London: H. K. Lewis, 1960.

The Wechsler Intelligence Scale for Children (WISC) (Performance Section). Intelligence, according to Wechsler, is the capacity of the individual to act purposefully, to think rationally, and to deal effectively with his environment. Intelligence, in his view, is global and subsumes personality.[12] In the construction of *WISC* it is apparent that he has been successful in developing such a concept. *WISC*, in its entirety, consists of ten subtests (and two alternates) divided into the subgroups *verbal* and *performance*. The IQ on performance can be derived separately and by translation of the raw score to a scaled score can be established for each age. Wechsler uses the traditional classification for intelligence (Table 8-1).

Table 8-1.

IQ	Classification	Percent Included
130 and above	Very superior	2.2
120-129	Superior	6.7
110-119	Bright normal	16.1
90-109	Average	50.0
80-89	Dull normal	16.1
70-79	Borderline	6.7
69 and below	Mental defective	2.2

SOURCE: D. Wechsler, *WISC manual.* Reproduced by permission. Copyright © 1949, The Psychological Corporation, New York, N.Y. All rights reserved.

The performance items are more useful in diagnosing linguistically handicapped children but one understands more clearly the global nature of the measure by noting the sweep both in the verbal and performance sections. In the verbal section the tests include (1) general information, (2) general comprehension, (3) arithmetic, (4) similarities, and (5) vocabulary. In the performance section, the subtests involve (1) picture completion, (2) picture arrangement, (3) block design, (4) object assembly, and (5) coding or mazes. The tests cover nearly all the discriminative and integrative functions associated with intelligence. In picture completion, a child must exercise visual discrimination, recall, and closure if he, for example, is to identify the missing spokes in an umbrella or the empty mercury bulb of a thermometer. Picture arrangement (cut-up pictures of dog, mother, train) demands accurate perception of the meaning of the figure, spatial relations, form, direction, and motoric skill. Block design requires all these aspects of intelligence plus discrimination, depth perception, and perceptual-motor proficiency. Object assembly is made up of a manikin (favored by all test makers), horse, face, and car. In the final subtest in this section, coding (or mazes), atten-

[12] B. A. Maher, Intelligence and brain damage. In N. R. Ellis, Ed., *Handbook of mental deficiency.* New York: McGraw-Hill, 1963. P. 232.

tion, spatial relations, reasoning involving analogy, and recall are all being assessed.

As one would expect, there is a greater tendency for rural children and children from lower socioeconomic groups to obtain higher scores on the performance than on the verbal scale. The test has been carefully standardized, and the established norms have won general acceptance. Because it is a timed test it poses a special problem for the child afflicted with perceptual-motor problems. Yet in itself this discovery of areas of deficit should be helpful in diagnostic teaching.

Tests of Perception of Nonverbal Stimuli

In our study of neural integration mediating perception we found no evidence of a separation of modalities, and conversely much evidence that visuomotor, auditomotor, and motokinesthetic systems operate as a unit in the CNS in mediating perception (pp. 97–105). Further confirmation comes from those workers in the field who find that many dysphasic children also are dyslexic.

Because perception is a unit, it is difficult to analyze its components. The tests purporting to assess visual perception, with the possible exception of the Columbia Scale (p. 288), really involve visuomotor tasks. If coding is unitary, then a disturbance or deficit must also be unitary in its effect. Of course it may strike certain systems more forcefully than others but all will bear some effect. A correlative question is the relation between verbal and nonverbal behavior. We believe that diminution or disturbance of synaptic power is not specific either with respect to modality or the dimension of behavior. Just as a child who recognizes only dimly the correct spatial relations of a design may not be able to execute it, so a language-retarded or language-different child may not be able to reproduce the correct articulatory form of a sentence although he may have some fuzzy perception of its spatial relations.

Visuomotor Perception

One day it may be possible to develop age norms for all perceptual processes, thus distinguishing perceptual deficits arising from developmental lag and those caused by injury to the CNS. Visuomotor perception is one area in which we have some normative data. Present studies are focused on such aspects of perception as eye-motor coordination, constancy of form, spatial relations, closure, and figure-ground perception. At first blush it might seem that visuomotor abilities pertain only to reading, but we know that the baby learning oral language depends heavily on *speech as he sees it,* on the visuomotor patterns (p. 54). If his eye movements are not well directed (eye-motor coordination), or if he cannot distinguish movement patterns of sounds in sequence (figure-ground), or if he confuses the order of sounds and syllables (spatial relations), we suspect that visuomotor perception is one area of deficit. The special language teacher usually is familiar with the materials used in assessing visuomotor perception—wood blocks, form and marble boards, paper and pencil designs, and objects or pictures for matching.

Developmental Test of Visual Perception, 4–8 Years. This test [13] seeks to measure five operationally defined perceptual skills: eye-motor coordination, figure-ground perception, form constancy, position in space, and spatial relationships. The child's raw score for each subtest may be translated into a perceptual age equivalent. The perceptual quotient then is a deviation score obtained from the sum of the subtest scale scores after correction for age variation. The percentiles for each age group are constant, with a median of 100, upper and lower quartiles of 110 and 90 respectively, and other percentile ranks consistent with IQ values of *WISC.* Perhaps even more important than the perceptual quotient is the opportunity to define more precisely the nature of a child's perceptual difficulties and to measure their severity.

The task in the *Eye-Motor Coordination* subtest is to draw continuous, straight, curved, or angled lines between boundaries of various widths, or from point to point, without guide lines. Spatial position and spatial relations are assessed in subtests IV and V. In subtest IV, *Position in Space,* the subject picks from five figures the one that is differently oriented from the other four, or from four figures the one that matches the test figure. In subtest V, *Spatial Relations* (Figures C-1 and C-2 on p. 402), the child analyzes simple forms and patterns. On the left hand side of the page is a line pattern drawn over dot guide-points. The child makes the same pattern on the right hand side using the dots as guide-points.[14]

Constancy of Form. The simplest test serving this purpose in visuomotor perception is the form board employed with children from 2 to 8 years. At the 2-year level, the blocks are a square, circle, and triangle. If the child does not start at once after the demonstration, he is handed the round block and asked, "Where does this one go?" He must be successful in one of two trials in order to score. The *Seguin Board* consists of ten geometric forms; after stacking them the examiner tells the child to put them back as quickly as he can. His score is the

[13] M. Frostig, *et al., Developmental test of visual perception; administration and scoring manual.* Chicago: Follett, 1964. P. 5.

[14] Ayres also has standardized a performance test for children, 3–10 years, which purports to measure perceptual deficits in spatial ability, perceptual speed, directionality or position in space. A. J. Ayres, *Ayres space test.* Los Angeles: Western Psychological Services, 1965.

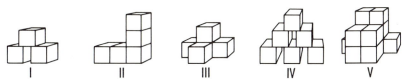

Figure 8-1. Block patterns.

SOURCE: M. S. Hiskey, *Hiskey-Nebraska test of learning aptitude.* Lincoln, Nebr.: University of Nebraska, 1966.

shortest time period in three trials. As Wood has pointed out,[15] the form board gives the examiner an opportunity to study many facets of the child's behavior. He observes trial and error placement, persistence in unsuccessful trials by pounding and forcing blocks, change in attack, resistance to help, the exclusive use of the left hand during performance, incessant turning of inserts before placement in recesses, a need to fit pieces together before placement, and the amount and kind of vocalization employed by the child while working.

Spatial Relations: Other Tests. Many visuomotor tests seeking to assess spatial relations are adaptations of Kohs' Blocks[16] (p. 403) and call for the reproduction of two-dimensional designs. Different colored blocks must be assembled so that their top surfaces make a colored pattern to match a diagram. The difficulty increases with the number of blocks, complexity of pattern, and degree of similarity of the diagram to the construction. Block patterns used in the *Hiskey-Nebraska Test of Learning Aptitude* are reproduced in Figure 8-1. Block pattern I falls at the 4.0-year level, pattern II at 5.0, pattern III at 5.6, pattern IV at 7.0, and pattern V at the 8.0 level.[17] Bortner and Birch[18] have explored the difference between visual and visuomotor perception in block designs. They found that some children could recognize the correct design among a group of designs but could not reproduce it. A *WISC* stimulus card as test item and three block designs as multiple-choice items were presented as a perceptual test to subjects who had failed to make a correct construction from the stimulus card. One block design was a correct construction of the stimulus card pattern, one a copy of the subject's incorrect construction, and the third a different incorrect construction. Subjects were asked to choose the construction that looked like the design

[15] N. W. Wood, *Communication problems and their effect on the learning potential of the mentally retarded child.* Cleveland: Western Reserve University, 1960. P. 40.

[16] S. C. Kohs, *Intelligence measurement.* New York: Macmillan, 1923. Pp. 66–67.

[17] M. S. Hiskey, *Hiskey-Nebraska test of learning aptitude.* Lincoln, Nebr.: M. S. Hiskey, Ph.D., University of Nebraska, 1966.

[18] M. Bortner and H. G. Birch, Perceptual and perceptual-motor dissociation in cerebral palsied children. *J Nerv Ment Dis* (February 1962), 134: 103–108.

on the card. Here the test object is a diagram of the actual object which is to be sought in the multiple choice set. We have reservations about this test because we believe that choosing the correct design from among several requires less perceptual power than production of a design from a model. Had the perception been clearer, would not the child have been able to produce the design?

The *Columbia Mental Maturity Scale* [19] is frequently employed, not as a measure of mental ability but as an exploratory technique to assess form constancy and spatial relations in visual perception. Designed for cerebral-palsied children, 3 to 12 years of age, it is particularly well adapted to the linguistically and/or motorically handicapped child. It does not require a specific motor response. The child identifies the drawing that "does not belong with the others" by any signal at his command. The test comprises 100 items, each consisting of a set of three, four or five varicolored drawings printed on a 6×19 inch card. The task involves only one dimension, the visual perception of similarities and differences. Categorization of the drawings is based on color, size, and form. The score is obtained from each subject by counting the number of correct responses. It can be converted to a mental age, which might more accurately be called a developmental quotient of visual perception. A score of 30, for example, gives a "mental age" of 53 months; a score of 40, 59 months; a score of 80, 120 months.

Closure. A defect of closure, whether it is in the visual or auditory field, is reflected in the individual's inability to perceive readily the elements that go into the completion of a percept. Its neurological correlate may be an impairment of the mechanism of facilitation and inhibition (pp. 36, 75). A rudimentary appraisal of closure in the visual perceptual field can be made by employing three widely used psychological measures. The *Healy Picture Completion Test I* [20] is a rural scene from which ten squares have been cut (see Figure C-4, p. 404). The child selects the square that best completes each part of the picture from a large array of pieces and puts it in the proper place. A second measure is the completion of drawings from the *Hiskey-Nebraska Test of Learning Aptitude* [21] (Figure C-5, pp. 405–406). It is designed for children from 4–10 years but the subtest is more appropriate for children from 6–10 years. A third measure is the jigsaw puzzle-type test that appears in several general classification scales. The form of a man, horse, face, or car, made of thin wood, is cut into pieces. In order to assemble the pieces the child must have a visual percept of the completed figure. Scores are

[19] *Columbia mental maturity scale* (1959 Revision). Copyright 1959, 1954 by Harcourt, Brace & World, Inc., New York.

[20] *Healy picture completion test I,* from Pintner-Paterson performance scale. Chicago: C. H. Stoelting, 1917.

[21] M. S. Hiskey, *op. cit.*

computed on the basis of elapsed time. Abercrombie [22] finds this test useful in studying deficits both in spatial position and closure in cerebral palsied children. Samples of her results are included in Figure C-6 on p. 407.

Figure-Ground. Among the many tests for probing the child's stability in differentiating figure and ground are two standardized tests: *Southern California Figure-Ground Visual Perception Test* [23] and Subtest II of Frostig's *Developmental Test of Visual Perception.* [24] A *Marble-Board Test* and *Mixed Figure Tests*, exploratory measures, are described in Appendix C and illustrated in Figures C-7 to C-11 (pp. 408–410).

The Southern California Test by Ayres, designed for children from 5–11 years, is comprised of two series of figure-ground designs. The examiner directs the child's attention first to the *multiple-choice plate* on which there are nine line drawings of common objects or forms, and then to the embedded plate of three objects (or forms). The child is asked to find the three objects (or forms) in the *multiple-choice plate*. A trial plate from the test is reproduced in Figure C-12 on p. 411.

Frostig's task also demands shifts in perception of figures against increasingly complex grounds. Intersecting and "hidden" geometric forms are used. The child is told, for example, to outline an intersecting figure or figures on a structured background. In the items reproduced in Figure C-13, on p. 412, the child outlines two stars in the first figure; in the second, the kites.

Tactile-Kinesthetic Perception

Tactile-kinesthetic modalities cannot be separated easily from other modalities for assessment. Their *modus operandi* is feedback and hence they operate in conjunction with other systems. Tests of discrete function that exclude vision and audition are hard to come by. All visuomotor tests also involve kinesthesis. Motor skills tests similarly are dependent on this form of feedback.

In the literature, tests of two-point discrimination are frequently described, but they are difficult to administer and their results inconclusive. Application of stimulus points by electronic means is not advisable because it produces undue apprehension and fear in children. One can stimulate the child's lips, tongue, and facial muscles with bristles, wood picks, ice, and chalk, thereby gaining some concept of responsiveness in these areas, but they are gross measures. Tests of stereognosis

[22] M. L. J. Abercrombie, *Perceptual visuo-motor disorders in cerebal palsy.* London: Heinemann, 1964. Pp. 1–19.

[23] A. J. Ayres, *Southern California figure-ground visual perception test.* Los Angeles: Western Psychological Services, 1965.

[24] M. Frostig, *et al., Developmental test of visual perception: Administration and scoring manual.* Chicago: Follett, 1964. P. 5.

(p. 118) are still in an embryonic stage of development but have promise. Several tests employing other muscle sets, however, are being used in the study of perceptual deficits in children handicapped by CNS injury or deficit. Two standardized measures of haptic perception are the *Southern California Kinesthesia and Tactile Perception Tests* by Ayres [25] and Werner's *Tactile Figure Background Blocks*.[26]

Ayres' test consists of a battery of six tests to evaluate dysfunction in somesthetic perception of children ranging in age from 4 years to 8 years. It includes tests of kinesthesia, manual form perception, figure identification, and double tactile stimuli perception. Werner uses three basic patterns in testing small children: rectangle, triangle, and oval in two sets. They are presented in a shadow box to the child who follows the outline with his fingers and then draws the pattern. Set 1 consists of a background of flat enameled thumbtacks with the patterns made of hemispherical upholsterer's tacks. Set 2 presents a plain background with the patterns made of 4/0 finishing sandpaper and mounted on smooth cardboard. The test should be completed successfully by a child, 7 to 8 years of age. Talbott [27] points out that the examiner may learn much about the child by reporting his mode of operation in the test. In her experimental group the children's movements were nonpurposive and disorganized; in the control group they searched the board methodically, exhibiting few random and repetitive movements which were characteristic of the experimental group.

Cross modality matching is a technique employed by Abercrombie and others in the tactile-kinesthetic appraisal of cerebral-palsied children.[28] A description and illustration of Abercrombie's test is contained in Appendix C.

Auditory Perception

It is relatively easy to find measures that assess visual perception, less easy to find reliable tests of auditory perception of *verbal sequences,* and difficult indeed to locate a single objective measure of nonverbal stimuli. Perhaps we do not have such tests because discrimination of nonverbal stimuli is poor, so poor in fact, that psychoacousticians believe discrimination of speech to be a learned phenomenon.[29] If pure-tone audiometry measured perception of the order required for meaningful

---

[25] A. J. Ayres, *Southern California kinesthesia and tactile perception tests.* Los Angeles: Western Psychological Services, 1965.

[26] A. A. Strauss and N. C. Kephart, *Psychopathology and education of the brain-injured child.* New York: Grune & Stratton, 1955. II: 156.

[27] R. B. Talbott, A study of the perceptual abilities of the child retarded in language. Unpublished master's thesis, Rockford College, 1962. Pp. 117–118.

[28] M. L. J. Abercrombie, *op. cit.,* p. 53.

[29] A. M. Liberman, *et al.,* The discrimination of speech sounds within and across phoneme boundaries. *J Exp Psychol* (November 1957), 54: 358–368.

interpretation of verbal signals, it might be employed as an index. Several subjective techniques, including play audiometry, reward audiometry and noisemaker tests, are useful adaptations in assessing *aural activity* in very young children. Presumably if the conductive mechanism of the ear is intact, the sound will reach the cochlea and *primary discrimination* of the sound results. But is this order of discrimination sufficient for meaningful interpretation of sound? Carhart suggests that "recognizing the occurrence of a pure tone is somewhat analogous to perceiving a color." [30] Is not a higher order of discrimination needed for complex sound sequences involving fusion, rhythm, pitch-stress, and signal-ground? The discriminatory processes, moreover, can be inhibited or distorted by deficit or injury to the CNS or by psychoemotional disturbances (p. 102). Sometimes language-handicapped children also evince transitory deficits in auditory perception.

The *Familiar Sounds Test* [31] employed in detecting *hearing loss* in children 3–5 years of age more nearly answers the requisites of meaningful interpretation in that it requires the child to point to a picture representing the sound stimulus. Sounds familiar to a child—such sounds as a *dog bark, car horn, bird song, cat meow*—were recorded after certain frequencies in each sound were removed by electronic filtering. Before the familiar sound is presented to the child, he is shown a plate of pictures representing the sounds. After he hears the sound he is asked to point to the appropriate picture.

Since definitive measurements of nonverbal stimuli are not available, the language clinician or teacher may have to return to direct observation and study of the aural behavior of the child. For this purpose the student is referred to the materials in Chapter 6.

Tests of Motor Development and Skills

From the longitudinal study of the motor behavior of the child (pp. 205, 219), the special language teacher will have identified those areas of motor function that seem to be deficient and should be subjected to further testing. Perhaps he has observed the child's lack of manual dexterity in holding and guiding the scissors. Or he may have noted the atypical gait, stance, sitting posture, or stair-step coordination. In the psychologist's report of *Draw-A-Man* test, the teacher's attention may have been called to the child's distortions in self-image, a factor closely related to motor incoordination (p. 52). From the reports on certain

[30] R. Carhart, Audiological assessment of the deaf child. In P. V. Doctor, Ed., Report of the *Proc internat congress educ deaf.* Washington: U. S. Govt. Print. Off., 1964. P. 147.
[31] M. Downs, Familiar sounds test and other techniques for screening hearing. *J Sch Health* (March 1956), 26: 77–87.

subtests of Stanford-Binet and Wechsler scales, he also may have other evidences of perceptual-motor dysfunctioning.

These reports and observations raise basic questions in the teacher's mind. Is the child's problem in speech fundamentally the result of imperception of the body position from which movement patterns emerge, so that walking, manual dexterity, and articulatory skills all are adversely affected? As a result, are the perceptual patterns mediating these skills so enfeebled or distorted that the child is unable to sequence the requisite synergies of movement? "Power failure" or disturbance in tactile-kinesthetic feedback, for example, may account, both quantitatively and qualitatively, for the poor speech of the linguistically impaired child (p. 56). Here again we are reminded of the sensory-motor unity in all linguistic processes (p. 93).

When the special language teacher or clinician goes searching for tests that answer his questions, he will find useful measures in certain areas of general motor development and skills but very few reliable means of assessing ideokinetic factors in speech. In lieu of such tests he will have to extrapolate his findings on general motor development and skills and employ exploratory measures for the assessment of articulatory competence. The evaluative measures described in this section are of three types; (1) scales of motor development (birth to 4½ years), (2) scales of motor development and skills (4–14 years), and (3) exploratory measures to appraise articulatory motor function.

Motor Development, Birth to 4.6 Years

The most comprehensive test of early motor development has been developed by Bayley from two standardized scales.[32] The incremental change in observed motor performance with increasing age of the child is plotted against the norm of age placement. Scores for three trials on each of 80 items are translated into a cumulative score, absolute scale value, and age placement in months. In the test are included items pertaining to the development of stance, posture, walking, jumping, hopping, and manual dexterity. A sampling of items from the test may be found in Appendix C.

Motor Development and Skills, 4–14 Years

Tests in this age range appraise such factors of maturation and proficiency as balance and maintenance of posture, speed, range, and accuracy of locomotion (walking, jumping, running, skipping, hopping, rolling); contact through movement (reach, grasp, release); and receipt

[32] N. Bayley, *A scale of motor development*. Inst. Child Welfare, Berkeley: University of California, 1933.

and propulsion of objects in space (catching, throwing, batting). The tests may be scored in terms of motor age, but more important for the language teacher is the opportunity to answer these critical questions: (1) Is there evidence of psychomotor disturbances—tremors, overflow of movement, tics, astereognosis, and extraneous movements? (2) In alternating activities, is the alternation a true flow of activity from one side to the other (reciprocal innervation) or is it a discontinuous, disjointed activity? (3) Are the first movements a definite part of the prescribed pattern? (4) Does the child perceive clearly the position of his body in space, by means of which his movements must be guided?

Adaptations of the Oseretsky Motor Development Scale, 4–14 Years

There have been many revisions and translations (from the Russian) of the *Oseretsky Tests of Motor Proficiency*. The original scale was composed of 85 items contained in six subtests at each age level from 4 to 16 years. The tests are arranged in year levels, as in the *Stanford-Binet Scale,* and a motor age may be computed by a procedure similar to that followed in the Stanford-Binet. The Oseretsky scale is designed to cover all major types of motor behavior, from postural reactions and gross bodily movements to finger coordination and control of facial muscles. Each age level includes six tests intended by Oseretsky to measure the following aspects of motor development: General static coordination, dynamic coordination of the hands, general dynamic coordination, motor speed, simultaneous voluntary movements, and asynkinesis (ability to perform without associated involuntary and superfluous movements). Several authorities on motor development have questioned Oseretsky's scheme for the categorization of behavior and the age placement of certain items on both the Oseretsky Scale and the Vineland revision of it.[33] Some items have been found too difficult at the designated age level for the American and European groups we have tested. A second criticism pertains to the demand for understanding of difficult instructions. The instructions often are too complex and too lengthy for the level of comprehension and recall of language-handicapped children.

The Vineland-Oseretsky Tests (translated from the Portuguese and standardized by E. A. Doll, 1946)[34] contain six items for each age level. The administration of the subtests requires such materials as spools, thread, paper, boxes, match sticks, rope, balls. Directions are given orally but one also may demonstrate the activity. When we have administered the test, demonstration has been mandatory because the child found the

---

[33] L. Malpass, Motor skills in mental deficiency. In N. Ellis, Ed., *Handbook of mental deficiency*. New York: McGraw-Hill, 1963. P. 617.

[34] E. A. Doll, *The Oseretsky tests of motor proficiency*. Minneapolis: Educational Test Bureau, 1946.

instructions too complex and too long. The child either must pass one of two, or one of three trials in order to score. In the age range 4 to 9 years, the following tests are illustrative:

4 years:
1. Remain standing for fifteen seconds with one foot advanced and eyes closed
2. Hop in the same place, feet together, seven times
3. Put twenty coins in a box in fifteen seconds

5 years:
1. Balance on tip-toe for ten seconds
2. Roll two meters of thread on a spool
3. Clench and bare the teeth

6 years:
1. Balance standing on one leg for ten seconds
2. Jump over a rope twenty centimeters high
3. Draw perpendicular lines, twenty with right hand, twelve with the left hand, in ten seconds

7 years:
1. Walk a line two meters long, while eyes are open
2. Distribute 36 cards in four piles in 30 seconds (right hand)
3. Knit eyebrows

8 years:
1. Wrinkle forehead without executing other movements
2. Touch thumb to all fingers (of the same hand) in five seconds
3. Kick a box a distance of five meters while hopping on one foot

9 years:
1. Balance standing on one leg, eyes closed, for 10 seconds
2. Tap floor rhythmically with alternate feet, simultaneously tapping with index fingers of both hands (as the right foot taps the floor) for twenty seconds
3. Leaf through a book for fifteen seconds

The Lincoln-Oseretsky Motor Development Scale.[35] This test includes only 36 items in the age range 6 to 14 years and represents a distinct advance over other scales in that it does not require elaborate test materials, permits reliable scoring, minimizes cultural bias, and has a significant positive correlation with age.[36] Separate norms are provided for boys and girls because scores for the girls' items are based on a different standard from that for the boys' items. This scale is used widely and is considered to be the best standardized motor development scale available. The Score Sheet (Appendix C) lists the items included in this modification of the Oseretsky Scale.

[35] W. Sloan, *The Lincoln-Oseretsky motor development scale.* Los Angeles: Western Psychological Services, 1955.

[36] W. Sloan, The Lincoln-Oseretsky motor development scale. *Genet Psychol Monogr* (1955), 51: 183–252.

Measures of Particular Skills

Balance and Locomotion. The most widely used measures to assess these special abilities are railwalking tests, of which the *Vineland Rail-walking Test* [37] is representative. It requires three wood rails varying in width from one to four inches. The rails are six, nine, and ten feet long. The child is required to take ten steps, heel to toe, hands on hips, without support. He is permitted three trials on each rail. Equal in importance with the score is the observation of atypical motor patterns: (1) overflow of movement; (2) rigidity of movement; (3) failure to alternate movement; (4) compensatory efforts to balance body; (5) frequent loss of balance; (6) watching of feet; (7) excessive hesitation; and (8) use of one side of the body more than the other. Age equivalents have been computed, based on scores of each subtest.

Dextrality, Manual Strength, and Dexterity. Tests of these motor abilities generally are measured by the comparative superiority of one hand over the other and consequently hinge on the development of dextrality. Dextrality has been a controversial domain for centuries, as Sir Thomas Browne implied when he wrote, "Whether Eve was formed out of the left side of Adam, I dispute not; because I stand not yet assured which is the right side of a man, or whether there be any such distinction in nature. . . ." [38] Although we have cleared certain corners of this domain much uncertainty about the central field remains. Delayed or confused laterality, we believe, adversely influences one's capacity to deal competently with simple motor tasks involving spatial orientation and the reconstruction of simple patterns from memory. The establishment of unilateral dominance is neither constant with age nor absolute at any stage of development. By the age of 4–6 years, as we have noted in Chapter 6 (Table 6-3, p. 219), the child "shows preference for dominant hand usage," but this does not mean that dominance is fixed. Many children have bimanual predilections at 7 years and are unimanual again at 8.6 years in the major portion of their motor activities. Belmont and Birch believe that the child is not consistent in handedness until he is 9 years old, although he has stabilized right-left discrimination with respect to his body by the age of 7 years. Apparently the preferential foot is established by 6 years. [39] (See p. 41 for discussion of cerebral dominance and laterality.)

Strength of Grip: Dynamometer Test. There are no established

---

[37] S. Heath, Railwalking performance as related to mental age and etiological types. *Amer J Psychol* (April 1942), 55: 240–247.

[38] Browne, Sir Thomas, K.T., M.D., *Religio Medici* Part I. 5th ed. Boston: James R. Osgood & Co., 1872. P. 46.

[39] L. Belmont and H. Birch, Lateral dominance and right-left awareness in normal children. *Child Develop* (June 1963), 34: 257–270.

data for very young children in this motor function. Francis and Rarick [40] have provided a chart (Figure 8-2) of their findings of strength of grip using the dynamometer for older children, 8 to 14 years of age.

Tests of Manual Dexterity and Dextrality. The purpose of these measures is to assess the comparative accuracy, steadiness, and speed of each hand in timed tests of assembling and placing objects or in such ordinary manual activities as drawing and writing.

Purdue Pegboard Tests. In one part of this test, pins are inserted individually in small holes with the right hand, left hand, and both hands together, in successive trials. In another part, the subject must use both hands simultaneously in assembling pins, collars, and washers in each hole.[41]

Iowa Performance Test of Selected Manual Activities. The test items are included in Figure 8-3. Directions for administration and

[40] R. Francis and G. Rarick, *Motor characteristics of the mentally retarded.* Washington: U. S. Office of Educ. Coop. Res. Program, Monogr., No. 1, 1960.

[41] J. Tiffin, *Examiner's manual for the Purdue pegboard.* Chicago: Science Research Associates, 1948.

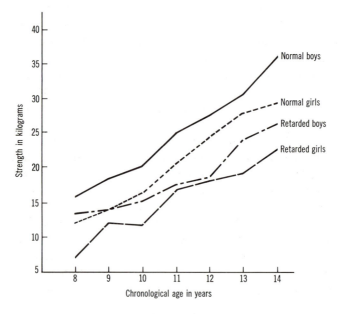

Figure 8-2. Mean strength of right grip for normal and mentally retarded boys and girls.

SOURCE: L. F. Malpass, Motor skills in mental deficiency. In N. R. Ellis (Ed.), *Handbook of mental deficiency.* New York: McGraw-Hill. 1963. P. 612.

```
    SCORE SHEET

Name _____ Age _____ Sex _____

Examiner _____ Dextrality Quotient _____ Date _____
```

Place a check mark in appropriate spaces below to indicate whether activities listed
were performed by the right hand (R), the left hand (L), or both hands (B), neither
hand predominating.

	R L B		R L B
1. Pull down curtain.	___ ___ ___	33. Pick up card.	___ ___ ___
2. Pull down curtain.	___ ___ ___	34. Pick up card.	___ ___ ___
3. Take article from desk.	___ ___ ___	35. Lay down card.	___ ___ ___
4. Take article from desk.	___ ___ ___	36. Lay down card.	___ ___ ___
5. Tear paper from tablet.	___ ___ ___	37. Tear paper from tablet	___ ___ ___
6. Turn over paper.	___ ___ ___	38. Turn over paper.	___ ___ ___
7. Sharpen pencil.	___ ___ ___	39. Fold paper.	___ ___ ___
8. Write with pencil.	___ ___ ___	40. Sharpen pencil.	___ ___ ___
9. Erase with pencil-tip eraser.	___ ___ ___	41. Turn page of book.	___ ___ ___
10. Write with pencil.	___ ___ ___	42. Turn page of book.	___ ___ ___
11. Draw a picture.	___ ___ ___	43. Draw a picture.	___ ___ ___
12. Put pencil in desk.	___ ___ ___	44. Put pencil in desk.	___ ___ ___
13. Take crayon from box.	___ ___ ___	45. Pick up scissors.	___ ___ ___
14. Take crayon from box.	___ ___ ___	46. Put scissors in desk.	___ ___ ___
15. Color with crayon.	___ ___ ___	47. Pick up pen.	___ ___ ___
16. Color with crayon.	___ ___ ___	48. Take top off pen.	___ ___ ___
17. Put crayon in box.	___ ___ ___	49. Take top off ink bottle.	___ ___ ___
18. Put crayon in box.	___ ___ ___	50. Fill pen.	___ ___ ___
19. Close crayon box.	___ ___ ___	51. Write with pen.	___ ___ ___
20. Close crayon box.	___ ___ ___	52. Put top on pen.	___ ___ ___
21. Pick up scissors.	___ ___ ___	53. Erase with pencil-tip eraser.	___ ___ ___
22. Put scissors in desk.	___ ___ ___	54. Fold paper.	___ ___ ___
23. Point to block.	___ ___ ___	55. Pick up pen.	___ ___ ___
24. Point to block.	___ ___ ___	56. Take top off pen.	___ ___ ___
25. Pick up block to pile.	___ ___ ___	57. Take top off ink bottle.	___ ___ ___
26. Place block on pile.	___ ___ ___	58. Fill pen.	___ ___ ___
27. Pick up block to pile.	___ ___ ___	59. Write with pen.	___ ___ ___
28. Place block on pile.	___ ___ ___	60. Put top on pen.	___ ___ ___
29. Pick up block to carry.	___ ___ ___	61. Pick up chalk.	___ ___ ___
30. Pick up block to carry.	___ ___ ___	62. Write with chalk.	___ ___ ___
31. Point to card.	___ ___ ___	63. Pick up chalk.	___ ___ ___
32. Point to card.	___ ___ ___	64. Write with chalk.	___ ___ ___

Totals: R _____ L _____ B _____

Dextrality Quotient (DQ) = $\dfrac{R+B/2+}{N}$ = _____ = _____

R = Total for column R
B = Total for column B
N = Total number of items performed

Figure 8-3. Iowa performance test of selected manual activities.

source: W. Johnson, F. Darley, and D. Spriestersbach, *Diagnostic methods of speech pathology.* New York: Harper & Row, 1963. P. 324.

scoring and the norms are found in Appendix C. Other tests of laterality by Blau [42] and Harris [43] are described in Appendix C.

Articulation. Sometimes a child passes tests of motor skills involving the large muscles and yet is unable to execute the fine movement patterns of speech. Whether the difference in task can be attributed to superior overloading in general motor skills, to the speed and complexity of articulatory patterns, or to excessive interference in feedback in verbal skills, we do not know. Articulation measures that assess the child's ability to produce phonemes in various positions have been standardized and are widely used. They have been discussed in the preceding chapter (p. 273). We are interested, however, in a different kind of assessment, *viz.,* in testing the motokinesthetic basis of articulatory skills. In the preceding section we have described rudimentary tests of kinesthetic feedback, but they do not assess the role of feedback in the execution of motor patterns of speech. Attempts have been made to measure operative sensitivity of the articulatory organs by electronic means but these attempts are purely experimental. By asking the child to think the sentence (but not say it), feedback strength presumably can be calculated. Another exploratory technique employs a sylrater (an electronic device by which one may measure the speed and repetitive skill of the lips and tongue in articulatory movement) to record diadokokinetic rates in articulating sounds or syllables.[44] Since repetitive movement depends largely or exclusively upon tactile-kinesthetic feedback, it may become a fair measure. The child closes his eyes and articulates first p-p-p-p-p, then t-t-t-t, as rapidly as he can until one minute has elapsed. The examiner notes such behavioral manifestations as a complete block after two or three repetitions; irregular, spasmodic rhythm; and weak approximation of lips in the production of [p] and of tongue with lingual alveoli in articulating [t]. The results of a sylrater study of the rate of repetition of three syllables by a group of 70 children are shown in Table 8-2.

A third exploratory technique employs the *delayed feedback test* (p. 122). If the child responds to a delay in feedback by an increase of pitch and intensity and marked disintegration of morphemic sequences, we may assume that synthesis of feedback (auditory-tactile-kinesthetic)

[42] A. Blau, Objective test of laterality. In H. Bakwin and R. Bakwin, Eds., *Clinical management of behavior disorders in children.* Philadelphia: Saunders, 1953. P. 297.

[43] A. J. Harris, *Harris tests of lateral dominance.* New York: The Psychological Corporation, 1955. Pp. 12–13.

[44] J. Irwin and O. Becklund, Norms for maximum repetitive rates for certain sounds established with the sylrater. *J Speech Hearing Dis* (June 1953), 18: 149–160. M. Patrick, Common denominators in school children with articulatory defects. Unpublished masters thesis, Rockford College, 1953.

Table 8-2. Diadokokinetic rates determined by the sylrater.

Age	No. Tested	Mean Number of Syllables per Second					
		[pǝ]		[tǝ]		[kǝ]	
		Girls	Boys	Girls	Boys	Girls	Boys
6	30	3.67	3.49	3.51	3.33	3.28	3.18
7	20	4.38	4.34	4.33	4.14	3.88	4.02
9	20	4.40	4.56	4.32	4.49	3.94	4.19

SOURCE: J. Irwin and O. Becklund, Norms for maximum repetitive rates for certain sounds established with the sylrater. *J Speech Hearing Dis* (June 1953), 18:157.

is a positive factor in language learning. If these disruptive influences are not present or are minimal, the assumption is that feedback is less important in the child's language learning than in that of other children. Perhaps when norms have been established for time periods within which kinesthetic feedback occurs in articulating a series of sentences, it will be possible to determine variance in the temporal interval of feedback when they are uttered by the language-retarded child.

A final exploratory technique used in feedback studies has been called a differential test. The child is instructed to speak the rhymes (below), the first time in loud, rapid speech, the second and third times with diminishing volume but increased duration and precision of the morphemes. If after an interval of five minutes the child repeats the rhyme with greater articulatory skill than the first time, monitoring by feedback presumably was effective. If the last repetition is no better than the first, we conclude that feedback is not a measurable factor in this child's learning and retention. The rhymes employed were:

1. Woe, woe, woe	2. Cling Bing Ding Ding!
for Joe, Joe,	Hear the fire engine sing!
Who couldn't say	Cling Bing Ding Ding!
Whoa, whoa, whoa	The bell has got to ring!
To the horse named Zoe.	

"Soft Signs" of Neuromotor Impairment. The **Romberg Test** often is used to test the child's balance. The child is instructed to put his feet together, close his eyes and extend his arms, and to maintain this position for fifteen seconds. If he sways noticeably in a lateral or forward direction within the time interval, one suspects neuromotor impairment of the great sensory-motor systems mediating posture and locomotion.

A failure in inhibitory feedback of finer motor patterns may be demonstrated by two tests of reflex response of the facial muscles. If the child blinks repeatedly following a tap on the forehead or responds with a jerk of the jaw when the examiner taps it, one suspects that the inhibitory mechanism is not intact.

Tests of Socioemotional Maturity and Adjustment

Some of the tests which we shall describe can be scored objectively. Norms of *social age* and *social quotients* have been established and, in some instances the social age has been equated with intelligence. The validity of these data and comparison with IQ have not been established.[45] More important than numerical results to the student of language disorders is the description of the child's behavior and his manner of dealing with test items. Numerical test results generally are unreliable and render a minimum service unless the teacher administering the test has a "way with children," and is sufficiently intuitive to establish a comfortable relation with the child. The child's failure may be the teacher's failure. Again we are prone to place more reliance on the longitudinal study of socioemotional maturation (see Chapter 6) than on any single test.

The dependence of language learning on socioemotional maturity and stability almost every student recognizes. The development of the child as a person is as important as the development of language, but what is not said as frequently is that language and personality are interdependent. They develop together. Tests of this type generally serve two purposes, developmental measurement and the detection of maladjustment. The first category to be described is developmental schedules.

Socioemotional Maturity

Vineland Social Maturity Scale.[46] This developmental schedule is so widely used with children that its administration has become standard procedure in speech, hearing, and language centers. Maturity is judged in terms of the individual's ability to look after his practical needs and to take responsibility in his daily life. The required information for young children must be obtained through interviews with the parent; older children sometimes can be relied upon for accurate responses to the questions. The statements on administration in the *Manual of Directions* are especially valuable. It is important, for example:

to avoid asking whether the S *can* do so-and-so, but rather (to ask) *does* he *usually* or *habitually* do so. These answers are then checked by detailed questioning until the examiner is able to score the item as a whole. It also is important to avoid leading questions and to follow up all general answers with detailed questions.[47]

[45] A. Anastasi, *Psychological testing.* (3rd ed.) New York: Macmillan, 1968. P. 258.
[46] E. A. Doll, *Vineland social maturity scale.* Minneapolis: Educational Test Bureau, 1947.
[47] E. A. Doll, *Vineland social maturity scale; Manual of directions.* Minneapolis: Educational Test Bureau, 1947. P. 11f.

Important details relate to *what extent, how much, what ways,* and *what kind.* There is no substitute for finding out just what the child *actually and habitually* does in respect to each item. The items fall into eight categories: (1) general self-help, (2) self-help in eating, (3) self-help in dressing, (4) self-direction, (5) occupation, (6) communication, (7) locomotion, and (8) socialization. A social age (SA) and a social quotient (SQ) can be determined. Test items and the categories they represent for age levels 0–8 years are included in Appendix C.

Behavior-Maturity Inventory. A second developmental measure is the Haggerty-Olson-Wickman Rating Scale.[48] In this test, norms of behavior-maturity age have been established for children from 19 months to 7 years. Each of the 120 items has a weighted score and an age equivalent. The structured interview with the parent follows the Vineland form but the categories to which items are allocated and the probing procedures are different. There are only two major categories, *routine habits* and *emotional maturity.* Subcategories of *routine habits* are concerned with everyday problems of eating, rest, toilet, washing, and removal of wraps. The second major category, *emotional maturity,* begins with a direct question to which are affixed fifteen subordinate questions. With each subordinate question are listed possible answers. For example, the first subordinate question to the main question, *Is he learning to live with himself?* is: *Did his initial adjustment to the school indicate emotional maturity?* Other subordinate questions are: (1) *Does his usual mood show a state of satisfactory adjustment?* (2) *How does he face difficulties (for example, when crossed)?* (3) *How long can he be absorbed in an activity?* (4) *Can he play by himself?* (5) *Is his emotional expression adequate (directed) or diffuse (irradiating)?* (6) *Does he take responsibility for his actions? When punished?* (7) *How does he control himself in a minor injury?* (8) *How does he behave in the face of a difficult task?* (9) *Does he show initiative?* (10) *What degree of social maturity is shown in his play with other children?* (11) *How much strain can his social attitude bear?* (12) *Does he see another's viewpoint?* (13) *How does he react to unfriendly advances of other children?* (14) *What is his place in the group?*

The test has proved to be a valuable supplement to the Vineland Scale and is particularly useful because of the extensive interpretive data, predictive of types of behavior, which follow each item.

Emotional Adjustment

The second category of tests deals with the detection of common preneurotic and psychoneurotic symptoms contributing to maladjust-

---

[48] *Haggerty-Olson-Wickman Rating Scale.* New York: The Psychological Corporation, 1952.

ment. They are valuable tools when used by clinical psychologists. Such behavioral deviations as fears, obsessions, sleep disturbances, fatigue, imagined illnesses, sensory failures, feelings of unreality, aggressive behavior, and family and school relations are probed. These tests offer only rough indices since the responses are scored in terms of their empirically established behavioral correlates.

Personality Inventory for Children, 9–14 Years.[49] This inventory comprises eighty questions which require only yes-no answers. No account is taken of behavioral inconstancy or invisible patterns of behavior. The following questions are typical:

1. Are you always having bad luck?
2. Do you ever feel worried when there is nothing to do?
3. Do you always have the feeling that something bad is going to happen?
4. Are your hands and feet usually cold?
5. Do you sometimes throw up after eating?
6. Do you ever have pains which move from one part of your body to another?
7. Do you always feel tired?
8. Have you ever been unable to hear or see for a while?
9. Do your parents like your brother or sister better than they do you?
10. Have you ever dreamed that your father died?
11. Do you usually have bad dreams at night?
12. Have you ever dreamed that you were locked in a room and could not get out?
13. Do you ever dream that you are trying to run away from someone who is trying to harm you?
14. Do you ever start thinking about yourself and forget where you are?
15. Is it hard for you to calm down after being angry?

Children's Manifest Anxiety Scale (CMAS).[50] Originally this test was designed for adults in order to measure the rubric, drive, of which anxiety states are the sequel. The test later was scaled for use with children.[51] Although originally the test presupposed some ability to read, it can be administered orally by the examiner without invalidating the test. Some questions have been raised about the influence of the response set and situational variables, but if it is used as an experimental procedure in connection with other studies of emotional adjustment, the instrument has value.[52]

[49] F. Brown, A psychoneurotic inventory for children between nine and fourteen years of age. *J Appl Psychol* (August 1934), 18: 566–577. F. Brown, *Personality inventory for children.* New York: The Psychological Corporation, 1935.

[50] J. A. Taylor, The relationship of anxiety to the conditioned eyelid response. *J Exp Psychol* (February 1951), 41: 81–92.

[51] A. Castaneda, B. McCandless, and D. Palermo, The children's form of the Manifest Anxiety Scale. *Child Develop* (September 1956), 27: 317–326

[52] M. Mueller, Mental testing in mental retardation: A review of recent research. *Train Sch Bull*, Vineland (February 1964), 60: 162.

Taylor's original interpretation of anxiety has been supported by Goda and Griffith who carried out a correlative study with measures of articulation and linguistic form.[53]

Projective Tests Employing Pictorial Techniques

As was true of the preceding group of tests these projective measures also are administered by clinical psychologists. The projective test sometimes has limited use in the evaluation of the language-handicapped child. Success in these tests is dependent upon verbal production and upon continuous attention to stimuli, in both areas of which the language-handicapped child is disadvantaged. One's faith in the results of the test also must rely upon the accuracy and skill of the clinical psychologist administering and interpreting it. In the hands of certain interpreters, the level of inference often has seemed far removed from the protocol; the examiner's production was imaginative but it bore little relation to the child's performance. Competence will depend upon the psychologist's knowledge of personality and its theoretical implication, his experience with types of behavioral deviations and his knowledge of test techniques and results. At best, reports of projective tests are useful to the language clinician only as corroborative evidence of the extensive observations of trained clinical language teachers.

Children's Apperception Test (CAT), 3–10 years.[54] *Apperception* by definition is "the integration of a percept with the individual's past experience and current psychological state." [55] The test employs pictures of animals on the assumption, now challenged, that young children identify themselves more readily with animals than with people. The animals are portrayed in typically human situations in the anthropomorphic style of a child's picture book. The pictures provide the stimulus for evocation of fantasies pertaining to oral activity, toilet habits, parent-child relationships, sibling rivalry, and aggression. Among the apperceptive variables to be tapped are (1) motive strength, (2) perception of the world, (3) defensive tendencies and conflict, and (4) cognitive-expressive styles.[56] The analysis sheet, together with an exemplary summary, on pp. 425–426 suggests the scope and results of this test.

The Blacky Pictures, 4–14 Years.[57] Twelve cartoon drawings of

---

[53] S. Goda and B. Griffith, The spoken language of adolescent retardates and its relation to intelligence, age and anxiety. *Child Develop* (September 1962), 33: 489–498.

[54] L. Bellak and S. Bellak, *Children's apperception test, revised edition: Manual.* Larchmont, N. Y.: C. P. S. Inc., 1954.

[55] J. Kagan, Thematic apperceptive techniques with children. In A. Rabin and M. Haworth, Eds., *Projective techniques with children.* New York: Grune & Stratton, 1960. P. 105.

[56] *Ibid.*, pp. 106–108.

[57] G. Blum, *The Blacky pictures: A technique for the exploration of personality dynamics: Manual.* New York: The Psychological Corporation, 1950.

anthropomorphic animals are utilized in this exploration of personality dynamics. The cartoons are designed to reveal a coherent summary of the underlying psychosexual aspects of personality or a type of object relationship within that development. Its clinical orientation is toward therapy rather than toward classificatory diagnosis (autism, hysteria). The pictures portray the adventures of a dog named Blacky. The first cartoon introduces Blacky, Mama, Papa, and Tippy, a sibling figure of unspecified age and sex. After the child has been motivated to use his imagination and express his feelings, he makes up a story about each picture. The examiner is provided with "inquiry cards," questions to the child about Blacky's activities and feelings. Children's responses have been interpreted as portrayals of such things as oral eroticism, oral sadism, oedipal intensity, sibling rivalry, guilt feelings, ego ideal, and love object.

Make-A-Picture Story for Children (MAPS). This measure is a variation of the principle of *CAT* and often is used in combination with it. According to the experience of the test maker,[58] *MAPS* has special usefulness with children, eliciting in some cases good rapport and interesting protocols. In this test the backgrounds and figures are separated so that the child's task is to select one or more cut-out human-like figures from among many such figures, populate a background picture, and then tell his story. Essentially it demands that the child respond to a stimulus situation which he himself has created in part, using *dramatis personae* of his own choice. There are 22 background pictures, printed achromatically on this cardboard. With two exceptions, there are no figures in any of the pictures. The set includes unstructured or ambiguous backgrounds such as the *Blank* card, the abstract *Doorway,* and the *Dream* background; semistructured backgrounds such as the *Stage,* the *Forest,* the *Cave,* and the *Landscape;* and definitely structured backgrounds such as the *Living room, Street, Bathroom, Bridge, Bedroom, Closet, Schoolroom, Camp, Cemetery,* and *Attic.* The background pictures are designed to tap specific problem areas and dynamics. The possible approaches to interpretation are listed as follows: normative, hero-oriented, intuitive, interpersonal, and formal. The test designer recommends no single approach but a combination of all of them.[59]

[58] E. Shneidman, The MAPS test with children. In A. Rabin and M. Haworth, Eds., *Projective techniques with children.* New York: Grune & Stratton, 1960. Pp. 130–148.

[59] *Ibid.*

IV

Children With Disorders of Verbal Communication

9

Studies of Profiles, I

The language profiles of these children do not fit neatly into definite etiological frames. Despite the perennial aspiration of the student for tidy categorization, linguistic behaviors of this group remain in the unclassified drawer of knowledge. Some fields may suffer from rigid categorizations, but disorders of language have not been afflicted in this way. Categorization is difficult because deficits or injuries of the CNS produce subtle and unpredictable disturbances in linguistic behavior, disturbances that vary with the age of acquisition and extent of involvement. Behavioral manifestations in one child often are very different from those in another child, although the cause and clinical pictures presumably are the same. In some cases it would seem that we are dealing not with one specific entity or syndrome, but with a component common to several syndromes attendant upon multiple handicaps. So we have to cope with a multiplicity of symptoms, some of which may be only tangentially related to the CNS deficit.

Psychosocial elements also are significant in disorders of oral language (Chapter 4). They affect many dimensions of the disorder. Questions pertaining to general mental ability, motivation and reinforcement, adaptive lability, attention, and memory frequently remain open-ended. The family, the economic group, the culture to which the child belongs may not be etiological determinants *per se* but they influence greatly his adaptive and compensatory abilities to cope with the handicap.

The treatment of children with communication disorders is always incomplete. So instead of a neat categorical listing of syndromic features, profiles are presented of children whose problems we have studied and evaluated. Although some formal tests have been administered, they do not weigh heavily in the evaluation. The profiles are really derived from observation and exploratory studies of the children's responses to diagnostic teaching covering a period of several years. The children have one common handicap—verbal communication—but its manifestations vary widely. Some differences are subtle and elusive, others gross and definite. In each case, the etiological summary must be qualified by the tenuous state of knowledge of these disorders. There is always an X factor that cannot be disallowed.

The Profile of David: Language Disorder Associated with Genetically Determined Deficits of the Nervous System

Physical Appearance. David entered the Center at 4.0 years, referred by a pediatrician for "delayed speech." From David's general appearance one would not assume any atypicality. He was a handsome, well-nourished youngster who seemed somewhat apprehensive in the environment of the Speech and Hearing Center. His facial expression was a stereotyped, "anxious smile." As his mother talked with the director, the child fidgeted with the pages of a picture book, but he did not really look at the pictures. His gait was and still is somewhat strange but not remarkably so.

Birth and Developmental History. David's pre- and perinatal histories were essentially normal. Delivery occurred two weeks prior to term and was uneventful. His birthweight was slightly over 7 pounds. He cried lustily at birth. No feeding problems were encountered. The baby left the hospital with the mother on the fifth day.

During the first four years of life, David suffered only from minor colds and a very light case of chicken pox. He slept and ate well, displaying few food idiosyncrasies. The mother observed that the child did not progress as rapidly in general development as her three daughters but was told by her pediatrician that girls develop at a faster rate than boys in the first year or two. David sat up alone at 6 months and took his first steps without support at 18 months. Although the mother acknowledged that such development was not atypical, his failure to meet other developmental criteria on time disturbed her. (Her major interest in college had been child psychology.) When pressed to discuss her misgivings, she spoke particularly of the child's lack of security in his environment. She reported that in the third month he still did not recognize her voice if he could not see her when she entered his bedroom at night. He was as apprehensive of her as of a stranger until she had taken him from his crib. Was this a signal of slow perceptual maturation? He took the same apprehensive approach to his sisters and his father. On one occasion when David was 10 months old, his mother transferred his high chair from the kitchen to the dining room for breakfast. He cried and refused to eat until he was returned to the kitchen. On his first birthday she recalled that she playfully threw a light silk scarf over his head in playing peek-a-boo. He screamed with fright and could not free his head. Later when one of the sisters repeated the game, the mother noted that David seemed to "take the long way" to remove the scarf.

The child's confusion in orientation and directionality were evinced in other ways. When David was 3 years old, the mother would ask him as they approached their home if they were close to their house. And despite the fact that she had pointed out the clubhouse and the flags on the golf course near their home on several previous occasions, he did not associate them with the approach to his home. In the house she also had noted that he often opened the door to the front hall closet when he wanted to open the main door to the outdoors.

Attempts at Oral Communication. David's babbling, the mother thought, appeared at the proper time but she began to fear impairment of hearing because the sounds which he made were strange sounds, unlike those of speech. We assured her that the initial sound vocabulary may contain few or none of the phonemes of speech. Yet she insisted there was something very different about the baby's babbling. Finally she concluded that the quality was "dead, impassive"; it bore no resemblance in intonation or rhythm to the normal patterns of speech. Apparently there was almost no jargon-like prespeech to which the family might respond. When asked how David communicated at 2 years in order to satisfy his wants, the mother said that he used "oral noises" and simple, rather generalized pantomime.

When David's first words, *m-m-m* (mama) *bə-bə* (bye-bye) appeared at 30 months, the mother stepped up speech stimulation by talking to him constantly during his waking day. His sisters talked too rapidly and excitedly to him, she said, so she used the approach of slow, quiet speech. There was an interval of a year between first words and two-word sentences. And unlike first or second words in the normal development of speech, David's first words did not mean "sentences." The expressions were not complete percepts—expressions which demanded attention or explored his relation to his environment. And these embryonic sentences did not sound like communicative speech. The mother said that the child might try to copy a phrase occasionally but he made no attempt to replicate intonation and stress patterns or expressive gestures. This is particularly strange in view of the mother's lively voice and dramatic facial expression. When he entered the Center at 4 years, he had very few two- and three-word sentences. They were: [ɔ-baɪ] (go bye); [ɔ-eɪ] (O.K.); [dɑ-bɑ] (Daddy bye); [mʌm:kɑ] (This is mama's car); [i:i] (T.V.); and [u:ʔeɪ] (see you later). The long interval between steps in his speech progress would indicate that for David learning did not proceed by steady increments. There were excessively long holds in the countdown.

Family History. David was born into a closely-knit, happy family, the fourth child and first boy. His parents are university graduates and enjoy a middle to high economic status. The sisters are attractive and lively. Two have clear but rapid speech and are excellent students in a private school. The youngest child (8 years) has cluttered, unclear speech, is reported to be ambidextrous, is a slow reader in the second grade, and went to a speech and reading clinic during the past summer. The father insists that he is still ambilateral in many activities and that he has two brothers who also are ambilateral. When the father had completed two years of architectural training, he transferred to a graduate school of business where he specialized in accounting. We asked him why he had decided to transfer. "I could do the math in architecture but courses in advanced design were difficult for me. Accounting is pretty much all figures; I like it." When we asked him about his own language and speech development, he thought that he did not speak clearly when he entered the first grade. Although he had no special or remedial training in speech, he remembers that words containing /r/ and /l/ still were difficult for him in the third grade. His parents had paid no special attention to his articulatory problems probably because they were greatly concerned over his two older brothers, both of whom were severe stutterers. To a casual observer the father's communication probably would be called different but not abnormal. This interviewer was struck particularly by the staccato, nonmetrical rate and the atypical intonation and stress patterns. We suspect that he tried unconsciously to compensate for his verbal eccentricities by a smiling countenance and frequent laughter.

The mother's speech was excellent and served David well as a model. She believed that children learn speech more easily from adults than from other children so she bombarded David's ears with her speech. She was an affectionate, outgoing person and should have afforded excellent motivation to her son. No external pressures creating tension or frustration were evident in David or the family. He was surrounded by cultural and social advantages that also should have provided excellent motivation for language growth. He played occasionally with somewhat younger neighboring children, but he preferred activities with his own sisters who, his mother repeated, undoubtedly pampered him.

Evaluation of David's Communication Problems Based on Longitudinal Study

Initial Status.   One is struck immediately by the meager quality and quantity of oral expression of 4-year-old David. He can identify objects easily but only with single words. When we ask, "What does the train do, David?" he is verbally silent but he will push it along the track and wave his hand to indicate the direction of the movement. He was fascinated by the trains and track set, by toy cannons, missile sets, but even under this kind of obvious motivation, we could not get him to combine noun with verb: *train runs, whistles; airplane goes zum; shoot* (the) *cannon.* The mother asked repeatedly, "Why doesn't David use phrases or sentences?" We suspect that he does not do so because he does not perceive morphemic sequences as meaningful units. Apparently when he listens to speech, he extracts a few word cues but they do not have fixed meaning. Even in the initial stages of language use—satisfying wants, giving directions, and relating himself to his little world—his words and phrases subtend vague, diffuse percepts. The profile of David's oral expression at 4 years is meager. He is a silent boy relying largely upon smiles mixed with expressions of anxiety for communication.

Sequencing and Articulation of Morphemic Units.   There was little opportunity to evaluate this phase of David's verbalization until he was 5.6 years. The amount of speech was increasing slowly but perceptibly. Without his knowledge we secured several taped records of his talk while operating the trains and "firing the missiles" with another child in the playroom. David scrambles the sounds within the word and words within the phrase. He says, [t²ẽɪ go noʊ] (train go now); [tẽɪ uːuːmɑ] (train whoo, whoo, make); [ɛnəpaɪ] (airplane fly). Later the two were playing picture-lotto. We could not comprehend much of David's speech because we could not associate it with particular picture cards. Here are some extracts which we did decipher: [nɪbo] (robin); [tɪpɪdʌg] (pretty good); [ʌbɛlə] (umbrella); [ɛfə²] (elephant); [ʃəs] (fish); [bʊs] (soap); and [gaɪdə] (tiger). Obviously David is in trouble because he cannot sequence sounds or morphemes, and this no doubt is basically a perceptual difficulty. When he was asked to imitate separate phonemes, he did fairly well. The integration of movements into complicated patterns of normal speech, however, is too difficult a task at present. He cannot comprehend the whole unit or sequence, so of course the oral musculature does not respond as a unit.

We have indicated that David's dyslalia is rooted in deeper, more basic problems of perception. He is unable to recognize the phonemic sequences quickly and to synthesize them into meaningful wholes. His recognition of phonemic structure is diffuse, unstable. When urged to repeat exactly what has been said to him, he improves the intonation and stress patterns of his response but the articulatory skills remain poor. He does not understand the morpho-phonological structure of language. We do not agree with those who might say that his phonemic structure is that of a much younger child. His articulation is not infantile; it is different. It is more primitive than the English paradigm. If he is to learn by imitation he must have the analytical tools, the phonemic and morphemic rules which must be employed in coding. At present the tools are too dull to be effective in carving language. The failure in unitary perception, in morphological sequencing is reflected also in his staccato, jerky speech. He codes "in tandem," rarely "perceiving all at once and nothing first."

Vocabulary at 7.6 Years. David actually knows the meaning of many words. If he could talk about their meaning, he might reach low average ability. His vocabulary is not very useful to him because he cannot order the words into sentences. The words he uses are mainly in the nominal and verbal categories. He omits functor words. General words are substituted for specific words. He introduces neologisms, words which are largely unrelated to sentence meaning which neither his family nor his teacher comprehends. He has overlearned many automatic and interjectional phrases which do not help him materially in the vocabulary he needs for propositional speech. Yet one is inclined to believe that his comprehension of single words is superior to all other aspects of his development in language. On the *Peabody Picture Vocabulary Test* his vocabulary age was 6.1 (CA 7.6). When we attempted to give the *Vocabulary Definition Test* he tried to describe meaning but he became lost in a mass of unstructured verbiage.

Grammar and Syntax, 6.0–7.6 Years. When David was 6 years old we tried an exploratory measure which required him to repeat sentences in scrambled and in correct order (p. 230). He did practically as well in recalling sentences with scrambled word order as with the correct order. Further exploration has confirmed our belief that grammar and syntactic form are great obstacles to him in learning language. In order to reproduce the sentence he hears, he has to recognize the pattern, and this is tantamount to saying that reproduction presupposes a knowledge or sense of the pertinent rules. It also presupposes a sense of prosody or *motor syntax,* an ability also predicated upon tactile-kinesthetic skills. Motor syntax embraces not only the morphemic sequences in a time-space order; it also demands a "feeling" for the prosodic qualities of language —rhythm, pitch, stress, and duration—a sense of the total effect of the sentence. David's ability in this subtle perceptuomotor function apparently is very limited. If he could learn or overlearn simple patterns so that integrative sequences are securely set in memory, he might have a basis upon which to build the language structure. Unfortunately there are few distinct patterns available to him for recall.

With another child whose evaluative study is reviewed below, we have attempted to aid the retrieval of patterns. In David's case, we suspect there are no patterns to retrieve. We often have tried to help him to learn very simple sentence patterns, insisting each time upon several repetitions. For example we have been experimenting recently with the passive voice in such a sentence as, "The baby is fed by Mama." Apparently David alters the linguistic form when he comprehends it for if we ask him to repeat the sentence, he says, "Mama feeds the baby." At other times he says, "I forgot one word in the middle." Usually the forgotten words are connective-tissue words (such as prepositions and conjunctions)—additional evidence of his inability to comprehend the whole sentence in grammatical form. If he understood syntactic forms, he would recall the code from principle cue words *and their connections.* Then he could recall and repeat without having to pay attention to sounds or syllables or even words. Recently the language clinician gave David our exploratory *Test of Comprehension of Grammar.* He was able to form the plural of three sentences and the past tense of two sentences. At 7.6 years his comprehension of linguistic form approaches that of a 5-year-old child. The language teacher gave up her plan to teach the order of negative sentences (e.g., *No, we are not going to the movie*). David needed help with simpler forms of grammar and syntax.

If David could clear this hurdle he would be able to take the next step, the creation of new combinations of stable, coded units. He would be able to experiment with language, turning verbs around, inverting subjects, introducing dependent clauses. Perhaps this hallmark will appear one of these days; we hope so.

Other Evidences of Perceptual Deficits. It is logical to assume that David's inability to perceive the temporal-spatial order of sequences, both phonemes and morphemes, would extend to other activities. It does. In finding the meaning of pictures on the *Binet* test (Dutch home, post office), he becomes absorbed with fringe areas of the picture and loses the meaning of the whole. In another series of picture tests a policeman is running after a small boy crossing the street against the light. David's attention is fixed on the gun in the policeman's holster. He saw little else so he said, "Man shoot." He overattends to and fixates on details, in part, out of anxiety. He fastens on one object or one symbol because he feels secure when he does so. David cannot see the forest for the trees.

On one occasion we accompanied David to the circus. It was almost a catastrophic experience for him. He tried to "take in" a mass of visual, auditory, tactile-kinesthetic, and olfactory details which did not meld. He could not make them into consistent patterns; he could not track them in complex succession. The result was that his perplexities and anxieties mounted until nausea overtook him. The game was over. When the subject of the circus was raised a few days later, David could recall only the most diffuse, tidbit-like perceptual experiences about the performance.

The perceptual problem is revealed in other clinical activities. On the marble board test he has difficulty with size, form, and space. He can remember three digits in a sequence but not five. Figure-ground distinctions perplex him. When objects are shown against backgrounds of various patterns, he has great difficulty in identifying the objects. He likes the security of one pattern and one orientation. When the form board is rotated he knows something is wrong but he cannot tell how to make it right—for him. His behavior in working puzzles betrays his anxiety and fixation on details. Feet and tongue twist as he turns the block and views it from every angle. On Frostig's *Developmental Test of Visual Perception* (p. 286) he reproduced accurately only one design. Then we placed an alphabet made of large felt letters in various positions, some upside down, some backward, many out of order, and asked him to "make them right." He had many trials, he worked hard, but he did not succeed.

Memory and Perception. We thought that retrieval of verbal sequences might be aided if we told him short classical children's stories, some of which he undoubtedly had heard at home, and then asked him to tell them immediately to us. In our telling we exaggerated the prosodic patterns believing them to be "sequence binders." David's responses were interesting. He would begin very safely "once upon a time" but the cue words and sequences soon failed him. Such difficult cue words as *goal-keeper* he turned into verbal hash (glo-peeka). He said, "Man ran downstairs" when he meant "upstairs." When he met a real roadblock, he either would ask, "What do you call that thing?" or he would begin a series of circumlocutions to get around the block until finally he was completely ensnared and gave up. The story trailed off into nothingness. In experimenting with intonational and stress patterns, we would ask him to imitate carefully the patterns we had used. Over and over he repeated the most dramatic, climactic sentences. The first replication was fair but with each repetition or with a short delay in time of repetition, the imitation failed; the vocal quantity of emphasis diminished and the old, monotonous, staccato rhythm reappeared. He seemed to have no way to set the pattern or to retrieve it from memory. When we asked him to tap out sequences of sound, he did fairly well in the first simple sequences and then the tapping pattern disintegrated completely. We then went back to the earlier simpler sequences which he had passed successfully but now he was unable to do them. Did the trouble lie in defective feedback or in the weak synaptic potentials of the reticular system, so that he could not focalize and sustain attention, or was the deterioration of response caused by power failure at the synapses of several integrative circuits? Perhaps the main power failure was in the reticular and limbic systems which produced a concatenation of failures along the entire track of comprehension and recall.

At 7.6 years David has learned to read the first pages of the pre-primer, *Dick and Jane.* After he had read it several times aloud to us, we took the book and asked him to tell us what he had read. Almost compulsively he snatched the book and read it again to us. When we closed the book, put it away, and said, "Now you know the story; tell it to us," he made verbal hash of the story. He could not order the words into a sequence because he does not perceive either linguistic form or the prosodic qualities of language.

Intelligence and Perception. Does David suffer from an intellectual handicap? If there are blocks in the integration of sensory-motor information, in the circuits serving feedback, memory, or motor-sensory projection, is it not logical to assume that they affect general intelligence? It may be argued that these deficits affect only verbal learning; the non-symbolic learnings of performance, for example, should be quite normal. We must remember, however, that performance activities demand internal verbalization so that one cannot say that nonverbal tests actually are nonverbal. Subvocal language or implicit language and language experiences influence nonvocal performance.

Tactile-kinesthetic Modalities and Perception. We already have alluded to David's lack of sensitivity to syntax, prosody, and articulation. You will remember that David's mother had noted confusion and fear in his early behavioral adjustments. Neither his voice nor facial expression gave evidence of keen proprioceptive feedback. David showed little evidence of listening even when we knew he was deeply interested in the story being told to him. The facial expression remained fixed in an anxious smile. The expression did not change as the story progressed. A child's venturesomeness, in part, determines his proprioceptive responses to another's speech. Believing that tactile-kinesthetic cues to articulatory *sequences* are very important in the comprehension of speech we urged him to copy articulatory movements. David seemed unwilling to copy articulatory and facial movements. When he tried to repeat a sentence in sharp, ballistic, rhythmic form, the tongue-jaw-lips synchrony simply failed him. The words were only two-syllable but he often could not "get his tongue around them." Since perception of speech depends, in part, on the proprioceptive stimuli which arise from the movements of articulation, much of David's difficulty may stem from inadequate comprehension of articulatory-motor sequences.

David's deficit in tactile-kinesthesis might be explained in several ways: (1) There is an actual deficiency, either in numbers or in potential, of the end organs of tactation and kinesthesis. This is a genetic variation which also may have been true of David's father and sister. (2) Unusual delays or distortions in the transmission of information via the tactile-proprioceptive routes may occur so that these impulses cannot be synchronized with auditory and visual impulses. They are at variance with the dominant wave form of other contributors to the sensory-motor fields. Parallel patterning does not take place. We know that there are critical time-periods within which the feedback accompaniments of a motor operation must be received in order to insure optimal control. If the interval is exceeded, then disorganization occurs. The tridimensional lattice, so to speak, has not been constructed properly. As a result, feedback is impaired so the critical self-monitoring system does not operate effectively. A bit of evidence to support this hypothetical cause of distorted feedback is David's increase of volume when he is asked to repeat a sentence that is not intelligible. This response is characteristic of delayed feedback. (3) David makes no spontaneous attempt to copy articulatory patterns mimetically. He does not watch the speaker's face; in fact, he seems to be disturbed by facial expression. Is it possible that visuotactile-kinesthetic cues are confusing because there are too many or because their timing does not accord with the arrival of other cues? Some scholars postulate that the perceptual pattern may arrive twice, once by the direct route and once via the indirect, reticular route, giving rise to the *déjà vu* effect.[1]

Hearing and Perception. Undoubtedly the reader has expected a consideration of David's auditory sensitivity and perception long before this juncture. His mother brought David to us in the first instance because she believed he was acoustically handicapped. Previously she had gone to several otologists who reported no discernible hearing loss, although they were unable to secure cooperation on pure-tone audiometric tests because of his age. The assessment of David's peripheral hearing by EEG audiometry in a medical center assured us that the child had no peripheral loss but he was inconsistent in his response both to pure-tone and to speech audiometry. David's auditory perceptual responses to speech were inconsistent. Could we account for these variances either by a defective attention-scanning mechanism or defective feedback in the reticular system or by diurnal neurophysiological shifts? We were inclined to think that the difficulty lay in feedback of his own speech since he could identify gross errors in the speech of others but he could not identify these same errors in his own speech. The feedback channels of the auditory system, direct and indirect, probably are impaired but the more serious difficulty may lie in the defective channels of the tactile-kinesthetic modalities. In the audiometric assessments made two years after the original tests of hearing, David did not respond to pure tones presented in a free field of intensities approaching the pain

---

[1] R. Efron, Temporal perception, aphasia and *déjà vu. Brain* (December 1963), 86: 403–24.

threshold but within that hour he responded to a whispered voice. Perhaps distortions through feedback may have been so confusing as to shut out the pure tones at one instant, and in the next the same feedback mechanism facilitated the cognition of the whispered voice. The feedback channels of the auditory system, direct and indirect, probably are impaired but the more serious difficulty seems to lie in defective tactile-kinesthetic perception.

Performance and Perception. There are, moreover, disturbances of other abilities which are manifestations of the basic problem, perceptual impairment. They, too, affect David's performance of nonverbal tasks. As he does not perceive the form of the language, so he has difficulty in perceiving form and direction in nonverbal activities. The spatial-temporal perceptive failures affecting his comprehension of language also extend to orientation and laterality. At 8 years David shows no unilateral hand preference. (Recall the father's report of his and his brothers' ambilateral expression.) In printing the child often cannot determine where the phrase ends; he has difficulty with sequencing in writing as in speaking. He is troubled by the same temporal-spatial difficulties in reading; he is dyslexic.

General motor dysrhythmia has been apparent particularly since his entrance in the first grade of school. One observes it in his gait; the arms do not swing in cross-pattern. He has trouble with left-right progression, becoming confused and shifting feet frequently when marching with others. The sequential patterns in running, jumping, and hopping are noncoordinated. Like his father and uncles, he is ambilateral, but unlike them, he is proficient with neither side, probably because he has not developed either hemispherical or cerebral dominance. When we consider these specific learning handicaps it is not surprising that on a series of "semi-verbal" performance tests at 8 years, his average IQ was 84. In the second grade general classification and achievement scales were administered. In the completely verbal sections of the test he stood at the bottom of his class. The examiner agrees with us that his responses were not typical of a mental retardate in many subtests. For example, when David was directed to "take this pencil, put it on the chair and bring me the book lying on the windowsill," he completed the first mission and then attempted to recall the second one. He looked finally in the direction of the window and with a sense of elation found the book and brought it to the examiner. The mentally retarded child completes the first mission and returns to his chair evincing no concern about the second direction. He is unaware of his error whereas David knew he had further direction and attempted to recall it.

In the performance tests demanding a measure of verbal skill, his learning quotient was 89. His response to one measure hearkens back to his inability to reproduce morphemic units which he apparently had comprehended for some time. After the original design in one of the Wechsler measures had been removed, the child could not execute the design yet he could select the correct design from a group of designs when they were presented to him. He could perceive its correctness but he could not make the necessary translation to the final stage of perception—motor execution of the design. Now can we say that David is mentally retarded? Probably the best answer is that he has grave perceptual deficits affecting all symbolic activities pertaining to language. We must remember, however, that this is but one face of mental retardation. There may be even more than three faces.

Psychoemotional Concomitants. The emotional strain and anxiety which we frequently observe in David's behavior has concerned his mother greatly. We have told the mother we are not convinced that these responses are abnormal for one suffering David's frustrations. We agree with her that his bearing, facial expression, and general attitude increasingly express anxiety, but we are not sure we would not exhibit the same behavior if we faced the daily disappointments and frustrations of David. On one occasion we realized too late that his nervous system was being overloaded by too many sensory-motor impulses. We were giving the *Comprehension Span Test* (p. 269). He brushed the pictures from the table onto the floor and struck his head with his hands. He could not organize the endless stream into meaningful configurations—into temporal and spatial patterns. The unfortunate sequel was that after these situations of stress had been experienced, retrogression in the comprehension and use of language occurred. Despite the mother's concern we regard the emotional disturbance as secondary sequela. Even at the age of 8 years, David realizes the social and economic liabilities of impoverished communication. He fears almost instinctively his destiny in a linguistic world for he is a child ill-equipped in the substance and skills of verbal communication.

A Neurophysiological Hypothesis: Summary. We believe that David's CNS deficit is genic, that from the paternal side he has inherited an atypical nervous system. His older sister, next in line, probably is an incomplete genotype of the same order. To be sure, these symptoms may not be restricted to genic causes. Some but not all of David's difficulties were apparent in a child, Ellen, an Rh baby, who suffered pre- and perinatally from anoxia and was severely jaundiced at birth. In other words the etiology may vary but many of the symptoms may be held in common.

We are concerned with the nature of David's neurological deficits. Apparently he is unable to develop the kind of tracking or pattern-making necessary for comprehension-use of language. Several hypothetical reasons may be advanced for his failure: (1) Chemical activity responsible for synaptic power may be relatively or absolutely deficient so that power failures occur in essential neuronal assemblies.

(2) The reticular activating system may fail to alert fully those cortical areas essential to perception of language. (3) As a result of power failures or idiosyncracies of synapses in cortical and brain-stem systems, visual, haptic, and auditory impulses may be distorted in their temporal-spatial relations. Even direct and indirect pathways mediating sensory-motor impulses of a single modality may not have the same temporal sequencing. The result is delayed or interrupted integration. (4) The feedback-scanning mechanisms may be impaired or they may be subjected to diurnal changes in synaptic power which temporarily interrupt the orderly sequence of patterned impulses. (5) The CNS may not be able to mediate morphemic sequences at the usual *rate* of presentation. Attempts to overload the system result in a breakdown of gating (facilitation and inhibition) in the integrative networks. (6) Retrieval of morphemic sequences is evanescent because the initial engrams were weak or distorted. In sum, David finds it difficult to establish, even by overlearning, those symbolic relationships that have meaning in experience. We fear that the pattern-making structure of the nervous system has irreversible deficits.

The Profile of Terry: Language Disorder Associated with General Learning Disability [2]

Family History. Terry is the youngest of six children of a family in the low economic group. They live in a rural suburb where the father works as a driver for a freight line. Two of the children have been "very slow" in learning to read, the mother reports, and their speech isn't "quite right." The father had eleven sisters and brothers, three of whom died in infancy. Among the sons and daughters of the mother's five brothers there are three who are in classes of "speech correction" and two who are enrolled in special education in the public schools. The father completed the ninth grade; the mother dropped out of school in the eighth grade. Both left school because of academic failure. The mother's speech is cluttered and sometimes unintelligible. The father's use of language and his speech, too, are superior to the mother's.

Pre- and Perinatal History. This child was the mother's ninth pregnancy, the seventh and eighth pregnancies having ended in miscarriage. Her pregnancy with this child was uneventful. The infant was full term; delivery was by breech presentation. The infant cried, breathed, and nursed as a normal baby. Terry weighed over eight pounds at birth; at present (7.1 years) his weight is 42 pounds.

Developmental and Health History. According to the mother's report, the child was content to lie in his crib. He balanced his head at

---

[2] Although language disorders caused solely by general learning disability are beyond the scope of this text, we present the profile for its value in differential diagnosis.

3.8 months but he made no effort to sit up before 7 months. He sat unsupported at 9.0 months. The first tooth erupted at 20 months. Terry walked with support at 21 months and at 4.6 years had gained voluntary control of the bladder and bowels. At 7 years, the child still is a thumb sucker and drools occasionally. Although the mother thinks the child is left handed, we find Terry's laterality to be ambiguous. The child had "roseola" at 8 months and suffered from a severe case of measles at 2 years. In the past two years frequent upper respiratory infections, followed by bilateral otitis media, have interrupted his attendance at kindergarten. In two attacks, the middle ear infections were accompanied by rupture of the tympani.

Language and Speech Development. As an infant Terry babbled little. The mother thinks he said [dɑdɑ] (Daddy) and [bɑ] (bye) some time after his third birthday. She was not so greatly concerned about the late appearance of speech as she was over his failure to understand her directions and commands. Unlike her other children, he would not come from play when called, did not follow her directions for dressing himself, and was invariably in trouble in outdoor play because he did not follow the rules of the game.

Following the appearance of first words Terry's speech did not advance materially for a long time. Not until after his fifth birthday did he use such two-word sentences as *ma-ma go bye; me go long;* and *tah-tu* (thank you). Terry has spent two years in kindergarten. Now, at 7 years, the child's language and speech are so retarded that he will not be accepted in the first grade. The mother came to the Center in the hope that "something can be done so that Terry can go to school."

On entrance to the Center, Terry (7.1 years) appeared as a phlegmatic, listless but fairly well-nourished and well-groomed, red-headed lad. When a toy was brought out in the playroom, his usual response was [aʔdæ] (What's that?). He used single words: [ʌfə] (whistle) and [əbu] (balloon), repeating them in echolalic fashion, but few two- and three-word sentences were elicited. Peripheral hearing had been tested prior to Terry's entrance to the Center and was reported to be "essentially normal." Subsequently a series of assessments was made. Acuity was diminished slightly in the range of speech frequencies; the greater loss in low frequencies was not significant for speech-hearing. Audiologists who administered the tests reported that Terry's responses were indefinite and often indicated a failure to focus attention on the task at hand.

Mental Maturation. From the initial period of diagnostic teaching, Terry's behavioral responses were indicative of a mild but general mental retardation. In successive measures both verbal and performance scales were employed. They included the *Stanford-Binet* test, *Raven's Progressive Matrices* test, and the *Wechsler Intelligence Scale for Children.* His scores on subtests of performance were only slightly higher than tests employing comprehension-use of speech. We had anticipated a greater differential.

Electroencephalometric studies of Terry also presented evidence of mental retardation. The alpha wave-pattern of 4–6 Hz was slow and irregular, an indication of an immature nervous system.[3] The sleep EEG pattern exhibited "extreme spindles" that have been correlated with mental retardation.[4] All assessments pointed strongly to mental retardation but we could not accept that as the sole cause of the child's incompetence in language. His speech was more severely retarded than we might have expected from the evaluation of general intelligence. We searched for other factors.

Maturation of Motor Patterns. There were other handicaps associated with general mental retardation which had specific adverse effects on Terry's language development. One was the retarded acquisition of motor patterns, both gross and fine. From the beginning of our association, we had been impressed with Terry's general hypotonic posture and movement which affected all his performances. On the first day in the Center we observed him on the playground. He did not walk with the easy coordination of a child of 7 years, who swings along, arms in opposition to the pattern of foot movement; who steps easily over obstacles; moves around blocks; hoists himself into the swing with a single boost and slide; or jumps onto the moving platform of the wheel. He stumbled often over his own feet, fell down, bumped into other children, and finally retreated to the sandbox.

In the Center we continued our evaluation of maturation, not so much of his fine motor skills as of his basic motor patterns. We concluded that the child did not have a clear picture of his own body and its position in space. Just as on the playground, so in the classroom he seemed to be "trying to squeeze himself through a knothole." Visual and haptic (tactile-kinesthetic) feedback did not guide him well in performance. We asked him, for example, to reach an object on the desk. He reached out with his whole body and fell over. When he was asked to hop, he did so but with clenched fist, closed eyes, and mouth open—a decidedly primitive pattern. The body image, the point of reference around which one organizes performance, was not distinct in this child's nervous system. We also noted his poor comprehension of laterality and directionality when we observed him on the playground the first day. He did not follow the directions of *in-out* and *right-left* in actions accompanying the song, *Looby-Lou.* Both dimensions (laterality and directionality) were poor, as one might expect because they are determined

---

[3] At one year in the normal baby, the alpha frequency is generally 5–6 Hz.

[4] E. Gibbs and F. Gibbs, Extreme spindles: Correlations of electroencephalographic sleep pattern with mental retardation. *Science* (December 7, 1962), 138: 1106.

first by internal awareness of bodily relationships and then by their projection in space.

In fine motor patterning, Terry experienced even greater difficulty but it was of a different kind. The tensions of fine muscles were too great for smooth, coordinated performance. He attempted to print his first name with movement so tense and disjointed that a tremor was noticeable. We also noticed these rigid and disjointed movements in his early efforts to duplicate articulatory patterns we had set for him. Diffuse percepts of fine motor activities also must have troubled him, for at 8 years he could not draw a circle without first naming it and repeating the word *circle* [səkə], as if to set the concept more firmly in his mind. On the Goodenough *Draw-a-Man Test* which he attempted at the same age, he continued to say [fə-mæʔ] (this is a man). On .the *Lincoln-Oseretsky Scale,* he reached a motor age of 5.8 years (CA 8.0). Specific tests of laterality repeated at 9.0 years confirmed our observation that right-left discrimination with respect to the body was still very unstable. In fine motor patterning—drawing, printing letters from copy, and imitation of simple articulatory movements, Terry's accomplishment sank to the 5.2 year level. He was able to protrude the tongue in imitation, for example, but he rarely could do so on command. He could produce four successive repetitions of the [tə-kə] sound units very slowly but no more. Although we demonstrated patterns of repetitive reciprocal movement, Terry was never able to repeat the sequence more than four times. His tongue was slightly large for the oral cavity but neither structural defects nor size could account for its failure in motor patterning.

Internal and External Motivation. As we continued our study we found additional factors of internal and external motivation that accounted, in part, for the difference between Terry's competence in the use of language and his general abilities. Low standards of language use and speech were quite acceptable in Terry's home and social environment. Both Terry's mother and sisters provided very poor models. Prior to counselling with the mother, we feel certain that the amount of speech which Terry heard was sparse. The mother repeatedly said, "We don't talk much at home." The father's use of language and his general speech patterns were adequate but he had little time for association with Terry. The cousins who played with Terry provided no better examples in verbal communication than did his sisters and brothers. The social age, measured by the *Vineland Social Maturity Scale,* was lower than his general mental age. The score on the Vineland reflected both the lack of normal extrinsic motivation from the family and the means of self-motivation. He had no skates, sled, wagon, game-toys, crayons or color books in his home. There was no table knife at his place. A few comic books were shared by the children. We found no other books or maga-zines in the home. To what extent a different environment might have influenced Terry's future progress is anyone's guess. Although we wished that we might find a way to effect such a change, we could not. Instead we persuaded a social worker to help us in counselling the family. Probably her work and the summer workshops for mothers of handi-capped children were as effective as our efforts in developing the right kinds of internal and external motivation.

Language Disability. The first difference we noted between Terry's language behavior at 7 years and that of others with psychoneurological language disorders was the boy's very *poor recognition and discrimina-tion of his environment.* Many of these language-handicapped children are aware of too many stimuli; they attempt to see too much, hear too much, feel too much. Their processing mechanisms at best are weak vehicles, easily overloaded, easily upset. Terry, on the other hand, takes in too little and what he does admit is often inaccurately recognized. For example, he was attracted to a book of folk tales about animals but because he had a previous acquaintance with the story of *Three Little Pigs* in which a wolf appears, henceforth all wild animals—foxes, bears, tigers, even lions—were wolves to him. He made other errors in gross discrimination. At table he did not readily discriminate between bread and cake, between salt and sugar. All meat was hamburger—but per-haps this is understandable. Although he drank various soft drinks, they all were "Cokes" to him. The same diffuse discrimination was evident in social exchange. He did not recognize the alternating roles of speaker and listener in verbal interchange. Only when he began to echo our questions did he show any sign of participating in the conversation.

The perceptual generalizations were made, too easily in fact, but they were not based on careful discrimination. The semanticist would say that Terry could not go down the ladder of abstraction, the poet that he could not see similarities in differences, differences in similarities. Both would agree with the psychologist that Terry was unable to dis-criminate quickly and clearly the experiences in his environment, both verbal and nonverbal.

Diffuse perceptual responses which were apparent in all language activities might be changed, we believed, if Terry could be taught to focus his attention on the centrum of the object or the idea. He must learn to *select* the proper cues. When we urged him to do so, fixation occurred so that he would not or could not move on. In preprimer reading, for example, we underlined words, the cue words with high perceptual content. But Terry could not get over peak words, move along and put the sentence together. He became stimulus-bound to components of the sentence but not to the sentence as a whole. We had better results when we urged him to read aloud more rapidly, to move ahead, but we recognized that we had made a kind of Hobson's choice for there were pitfalls in both courses.

From observation of behavior and tests of figure-ground in non-verbal functions (p. 285), we anticipated Terry's difficulty in separating oral sequences from a changing background of noises, sights, positions and movements. In order to perceive syllabic and sentence sequences he must be able to hold them in their proper *spatial and temporal relations.* Terry frequently was unable to establish the necessary stability of foreground. As a result he rarely perceived sentences as integrated, global percepts. He made a kind of piecemeal selection, sometimes of the first words of a sentence, sometimes of scattered words or parts of words. He wrote his name in the same piecemeal fashion: one letter, a pause, then another letter. But speech cannot be perceived piece by piece, for it is precisely the joiners, the "events between syllables and words," which provide the hallmarks of perception of oral language. This kind of piecemeal, unstable perceptive processing must also affect adversely the prosodic qualities of language. Sometimes Terry's voice sank to a whisper. Sounds and syllables often emerged in topsy-turvy style. Cluttered speech resulted. We believed that if Terry could learn to comprehend the order of morphemic sequences, and to hold them against a background, oral expression would improve.

Terry's failure to connect his learning experiences, (i.e., to find semantic relations), had also been anticipated through early exploratory measures, both verbal and nonverbal. At 7.4 years he completed only six of fifteen drawings in the subtest of closure in the *Hiskey-Nebraska Test of Learning Aptitude;* in the *Intraverbal Test* of the *Parson's Language Sample,* his oral response was correct only for five items (CA 7.5 years). Just as Terry had not learned to anticipate the end of a sentence so he did not anticipate the relation of ideas. Each phrase, each learning experience was a unit in itself. He did not look ahead; he did not predict. In much the same way he had not learned to weld more complex learning experiences. We were not keenly aware of this facet of his problem in the first months of diagnostic teaching, probably because we were mainly exploring his ability to learn new words and to find words similar in meaning—a comparatively simple exercise in semantic relations.

If we were to find the most productive means of education, we also needed to assess the comparative strength of the sensory modalities in language learning. Haptic feedback seemed to be even poorer than auditory feedback. One could anticipate this disability by observing the failure in reciprocal coordination of the phonatory and articulatory muscles, a function dependent on tactile-kinesthetic sensitivity and feedback. Terry's voice often faded out before the sentence was completed. The smooth coordination of lips, tongue, and jaw in such a rhyme as *Humpty Dumpty sat on a wall,* was very difficult. Terry did not mimetically copy the articulatory and expressive movements of his teacher, although every effort was made to teach him how to do it. We also tried to teach him to watch himself talk, an operation which he disliked. If he was to perceive proprioceptively the form and order of the sentence, he had to repeat it over and over again. Here again we noted the difference between Terry and other children with language disturbances. His difficulty began with a primary insensitivity to pertinent stimuli. In order to reinforce perception at its origin, he must follow a course of endless repetition. If he did not do so, he would not perceive rhythmic balances and duration of words and phrases; hence, he would not recognize that he had left out articles or prepositions. With reinforcement of perception, telegraphic style was less noticeable.

Certainly impoverished auditory sensitivity and feedback also were present. The whispered voice, lack of control of pitch and loudness, and the incoordination of phonatory and articulatory movements all point to diminished auditory sensitivity and feedback. In Templin's tests of auditory discrimination, he was successful at the 5-year-old level (C.A. 7.6) but he could not cope with more advanced measures either of word or sentence discrimination.

We gave no formal tests of articulation because we considered discrimination of verbal sequences the primary problem of oral expression. The feedback monitor was weak in part because there was so little coming in to scan, to integrate and transform into patterns appropriate for motor output. Believing that sensitivity and feedback might be reinforced by performance, both directly and indirectly, we explored Terry's ability to copy *pretended actions* (p. 229). Then we encouraged him to copy exaggerated, gross movements of the body accompanying speech as well as fine articulatory and phonatory movements. As a result of this training he developed a more alert posture, a louder and more inflected voice pattern, livelier facial expression, freer action of the head and arms accompanying speech, and more definite articulatory movements.

As the program of supportive education continued in the Center, Terry's success, however minimal, encouraged him. Immediate recall was seriously deficient but once he had overlearned a sentence, he remembered it. He held to the language he had overlearned with a tenacity that frequently resulted in rigid verbalization. He had learned certain sentences in a specific way and he must say them exactly that way. He could make no changes, either in the words or the form of the sentence. Hence he was not free to experiment either with vocabulary or syntax. Upon one occasion we decided to change the breakfast food which he always included in his description of his morning meal. When he returned to the first name he had learned, it came out as "Crice Rispies." The problem also was apparent in his clumsy replies to questions. When he was asked a question he would repeat it, using these echolalic means to reinforce feedback, and then would attempt to modify the question form slightly by way of answer. For example, "Why did you tear the Kleenex?" becomes in answer, "You tear Kleenex . . . fun." Echolalia probably served a secondary purpose. It expressed Terry's desire to sustain contact with his interlocutor. He wanted to answer the question and echolalic repetition kept the attention of the interlocutor.

Terry was fairly successful in this phase of learning. He could perform in the sense that he learned to give set responses and to recount very simple stories and events, but he could not integrate these language experiences with those outside the classroom. Possibly he did not comprehend them as clearly as we thought he did. We had not taught him to modify, elaborate, and relate the pattern. After a fairly successful first year, language development was slowing down; we could ascribe it only to this failure to comprehend and to relate the experiences. In some way we should have to stimulate the integration of language-learning experiences. We found that he had to meet certain language demands outside the classroom and we set about helping him to meet them. He wanted to say "two tickets please" so that the ticket-seller at the movies would understand him; to be able to repeat the Scout pledge; to call out the signals as a member of the school patrol; and to read the bus signs. To help him in developing prosodic qualities of speech, we intensified our efforts in rhythmic training. Terry enjoyed fitting words to the beat of the tom-tom and to marching rhythms. Our experiments in lip reading, a finer form of visual-haptic feedback, were not equally rewarding at this juncture.

Now at 9 years, Terry can communicate with others. His speech is fairly intelligible but articulation is not sharp or clear. He has learned to comprehend and use language, as he has learned to write and to draw—very slowly. What he has learned has motivated him to continue learning. The experience-producing drives are an intrinsic motivation in learning. His language has reached the descriptive level. He has not moved on to interpretation based upon relationships. Here is his response to the instruction, "Tell me all about this picture" (Wash Day, *Stanford-Binet, Form L-M*): "Mama hangs up wash. Doggie run away." When asked, "Why is the dog running away?" he repeated the question and then said, "Dog run away. . . fun." The significance and the relation of the woman's and dog's actions had escaped him. Perhaps he will get beyond the descriptive level one day and advance to the interpretive level. Then possessing the ability to discriminate and categorize his experiences, he will have a basis for interpretation. We do not mean to suggest that Terry has not made significant strides in the comprehension of semantic relations and linguistic form. He has. He also has made gains qualitatively and quantitatively in vocabulary and in the prosody and articulation of speech.

Continued development in the comprehension-use of language will depend upon the extent to which Terry can reinforce basic sensitivity, integration, and controlled feedback of impulses. By experience-producing drives, intensive stimulation, and overlearning we may step up the strength of synaptic potentials, thereby enlarging the population of the neuronal assemblies and increasing the effectiveness of coding throughout the reticular-limbic-cortical complex. When and if this is accomplished, we would expect the primitive patterning which now meets the requirements only of elementary language activities to give way to patterns mediating a more mature comprehension and use of language. The rate at which Terry accomplishes this goal will depend upon the degree to which he learns perceptual generalization based upon careful discrimination. It will be conditioned, in part, by the number and diversity of drives and reinforcements which can be realized in a culturally deprived environment. We have not attempted intensive training in general motor skills and in the special sensory-motor skills of phonation and articulation. Undoubtedly such a program now should be instituted.

We must view Terry's maturation, not in terms of the development of intelligence, but of the development of learning patterns. There are limits to Terry's achievement in learning and using a language: limitations imposed by neuronal assemblies meager in number and low in synaptic power; by extraordinary sensory-motor deficits affecting both nonverbal and verbal activities; and by psychosocial deprivation. To have explained the way by which a deficient nervous system may retard coding of verbal symbols in a sentence or two undoubtedly will not satisfy the student perplexed by the nature of mental retardation. If we should say that Terry's mental retardation is the result of a polygenic inheritance, we yet have not answered the question of cause. Genetically induced factors enter into this picture, but how do they conspire to inactivate or to limit the population of neuronal assemblies? In the most general terms we may postulate that the genetically induced electro-chemical balance which would establish potentials in a wide field of circuits is imperfect. The requisite neuronic potential at synapses is in deficit because these chemical balances are not maintained. Too many *perhaps,* too many *ifs,* are in the present dialogue to satisfy the positivist. The cause "doth tease us out of thought as doth eternity."

The Profile of Sandy: Language Disorder Resulting from Lesions in the Central Nervous System

The Cerebral Accident. Sandy, an attractive, brown-eyed lad, small in frame and stature for his age, 9.3 years, came to the Center with his parents three months after the boy had suffered a serious cerebral accident while visiting a neighbor. Sandy fell head first from the haymow into a feeding chute six feet below. In the fall he struck a cement frame of the feeding trough; it was a glancing blow to the posterior-inferior temporal and parietal areas of the skull on the right side. When he was admitted to a small nearby hospital, in a semiconscious condition, the attending doctor noted contusion and swelling in the right parietal and mastoid region. Blood mixed with cerebral-spinal fluid issued both from the right ear and nose. The tympanum of the right ear was punctured in order to relieve pressure resulting from splintering of the petrous portion of the temporal bone. X-ray examination revealed an extensive linear fracture in front of the right ear and extending upward into the parietal bone. There was marked rigidity of the neck. The semiconscious condition continued for eight days, during which he was able to take only a small amount of liquids. In this period, there was marked restlessness and moaning, twitching of the right arm, neck and back spasms, and incontinence. He occasionally opened his eyes but he was totally unaware of people around him. Drainage of spinal fluid continued for ten days. On the tenth day he responded to verbal stimuli by opening his eyes and frowning when his head was moved by the nurse. He apparently was aware of the presence of others in the room but he did not recognize them. The right arm moved in a spasmodic, involuntary manner. On the eleventh day, he appeared to be more alert; he looked around the room occasionally and took some fluids. His action in the next few days was irresponsible; he pulled the nurse's glasses from her face, threw the food offered him, struck at any one who came near the bed, and uttered strange, shrill cries at intervals. Thirteen days after the accident he made some verbal response to his mother and two days later made an obvious effort to talk to his sister. He responded, however, neither to questions nor noises. Spinal fluid drainage ceased on the eighteenth day and he was dismissed.

After he arrived home he began to take solid food, and gradually he became more perceptive of events in his immediate surroundings. He remained, however, without verbal or gestural communication. Encephalometric examinations one month after the injury "showed moderately slow alpha waves for the child's age with decreased amplitude of the waves in the *left occipital area.* There were a few 14 plus 6 per second positive spikes in the *right temporal and occipital area.*" You will remember that the alpha wave is a rhythmic, autonomous pattern of the resting cortex. The occipital-parietal-temporal areas, it also should be remembered, are concerned primarily with the organization of successive sensory-motor patterns.[5] The neurologist concluded that both hemispheres had been injured.

When Sandy returned to school three months after the accident, he had very little speech. According to his teacher, basic arithmetical skills of addition, subtraction and multiplication "returned much faster than speech." Since arithmetic was his favorite subject prior to injury, it is possible that the automatic use of number symbols was more deeply set in intermediate coding systems than verbal symbols.

Family Background. Sandy is the third of four children. Two older brothers do not resemble Sandy in physique and temperament. They have large frames, are outgoing, and less aggressive and less well motivated in school. Both boys, however, receive average to above average grades in their academic work. Sandy's sister was less than 3 years of age at the time of the accident.

The family lives on a large farm in a prosperous agricultural area. The home atmosphere has been secure and pleasant. Sandy's mother is. well motivated in the sense that she has set high goals for her children and works actively to help them to realize these goals. The father is more relaxed, quiet and less dominant than the mother. The father states that he himself always has been ambilateral and that Sandy and the next older brother "use either hand a great deal." The oldest brother's orientation definitely is sinistral in all major unilateral activities. The family enters actively into the social and cultural life of a small village and farm community.

Health and Developmental History. Sandy is a small-boned child, slight in stature, but very energetic. He has suffered the usual children's diseases: measles at 3.0 years, mumps and chicken pox at 7.0 years. As a very young child, he enjoyed puzzles, construction toys, and every type of mechanical play equipment. The mother reports that the child was clearly ambilateral but wrote with his right hand and held the fork in eating in his right hand.

The boy always has been highly motivated in everything that he undertook, both at home and at school. He was in the top quarter of his class (fourth grade) prior to the accident. He particularly enjoyed learning basic skills in arithmetic but was a consistently good student in all subjects. Possessed of a highly sensitive temperament, Sandy was easily upset emotionally even by gentle reproof. The mother found that the usual disciplinary methods she had employed with the older boys could not be used with Sandy.

Early Evaluations. Observation of the lad's general behavior and

[5] A. R. Luria, *Restoration of function after brain injury.* New York: Macmillan, 1963. Pp. 53–54.

exploratory techniques employed during the first six weeks provided us with an overview of the global nature of Sandy's handicap in language. Comprehension and use of all types of symbols were seriously impaired. His visuomotor responses indicated that he could not perceive visual sequences of letters, numbers, or designs. Although he used some speech, it was generally incomprehensible because of grave deficits in comprehension of vocabulary, linguistic form, and syntax. Sandy is an aphasic child, but this superficial diagnosis is feeble assistance either to Sandy's teachers or to the student of language disorders. What we need to know are answers to several questions that will ferret out specific dimensions of Sandy's linguistic—and intellectual—losses. Some questions are: (1) What sensory modalities have been most seriously affected or are they all equally affected? (2) How extensive are the perceptual losses affecting comprehension-use of language? (3) How seriously have retention and recall been affected? (4) Have motivation, drive, and personality been altered by the cerebral accident? (5) Is intellectual impairment—or the impairment in learning—limited to symbolic learning or does it also affect performance activities? (6) In what dimensions will he make greatest gains in relearning language?

Perception of Sensory-Motor Patterns. In evaluations made three months after the accident, visual, auditory, and tactile-kinesthetic cognition and feedback were equally affected. Sandy attempted to read a story in a second-grade reader. He made so many errors in recognition of nouns that the story was totally incomprehensible. Apparently he was not aware of his errors for he made no attempt at spontaneous correction. That he was unable to build and/or to retain any visual percepts of the letter-order of words was apparent when he attempted to spell simple words after studying them intently for several minutes. On these visual memory tests he was in the lowest percentile group. Prior to his accident he had been excellent in basic arithmetical skills. Now Sandy recorded 36 as the product of 9×6, and 64 as the result of 3×8. They seemed to be errors in visual recognition of the numbers to be multiplied. We noted other instances of impairment in visual recognition. He did not recognize, for example, abstract forms from pictures. He called a circle a bowl; a square was a box; to the triangle he made no response.

Before we attempted to assess auditory perception, the loss in peripheral hearing was evaluated. Hearing in the left ear was found to be essentially normal, although there was a consistent difference of 10 db between air and bone conduction at all frequencies, 125–8000 Hz. He had no usable hearing in the right ear. He responded to 250 cycle tones at 60 db and to 500 Hz at 85 db, but the audiologist could obtain no response for any frequency above 500 Hz when a 45 db masking tone was used.

In the oral vocabulary test Sandy frequently misunderstood words he was to define. He interpreted *lecture,* for instance, as *electric chair,* and *skill* as *skip.* In the *Templin-Darley Articulation Test,* Sandy looked at the word as the examiner said it, yet he made so many errors in visual and auditory perception that the test could not be scored. We had noticed that the boy looked neither at the examiner's face nor in the mirror at his own articulatory movements during speech. Before a retest was attempted we devoted several sessions to coaching Sandy in tactile-kinesthetic reinforcement of articulatory patterns. He made a somewhat better but still unacceptable record on the retest of articulation. As far as we could determine, all sensory modalities associated with language perception were seriously impaired.

Vocabulary. Coding, you will remember, is a continuous process. If circuits are damaged at any point, cortically or subcortically, the whole system is impaired. Evidences of damage to circuits mediating comprehension-use of language are clear in Sandy's case. He was unable to perceive the meaning either of words or sentences. We attempted to give the *Peabody Picture Vocabulary* and the *Picture Discrimination* tests. No basal score could be established for either test. We also tried the *Similar Sentence Exploratory Test* (p. 264). All sentence pairs were the same to Sandy. We could not establish a basal score on any test of vocabulary comprehension. Four months after these tests he had reached the 6-year level (C.A. 9.8) in vocabulary comprehension. He was so seriously handicapped in the *use* of vocabulary, however, that even when he was able to demonstrate the use of a simple object, he could not explain it verbally. His tearful, sometimes explosive question was: "I used to know; why can't I say it now?" The extent of ideokinetic apraxia can be seen in his responses to the picture absurdities subtest (*Stanford-Binet* VII): (1) "He took *that thing*" (umbrella) "and didn't put it *on* his head;" (2) *"that* should be *in* the bottom" (the cutting edge of the saw); (3) *"That stuff* . . . I don't see it this time" (dog chases rabbit; his remark in this instance is incomprehensible). The interpretation of the last picture highlights another problem. Perceptual and verbal accuracy declined together. At the beginning of a session, his percepts often were fairly clear and remarks comprehensible. But if the exercise extended beyond ten minutes, percepts became unstable or fuzzy. He worked at the fringes of perception and speech became equally unclear. Sandy often said words that had a vague resemblance *in sound* to the word he should have used. For example, he said *Ofaker* for *October, edel* for *elbow, ster* for *star, shubble* for *shoulder.* One might argue that Sandy perceived the word correctly but could not execute motorically the correct articulatory movements. A sounder explanation is that he could not say the word because sensory-motor pathways involving both integration and projection were impaired. The injury was apparent on the sensory side and continued over motor-sensory routes. Because he could not comprehend morphemic sequences of the word he could not order its motor execution. No weakness of the muscles of articulation was demonstrated. We tried to correct gross mispronunciations by direct stimulation. He would change his pronunciation slightly but he could not match ours. Whenever he was corrected, his facial expression became querulous. He made an effort to perceive the word more clearly but auditory, visual, and haptic patterns were so diffuse that he could not capture the percept.

Linguistic Form. The examples in the preceding paragraph illustrate another primary linguistic impairment. Sandy did not perceive the *form* of the sentence. In fact, we had to interpolate much of the connective tissue of the sentence. Obviously the man would put the umbrella *over,* not *on* his head. The cutting edge of the saw should be *on* the bottom, not *in* the bottom, although this correction still makes meaning ambiguous. The way in which the boy jumbled sentences because he could not perceive the *form* is apparent in his responses in the test of comprehension (*Stanford-Binet* VII). To the examiner's question, "What would you do if, on the streets of a city, you found a three-year old baby who was lost from its parents?" Sandy replied, "Try to get babies if one or two." To the question, "What's the thing for you to do when you are on your way to school and notice that you are in danger of being late?" Sandy said, "We get that when we get snow and got . . ." We think he wanted to explain his tardiness at school because of a recent snowstorm; he could not command either the vocabulary or syntactic form. Sentence comprehension had improved only slightly eight months after the accident. When he was asked to repeat this sequence: "I may go fishing on Sunday," Sandy said, "I to go to fish." Even in such automatic sequential measures as the repetition of the alphabet and the months of the year, he made several omissions.

Prosody. If Sandy's perception of grammar and syntax had not been so seriously disturbed, his relearning would have progressed much faster. It was further complicated by an impairment of the prosodic elements of speech. He did not perceive the melody of a sentence, the way in which a sentence begins and "swings along" to its terminus. In the early months of teaching Sandy, we often attempted to enliven his passive, dead voice and unnatural rhythm by the stimulation of lively facial and bodily gestures. We hoped that heightening tactile-kinesthetic feedback of certain motor-sensory patterns mediating speech might increase feedback in related patterns. It didn't work. Sentence melody did not improve. We were never able to reconcile this failure with Sandy's success in gross motor activities—basketball and baseball—which are also dependent on tactile-kinesthetic feedback.

Categorization. Impairment of categorization followed in the wake of diffuse perception. In the verbal subtest of similarities and differences (Binet VII), Sandy made no response to the questions, "In what way are an apple and a peach alike; iron and silver alike?" When asked about the similarity between *wood* and *coal,* Sandy said, "I don't know . . . coal." "In what way are a penny and a quarter alike?" (Binet VIII), asked the examiner. "Penny and quarter . . . 26," Sandy responded. Here he comprehended the meaning of the words but not of the sentence. He grasped instead at an arithmetical skill that had been largely automatic prior to the accident.

Recall. In every dimension the injury to perception was apparent. He was completely bested when he was asked to recall the meaning of a short oral paragraph. He could not remember the names of the characters or recall the events recounted in the passage. He was not able to remember words, word order, or object design in any of the objective measures we tried in the first months of diagnostic teaching. The writer still recalls his poignant self-rebuke: "I knew it once but now I can't remember it." The recall of the sequence of morphemes, words, and sentences—in fact, of all symbolic patterns—was to be his greatest roadblock to academic achievement. Although we have made separate designation of memory, it scarcely can be considered apart from perception. Loss of memory in Sandy's case simply meant the loss of what the word sequence looked like (visual memory); what it sounded like (auditory memory); what it felt like (tactile-kinesthetic memory). He must develop percepts again, albeit the pathways now are crippled.

Nonverbal Performance. If performance tasks depended on verbal direction, Sandy generally made many errors. When the task was demonstrated without verbalization, he was much more successful. We asked him, for example, to tap a rhythm with his fingers; he tapped it with his foot. When told to pound the table top, he polished it with his hand. On the *Stanford-Binet* scale that demands both comprehension and use of language, he achieved a mental age of 6.8 years (IQ 70; CA 9.4), but on the performance section of *WISC* (*Wechsler Intelligence Scale for Children*) his intelligence quotient was 103. In the latter test he had particular difficulty when the task depended upon the comprehension of verbal directions or cognition of spatial relations, as in block design and object assembly. Unfortunately for Sandy academic achievement will depend mainly upon his ability to relearn language.

Sandy's high motivation sometimes became a deterrent to learning. In comparison with his brothers, both of whom were older, Sandy was much more determined, energetic, and purposive. When he returned to school after an absence of four months, he was determined to regain his position in the top academic group in his class. His highly motivated and aggressive personality suffered under disappointment and defeat. He became impatient, angry with himself. He wept over his failures because he had "tried so hard." And indeed he had. He avoided confrontation particularly in communication. Emotional outburst followed by periods of sulking made relearning of language all the more difficult. Sandy's personality basically was the same as before the accident, but now he was not able to inhibit states of anxiety and frustration which followed thwarting of basic drives.

Final Evaluation. And now after nearly three years of special clinical education in oral language, speech and reading, carried along with general schooling, what assessment can one make of Sandy's gains in language learning? Sandy has come a long way—first because of Sandy, of his high motivation, tenacity, and his willingness to spend hours in overlearning and review. Secondly one must acknowledge the understanding and help of parents, public school teachers, and his special clinical teachers in speech, language, and reading. The problems in language learning, nevertheless, remain essentially the ones with which he started, although he has made greater gains in certain areas than in others. *Perception* has improved but it still is blunt, edgeless. There are three specific aspects of his perceptual problem which we might delineate: (1) Sandy cannot discriminate *quickly;* (2) he is unable to focus readily or certainly on the centrum of significance; and (3) the results are frequently inaccurate. If the lad is pressed to perceive quickly the order of phonemic or syllabic units in a word, or words in a phrase, he fails. He can proceed in coding only at one speed and that is slow. This loss in integration cannot be connected solely with the cortical lesion. A sounder explanation is the general electro-chemical disturbance, initiated by the cortex, which affects synaptic potentials throughout the entire coding process from periphery to centrum.

Disturbance of synaptic potentials also is related to his inability to focus readily on the *centrum of significance.* In other words, foreground and background become intermingled. The resulting percept is unclear, undefined. Sandy's mother reports that his conversation at the table reflects this lack of clarity. He begins to tell an incident but becomes entangled in numerous side-sallies and circumlocutions both in idea and phrase, until the significant centrum of the incident is lost. He cannot shut out irrelevant associations. In responding to the question, "What is missing in this picture?" (*Picture Completion* test; *WISC*) Sandy does not perceive that the band on the man's hat is missing. He points instead to the faint outline of the coat lapel and says, "There's no button-hole." When he was asked in the analogies and similarities test, "In what way are a piano and a violin alike?", he said, "They make sounds; they have strings." The response reveals both a fuzzy percept of the instruments and an equally fuzzy percept of the words to describe the similarity.

Sandy is relearning language but at a slow pace. Much work remains in training perception of sequencing, linguistic form, prosody, and vocabulary in oral language. In the *Picture Arrangement* test (*WISC*), Sandy missed four out of seven items. He did not perceive the sequence of events making up a logical picture story just as he did not perceive the proper sequence of words in a sentence. In the visual-motor sequencing subtest (*ITPA*) Sandy had considerable difficulty visualizing the task although the examiner had demonstrated the picture chips twice. In the *Object Assembly* test (*WISC*), it took Sandy four times as long to correctly assemble the pieces of the face as to complete the figure of a horse.

We have laid great stress in our teaching on the perception of morphemic and word sequences, and of grammar and syntax. Here the crux of the problem lies mainly in temporal relations. Sandy rarely speaks in complete sentences. Today in answer to the question, "What must you do to make water boil?" he said, "Heat water . . . something to put it on." In reading he said *quatity* for *quality*, *collasp* for *collapse*, *imagine* for *image*, *pilot* for *plot*. He tries to spell the word the way it sounds *to him*. Here are some samples from a recent test: *expelt* (expect), *berf* (purse), *serpise* (surprise). In a timed test of paragraph copying he ranked in the eighteenth percentile, a very low score, which might be accounted for by his poor perception and retention of sequences, both of letter and of word and phrase sequences. Basically these temporal and spatial deficits go back to a blunting of visual, auditory, and tactile-kinesthetic perception.

Realizing that the boy was not progressing in sentence building, his classroom teacher decided to teach him the rules of grammar. He was then in the seventh grade. Sandy worked diligently to learn and over-learn the rules. His teachers and parents believe that this technique brought gains in grammatical usage. Sandy's response to our praise of his knowledge of the rules of grammar was guarded: "It's O.K. I don't remember the rules sometimes." His score on vocal encoding in the *Illinois Test of Psycholinguistic Abilities* was 7.4 (CA 13.1). It reflects clearly his incompetence in vocabulary and in grammatical form. Although he plays basketball and baseball, when the examiner handed him a ball and said, "Tell me about this!" all he would say was: "A ball . . . rubber ring around it; hard . . . red." When urged by the examiner to "tell me more," he added, "It bounces." That was all. To be sure he knew much more about many kinds of balls but he probably could not command either the words or the linguistic form necessary for expression. Similarly, in the auditory-vocal sequencing subtest of *ITPA*, he reached only the language age of 7.4 (CA 13.1). In the digit-span test we observed that Sandy did not follow the usual practice of grouping numbers either in a spatial or temporal relation. When the series involved five digits, 2-5-4-9-9, he said them in a broken and inaccurate pattern in this manner: 2—5-4—9-9. The series 6-1-6-3-7 became 6—3—6—

1—7. His difficulties in getting the proper sequence in spelling, reading, and speaking, we must point out, are not caused chiefly by a failure to *retain* patterns of auditory-vocal or visuomotor sequencing but by the lack of clarity or accuracy of the original pattern.

The immediate and obvious effect of perceptual deficit in learning is reflected in the processes of memory. Sandy overlearns the weekly spelling list but since the percept is edgeless in the first place, he is unable to retain them. Sandy spends countless hours preparing for examinations. On one occasion a teacher lost Sandy's examination paper in mathematics, and without warning the boy, presented him with another set of questions three weeks after the first test. Sandy took the test, went to his grandmother's home near the school and cried during the whole noon hour. He realized that he could not pass the test successfully unless he had opportunity to review completely and *immediately* before he took it. At some time he will have to recognize limitations of the time he can spend on review of materials. If his short memory span were restricted to the auditory dimension, he might turn to visual and tactile-kinesthetic methods of learning. Unfortunately they also remain in serious deficit.

One wishes that this boy might find effective ways to stabilize his personality. He remains highly motivated but yet he is a boy of moods, often sulky and depressed. He still is quick to show anger, but the outbursts are less vehement. Manifestations of frustration caused by problems in learning and recall are constant. Perhaps as he faces more realistically the *fact* of a nonreversible injury to his nervous system, he will become more stable and patient with himself. He must learn to "hitch his wagon to a lower star."

The extent to which Sandy will develop competence in language again will be conditioned by many factors that we have discussed. The unknown factors are the plastic and homeostatic potentialities of the boy's nervous system. We certainly assume that it is more plastic than that of the adult, and hence nonspecific inactive cell assemblies yet may enter into active learning processes. We know that as various neuronal systems take on comparatively specialized functions they become less available for more general purposes, and the capacity of the brain to function in an undifferentiated way is reduced as functional differentiation proceeds. The high degree of focalization so characteristic of adult learning behavior could not have been well developed in Sandy's case. We must gamble on the take-over of "unoccupied cell assemblies."

10

Studies of Profiles, II

The Profile of Per: Language Disturbances of a Cerebral-palsied Child

Introduction

Terminology. Our use of the general term, *cerebral palsy* must be explained. Per had been diagnosed, as had many children in the orthopedic hospital where the writer was teaching, first as a spastic, then as an athetoid, and finally as an athetoid child with tension manifestations. In the protocols, the neurological diagnosis had changed as the child developed and as new personnel in neuropediatrics introduced additional criteria for appraisal. As it became apparent that lesions of the nervous system could not be determined by behavioral manifestations, ambiguities in description multiplied. Many a child whose muscles exhibit the "stretch reflex," characteristic of spasticity, also exhibits involuntary muscle movements that are athetotic in nature. Or the muscles may be quite unresponsive to manipulation; they exhibit a lead pipe rigidity. As the child grows older his lack of balance and coordination is noted; the neuropediatrician now adds ataxia to his diagnostic summary. In one individual the behavioral manifestations may be so mixed as to place him in no clearly identifiable class. As someone has said, "cerebral palsy affects individuals so differently that no one statement can apply to all of them, and all of the statements can apply to no one of them. Perhaps a few can apply to some of them."

The neurological syndrome in all manifestations of cerebral palsy must be related to a failure in function in sensory-motor and motor-sensory assemblies. Can the damage be traced to pathways mediating specific functions; to systems of neural integration; to chemical changes in neural substance? Some neurologists hold that the principal damage is in the sensory analyzers and their feedback complements. Others believe that the reticular activating and organizing systems or the limbic and thalamic systems are impaired. Still others interpret the injury as a result of destruction of the glial substance of the cerebrum. Some locate the damage in the parietal and temporal overlay in the cortex. And more recently researchers in the field have been studying chemical alterations of postsynaptic potentials. Answers may come from future research. Determination of loci of lesion goes a very short way toward the answer.

In view of the confusion in terminology and behavioral manifestations, we simply state that Per is cerebral-palsied, that he has suffered damage to the CNS resulting in moderately severe sensory-motor handicaps with sequelae in impaired intelligence, speech, and language. We regard cerebral palsy as a complex of symptoms and not a disease entity. Others define cerebral palsy as but "one component of a broader brain-damage syndrome comprised of neuro-motor dysfunction, psychological dysfunction, convulsions and behavior disorders of organic origin." [1]

Pre- and Perinatal History. Per was one of premature, male, monozygotic twins.[2] His twin died one hour after birth. According to the deceased twin's protocol, portions of his lungs were filled with fluid; the assumption was that the arterial blood was insufficiently saturated with oxygen. Anoxic anoxia was thought to have afflicted both neonates, one fatally. The mother was 30 years of age, the father 36 years at the time of the birth of the twins. Birth was precipitous. The mother reported that some measures were taken in the hospital to "hold back the delivery" until the doctor arrived. Per has one brother, six years his senior. Between the two pregnancies the mother had two miscarriages in the third month of gestation. Although the question of the Rh factor had been raised in medical conferences following the delivery of the twins, no conclusion on that point appears in the record.

Per was placed in an incubator for the first ten days of life. He suffered both from respiratory and feeding problems and did not leave the hospital for six weeks. The mouth reflexes of sucking and swallowing (which ordinarily follow turning of the head) were weak, and they were not coordinated with respiration. The child's weight at six weeks was 5.1 pounds. When the infant was 6 months of age, the mother re-

[1] W. M. Cruickshank and G. M. Raus, *Cerebral palsy.* Syracuse, N. Y.: Syracuse University Press, 1955. P. 2.

[2] In a study of 551 twin births it was found that 12 percent were afflicted with cerebral palsy in one member of the pair.

turned with him to the outpatient clinic of the hospital. She was dissatisfied with his development and reported that the baby cried a great deal, sometimes stiffening the whole body as he did so. He often choked even on liquids and seemed to have much difficulty in swallowing. At this time the neuropediatrician noted in the record the presence of *fisted hands, cat back* (rounded back), *tonic neck reflexes, extension of neck and spine,* the *grasp reflex* of a neonate, a *head lag* in being pulled up by the arms, and the persistence of the *Moro reflex* (startle response). Except in cases of CNS injury, tonic neck reflexes are abnormal after the first five months of life. The Moro reflex normally disappears within the first three months of life. The neuropediatrician gave a tentative diagnosis of "brain injury" but made no mention of spasticity or cerebral palsy at this time.

Developmental data. At 16 months Per was able to sit with the support of his less affected hand, but the mother reported that he usually collapsed in a forward position after a few minutes. At 2 years he could be pulled to a standing position but with dominance of the flexion pattern in his feet. Excessive tension of the whole body accompanied standing. Per took his first step at 3½ years but before that time the mother had noticed the flexed position of the child's right forearm and the inversion of the right foot. Although she was positive that the child understood some language at 3 years, he babbled very little beyond calling [ɑʔɑ] for *mama,* and made no attempt to imitate the speech of those around him until he was 4.6 years of age. The mother admits, however, that in their isolated home environment motivation of speech has been minimal.

Neurological Reports. When Per was 2.6 years old, he was hospitalized for neurological study. Both electroencephalography and pneumocephalography were employed. The EEG revealed epileptogenic foci, spikes, and slow waves in the left occipital area, and a general slow dysrhythmia of the alpha wave in both hemispheres. At 4.6 years the examination was repeated. In the pneumocephalographic study the third ventricle and upper lateral corner of the lateral ventricies were found to be enlarged. It was reported that such an incursion undoubtedly involved the reticulostrial and corticofugal networks of the central nervous system, and perhaps even greater atrophic changes in the striate bodies and thalamus. The second EEG revealed spikes in the left temporal-parietal area. The shift in rhythmic disturbance from occipital to parietal-temporal areas was considered a common neurological occurrence. In the protocol the pediatrician notes the presence of exaggerated stretch reflexes (the result of disturbance in the gamma spindles) and ankle clonus. The diagnosis of moderate spastic quadriplegia now is entered for the first time in the record.

Orthopedic Hospital School. Per was 5 years old when he entered the resident school operated by an orthopedic hospital. He walked with the right knee and hip noticeably flexed; the left was only slightly impaired. His gait could not be described as scissored; it was rather a plunging, unstable movement. Both in sitting and standing postures the head was carried in a forward position, shoulders rounded, the right forearm bent forward, right hand pronated, and fingers flexed. There was a weaving motion and considerable instability throughout the body, even when he was sitting. When he began to walk the head was mildly retracted and everted; tonic neck reflexes and athetotic movements were much more evident. In repose the mouth was open, the lips flaccid, and the tongue often protruded slightly. When performing any motor task, and particularly in speech attempts, facial grimaces replaced the mask-like expression. Sometimes the muscle tone was so great that the athetotic tremor no longer was evident. At other times there was a cogwheel rigidity caused by the locking and release of muscles. Three months after he entered the hospital school, a diagnosis of tension-athetosis was entered in the medical protocol.

Per appeared to be a frail child but the mother said he was rarely ill. He has suffered none of the usual childhood diseases, but in his hermetically sealed environment this was quite understandable. At the doctor's insistence the mother had begun to give the child solid foods. She insisted that he had great difficulty chewing and swallowing solid food but she also admitted that he had very little practice. He handled a spoon and a pusher adequately but awkwardly with his left hand. His sleep generally was restless, the mother thought, but since his father or brother had begun the practice of taking the child out of doors for a ride in his go-cart, sleep habits had improved. The mother was apologetic for her overprotectiveness, but the child was so easily upset, she said, even by the bark of a dog or the hoot of a train, that such protection seemed necessary. It was evident that the child did overreact to many situations. The writer upset a flask containing large wood beads. Per was greatly startled; his hands flew up and his head turned to the side. After recognizing the nature of the accident, he went into paroxysms of laughter, a response as uninhibited as was his startle reaction. Drooling was most evident during this episode.

Initial Evaluative Studies

Basic Motor Patterns. 1. *Motor infantilism.* In introducing this profile Per's general motoric behavior was described. Some characteristics are clearly the result of motor infantilism; others are compensatory motor abnormalities that have developed as a result of motor infantilism. The Moro, or startle reflex, for example, about which Per's mother had been concerned, is a set of reflexes in which selected musculature of the trunk and limbs responds to maintain security of the body. It precedes the development of equilibrium reactions that later emerge as a reorganization of the Moro pattern and are largely inhibitory in nature. In Per this set of reflexes appears as an independent functioning unit.

2. *Postural patterns.* Basic to Per's problems of posture and movement are the tonic neck reflex patterns. They too reflect a developmental failure in reciprocal innervation and control. The feedback mechanism that normally limits the reflex by stimulation of discharges in the antagonistic muscles has been impaired. As a result of this developmental failure, the disorganized reflex movements initiate a circular phenomenon of facilitation, hypertonicity, and inhibition or distortion of movement. The reflexes, in other words, operate as independent functioning units, uninhibited and disorganized. If Per sits, presumably unnoticed in his chair in the lounge, his head is forward, the shoulder girdle depressed and his right arm adducted and rotated inward. But when he hears my footsteps, the head is thrown back, the shoulders retracted, and hypertonicity of the neck and facial muscles occurs. Then very slowly mild athetotic writhing movements appear, first in the hands, and then throughout the entire upper body. The extension patterns of reflex presumably now are predominant. When he recognizes me, the facial mask breaks into laughter; he cannot smile. His gait also reflects the domination of disorganized reflex patterns. Now 6 years old, Per walks, aided by a walking stick, with a plunging gait, swinging the severely impaired right leg and foot in a semicircular movement. A twister is to be fitted which should stabilize and correct ankle deformity.

3. *Speech—Overlaid motor function.* The fact that speech is an overlaid function is significant when a child is handicapped by neuromotor disturbances. Because the production of speech is superimposed upon a breathing mechanism (power supply of speech), a part of which has been transformed into a complex tone generator, and upon deglutitory and air transmission channels (resonance and articulation), speech must take on all the disturbances peculiar to the visceral responses of breathing and deglutition. If the prespeech reflexes of salivary control and of chewing and swallowing have not developed, the mechanism cannot be easily adapted for learned patterns of articulation. It is difficult to impose controlled breathing patterns upon patterns already asynergic, and even more difficult to coordinate the phonatory and articulatory mechanisms for speech.

Sensory-Motor Disturbances. Language learning requires an integration of neuronal assemblies embracing several sensory modalities. Patterning of visual, haptic, and auditory stimuli in the CNS may be distorted if fluctuation occurs, either peripherally or at some point in the neural run. When haptic feedback produced by reflex postures of the head and neck is disturbed, for example, auditory or visual perception may be affected. The presence of dysrhythmic cortical waves suggests that sensory-motor impulses from several modalities also may be subjected to cortical interruption or distortion. Although we shall discuss modalities separately, we must remember that they are not independent operants in perception.

Auditory Disturbances. Per was referred to a national hearing center for auditory assessment. A moderate loss of acuity in the right ear for high-frequency tones was established. In a subsequent study made when Per was 7 years old, the audiologist suggested the possibility of other cochlear disturbances, namely diplacusis (the hearing of a tone as if it were two tones of different pitch), and a latency between stimulus and response. Whether diplacusis was the result of a peripheral or central disturbance was later questioned. The audiologist concluded that Per's disturbance in auditory perception might be caused by one or several factors: shifting thresholds, response latency, or faulty feedback.

In our initial study we thought that unilateral loss of high frequencies materially affected Per's ability to comprehend speech. Later we were less inclined to consider the loss significant and more inclined to place greater weight on the interruption of auditory perception by the involuntary movements of the head and neck. Auditory perception suffered not so much from a dearth of sensations as from distorted auditory patterns in the CNS.

Visual and Haptic Disturbances. Comprehension of language is not dependent solely, or even primarily, upon audition (Chapter 2). Visual signals, subjected either to peripheral or central fluctuation may produce distorted visual perception of the movements of speech. Tactile-kinesthetic learning may be interrupted in the same way. When Per tried to imitate subvocally the pattern we set for him, for example, lightning-like movements of the head and neck produced fluctuations in kinesthetic feedback. Disturbances in haptic feedback also are inevitable when articulatory movements are impaired; this was the case with Per. He was dysarthric because the muscles of the speech mechanism were constantly "misinformed" by distorted sensory-motor patterns in the CNS.[3] Per frequently said, "I can't remember where or how my tongue should go." He cannot perceive the sequential pattern of movements required for articulation because his nervous system is unable to integrate sensory-motor patterns into a chain activity resulting in accurate perceptual configurations.

Perceptual Processes. We were interested in studying the total effect of sensory-motor disturbances upon the perception of linguistic elements. What was their effect upon such elements of sequencing as selection of cues, syntactic form, closure, and prosody? We observed that

[3] H. Schuell, Dysphasia as dysarthria. *J Speech Hearing Res* (December 1962), 5: 366.

Per confused the sequence of morphemes, words, and phrases but once he had learned the correct sequence he would not change it. Just as he did not recognize his last name if a single letter was changed or omitted in writing, so he would not recognize a word or phrase if we introduced slight changes in order or in pronunciation. Occasionally we would print a word but write one of its letters in script; the word no longer was intelligible to him. He could cope with no variations, whether they were visual, auditory, or haptic.[4] When he learned a pattern, it was fixed, rigid. He knew how to order certain sentences, and he was not free to experiment with the form. The need for constancy of form also extended to nonverbal learning. Nonsignificant variations in shape, position, or color as in forms or letters made recognition difficult. In the early years of his training a square was a square only in terms of color or the material of which it was made. He found security in a very specific pattern and entertained no alterations in the percept. Would multi-sensory training employing verbal symbols in sequence be the best approach to the semantic and prosodic elements of language? We would try it.

A related problem in sequencing was his tendency to perceive words in isolation, not as part of a phrase or sentence. We observed that when he read a news headline, he attempted to "take it in" word by word. When he was asked to repeat the sense of the headline, he grabbed the paper and read it again, this time aloud to us. If he continued to perceive words out of context, certainly he would be handicapped in recall. He would have to set the cues in the phrase or sentence if he would turn the key to recall. This kind of piecemeal sequencing undoubtedly was related to disturbances in comprehending other linguistic elements: closure, figure-ground, syntactic form, and prosody. One problem rode upon the heels of others. Per was unable to use cues to anticipate what was to follow. In the perceptively normal individual all perceptual relations tend to be probablistic in the sense that anticipations determine his response. Per was not able to predict the next cue from those which had preceded it. Perhaps this difficulty was caused by the evanescent, slight distortions which he experienced in all cues. Disregarding the specific cause, we know that he perceived all cues as independent, isolated bits of information. The difficulty might be also related to a failure in general drive and set-to-attend mechanisms which generally enhance the organization of cues. Perhaps if Per learned to perceive more accurately the initial cues of a sentence, not only would his prediction of successive cues increase but he also might be able to perceive the sentence as a whole. The total pattern, no longer blurred and piecemeal, would approximate reality, and that is the aim of all perception—to make the percept veridical, to make it agree with reality. We knew that training in perception

4 W. F. Hull, Learning. San Francisco: Chandler Pub., 1963. P. 98.

of syntactic form also would improve perception of the whole phrase or sentence, but how could we teach it? The question was not answered very satisfactorily in the course of our teaching.

Per's perception was noticeably affected by shifting figure-ground relations. He was frustrated and irritated by low-level noises of his surround, particularly if they were strange or persistent noises.[5] He could not be taught in a group because certain noises inevitably were strange, at least to him. And if speech signals were to remain in the foreground, they also must be in the customary temporal relations. If we increased the rate he seemed unable to find meaning. What became of the speech signals? Were they confused with the surround? That this perceptual immaturity or disturbance applied to other modalities could be surmised from the way in which he identified pictures. Like a 3-year-old child, Per compared the figure carefully with the background. He did not distinguish automatically between foreground and background or study the particular characteristics of the outline of the figure, as 5-year-olds are wont to do.[6]

Dysrhythmia and meaningless intonation patterns combine to produce a kind of scanning speech, which again must result from reciprocal difficulties, peripheral and central. The melodic patterns of speech are disturbed in execution because the breathing-phonatory-articulatory triumvirate is asynergic. But Per also cannot comprehend the melodic patterns because he cannot follow them mimetically. Disorganized and discordant tactile-kinesthetic impulses flow in the nervous system but it is unable to form them into patterns which can be discriminated. The waves do not fit in with tactile-kinesthetic patterns previously laid down or with parallel auditory and visual patterns. As a result, Per has no firm imprint in the CNS of time, force, and direction—the analogues of rate, stress, and intonation. Anyone who has worked to modify a scanning rhythm in a cerebral-palsied child knows how difficult this is. The rhythm is perseverative probably because the nervous system cannot build up a positive after-potential in short order. The result is that there is created a closed self-reexciting chain of neurones which have no fixed circuits and serve to confuse rather than to heighten perception of the prosodic qualities of speech. Although we knew that this deficit contributed to Per's blurred perception, we decided to pursue less complex means of reinforcement.

Motivation. One's mind must be explored, if it is to develop. Like so many cerebral-palsied children Per's very early life was an

[5] L. Lerea, An investigation of auditory figure-ground perception. *J Genet Psychol* (June 1961), 98: 229–237.

[6] V. P. Zinchenko, *et al.,* The establishment and development of perceptual ability. Translations from *Voprosy Psikhol* (*Problems of Psychology*) (November 29, 1962), 3: 1–17.

egocentric fixation. Communication with others was rare. Until he entered the hospital school, he knew only the world of *Me*. In such an egocentric world, the drive to explore, to learn, rarely is exercised. Yet drive must be incited. Motivation, as we have pointed out earlier, has a psychological substrate (Chapter 4). If Per's environment remained "faceless"—and there are countless numbers of cerebral-palsied children who live in environmental deprivation— certainly motivation would wither on the vine. The solicitude of Per's parents had reduced early motivation. Social and physical isolation had dulled the drive to explore. His own distractibility and ineptness in blocking intrusive sights and sounds had diminished his power to attend. Upon his admission to hospital school, he was faced with frustrations and failures. Two vital objectives emerged in the first year: the development of an environment conducive to learning and the regeneration of drives and built-in incentives. Once Per learned to enjoy a barrage of sensory-motor experiences, verbal stimulation, and rewards, we expected the motivation in learning to mature despite his early faceless environment.[7]

Later Evaluations

As we continued our exploration of Per's language disability we began to experiment with more specific evaluative techniques. Very few were objective measures and few could be called entirely reliable, yet they were useful tools in our observation and diagnostic teaching. Many measures that we now employ were not available to us.

Mental Growth. The psychologist on the staff modified standard procedures of psychological testing to suit Per's needs. With the exception of the *Columbia Mental Maturity Test* and *Ammons Picture Vocabulary Test,* all psychological measures including *Wechsler Intelligence Scale for Children* and the *Stanford-Binet Test* (Terman-Merrill Revision, Form L) were adapted by the psychologist. Sometimes she gave the test first according to standard procedure, and then gave it later with modifications, a kind of controlled flexibility. She did not think that she had invalidated the results by making such changes as these: In stringing beads, Per placed the beads on the table according to the recalled design (Stanford Binet, Form L: Year VI:2). Instead of counting blocks (VI: 4), colored balls were drawn in a row on a long piece of paper and spaced well apart; Per was asked to make a mark on the ball indicating the correct number. When matching of outline forms was called for, the psychologist substituted greatly enlarged cards with solid color forms. Sometimes she used test items in a multiple choice situation though they are not standardized in that manner. She did not always ad-

[7] C. J. Phillips and R. R. White, The prediction of educational progress among cerebral palsied children. *Develop Med Child Neurol* (April 1964), 6: 167–174.

minister the tests in order. Because Per's abilities were scattered she did not follow the established rules with respect to cellar or ceiling. She rarely completed one test in a single session.

The first psychological evaluations were completed in his seventh year. On the *Peabody Picture Vocabulary Test,* which measures a facet of intellectual development especially important in language learning, i.e., the ability to comprehend words, Per had a mental age of 78. On the *Columbia Mental Maturity Scale,* his MA was 90 but one must remember that this test measures only one aspect of perception: categorization based on differences. The *Leiter International Performance Scale* was modified considerably because of Per's motoric handicaps; his score was 79. At 9 years he received a score of 86 on the *Stanford-Binet* (Form L-M), and on the *WISC* administered later the same year, he earned a score of 88. Were his gains to be accounted for on the basis of maturation, environment, or of consistent teaching by the entire staff? All three factors undoubtedly contributed to his mental development.

Auditory Comprehension. We were not concerned with tests of comprehension which measure a child's ability to comprehend phonemes or words in isolation because, as we have made clear earlier (Chapter 2), we believe that they do not measure the basic perceptual abilities of the child in comprehending speech units, the continuum of oral language. Selected spondee words may measure auditory acuity but they do not measure comprehension.[8] On the other hand, assessment of articulation of linguistic sequences does bear directly upon comprehension, for articulatory competence depends on accurate perception and recall of gestalten, the integrated patterns of tactile-kinesthetic, visual, and auditory patterning.

Evaluations of auditory perception were conducted informally in a teaching situation over an extended period. Commands such as the following were introduced casually during a learning session: "Here are three papers, a big one, a middle-sized one, and a little one. Take the biggest, rumple it up and throw it on the floor. Give me the middle-sized one. Put the smallest one in your pocket." (Pierre Marie's *Paper Test.*)

A test of comprehension span which required knowledge of a basic vocabulary was useful in the first period of evaluative teaching. Similar in design to the Rochford-Williams test (p. 269), it consisted of a set of cards, each bearing a series of three pictures. As we pointed to each picture, proceeding always from left to right, we asked such questions as, "Is this the ball? Is this the smallest book?" Per responded by nodding his head.

Later we tried a more formal *Token Test,* similar in design to the

[8] H. A. Grey, M. J. D'Asaro and M. Sklar, Auditory perceptual thresholds in brain-injured children. *J Speech Hearing Res* (March 1965), 8: 49–56.

test that de Renzi has developed.[9] Adjustments were made for his motor handicap, and confusion arising from a mass of stimuli was avoided by presenting only two lines at a time. In this test there ordinarily are four rows of five tokens each—large circles, small circles, large rectangles, and small rectangles—in each row there is a red, blue, green, yellow, and a white token. In the first four parts, commands are expressed in nonredundant, elementary grammatical and syntactical form: *verb-object*. In the fifth part, grammatical particles or other more complex syntactic structures are introduced. The test makes two kinds of demand upon comprehension: the necessity to identify a particular token by three independent features, and to grasp the semantic restrictions introduced by the "small instruments of language." One proceeds from the first level of comprehension: "Pick up the yellow circle" to the second: "Pick up the large blue rectangle," to the third, (large tokens only): "Take the red circle and the green rectangle," to the fourth: "Take the white large circle and the small green rectangle," to the fifth: "Put the red circle on the green rectangle." Per was not able to reach the fourth or fifth levels, even in the final period of diagnostic teaching.

Although the *Auditory-Vocal Automatic* Test (ITPA Subtest) was not available to us when Per was a student in the hospital school, we had devised similar test items to assess auditory perception. Again we are dealing with the comprehension of sentences, not words, and particularly with the perception of syntax and grammar. From behind a screen we would say, *Here is a flower; here are two* _____; *I have a sausage; you have two* _____; *All the apples are big but this one is the* _____; *Daddy likes to drink ale; now he is* _____. In auditory-vocal association, we employed such simple completion items as, *The bear walks; the fish* _____. To evaluate auditory-visual-motor discrimination, we presented a progressive series of pictures from the story of *Little Tin Soldier* (H. C. Andersen). As we told the story Per selected the appropriate picure for each event.

Haptic Perception. Several tests of general tactile-kinesthetic perception were available, but we found no way to appraise objectively the integrity of haptic control of articulatory muscles. In view of Per's low threshold for many stimuli, we could not explain his high threshold for touch. He never seemed to be aware of saliva dripping from his chin or a fly crawling over his hand. Two-point discrimination on both sides of the lips was very poor. The front tongue was superior to the lips in stereognostic perception but both were feeble sensory receivers.[10] From

[9] E. de Renzi and L. A. Vignolo, Test for aphasics. *Brain* (December 1962), 85: 665–78.

[10] Natadze has devised a test of oral stereognosis which he believes assesses the haptic control of the articulatory organs. R. G. Natadze, Studies on thought and speech problems by psychologists of the Georgian S. S. R. In N. O'Connor, Ed., *Recent Soviet psychology*. New York: Liveright, 1961. Pp. 304–326.

these informal measures and from observation we assumed that haptic perception must be poor, but we were not able to formulate reliable measures. When blindfolded, Per could not identify a tennis ball, or the box in which we kept the marbles for the marble-board test. He did promptly identify an apple and a piece of chalk but we suspect that the cue to the former object was smell and the latter, temperature. (The box of chalk was kept on the ledge of an open window.) We were not successful in getting him to approximate tongue movements in imitating our articulation of three-word sentences. He did somewhat better when we used his hand to describe the movements of the tongue as the sentence was articulated.

We learned more about Per's deficit in haptic feedback by observing his motor behavior in speech and other activities than by any tests. Per could not simulate the articulatory movements of a phrase without saying it orally. He could not go through the *pretended action* of drinking a glass of water. He often said that he knew what he should do but he could not do it. Muscle memory apparently was so weak that he could not articulate a phrase successfully a second time. The expressionless face and the absence of gesture (with the better hand) were further evidences of a disability in motor learning.[11] Sometimes we would ask him to copy our slow and measured articulatory movements of phrases very familiar to him. He practiced them diligently but the next day it seemed as if he began learning the pattern all over again. His kinetic memory of speech patterns remained blurred and insubstantial for a long time.

Spatial perception. As a factor in sequencing linguistic units, we already have been concerned with space perception, but we have not measured it as a separate entity. Indeed we cannot measure space perceptors because we do not possess them. We assess the perception of space by a series of relations among cues from visual, tactile-kinesthetic, and auditory modalities, and these relations are predicated upon the body image and one's sense of directionality or laterality which develops from it. That is to say, we locate objects laterally with relation to each other but also with relation to our own bodies. In the first stages of learning perceptual-motor matching, the modalities of taction and kinesthesis logically would precede the visual and auditory, both in time and in importance. The distortions of body image and posture which Per experienced certainly affected not only his sense of position but also his directionality. If we asked him to line up his body with the vertical line drawn on the long mirror which he faced, he would overshoot the mark, shifting from a right-sided tilt to the left. He often complained of dizziness and disorientation after a strenuous session in physical therapy.

[11] H. Goodglass and E. Kaplan, Disturbance of gesture and pantomime in aphasia. *Brain* (December 1963), 86: 703–720.

Perhaps his reaction was similar to ours when we look out from a tilted airplane and find the sky "in the wrong place." In other words, the effect may have resulted from an inability to relate parts, suddenly out of line, to the perceptual whole. The deficit is in perceptual integration. Space perception, moreover, is a relative judgment. Only by comparison with something else can we judge size, texture, or structure. We say that "it is longer than one's foot," "as smooth as velvet," "larger than a bread basket," "built like the Seattle 'Needle.'" An Italian lad, blind from birth, said recently when sight had been restored, "I always thought an elephant was as big as a house."

The right hand of Per was more seriously impaired than the left so one would expect him to establish the left hand as the dominant one. In view of his genetic history (twinning and sinistrality in the family), it is highly probable that Per was natively left handed. That he was clearly confused at 8 years in right-left orientation was evident from his responses to commands. A crossed command, "Put your left hand on my right shoulder" was not executed correctly until he was nearly 10 years old. If Per could develop a left-right gradient for the projection of dimensionality, we believed that the skill also should promote his perception of the other coordinates of space: up-down and before-behind. How to develop this sense of directionality within the body first as a part of its motor patterns and then to project them into outside space was clearly a problem. Although we do not hold that psychological integrity, the self concept, must be fully developed before any language skills can develop, we found that gains in language use proceeded apace with his gains in body image and position sense.

We did not investigate all dimensions of space perception—shape, texture, size, and structure—but we made many observations, both formal and informal, of perceptual deficits. Per regularly misjudged space and distance in reaching for or replacing toys on the shelf. In the first year of his schooling, we found that only a red square was a square; he would not identify a blue square of the same dimension as a square. He later modified this response but in a strange way: he counted corners before he named it a square. In his second year of schooling (now 8 years old), he understood letters only if they were in block print. He could not accommodate perception to any change in form, although the basic outline might not have been changed. Occasionally we would present the form board to him, rotated a half turn. He still could recognize where the block belonged but he could not fit it in without great twisting and shifting of himself and the formboard. His immaturity in visuospatial perception was further demonstrated in all exercises of figure-ground discrimination. We already have alluded to his practice of scanning the outline of the figure in detail before he could separate it from the surround. In the interpretation of pictures this practice handicapped him for he often would fix attention upon one detail of the picture. The result was that he was unable finally to integrate these piecemeal perceptions. Perception, you will remember, "takes place all at once, and nothing first."

On three tests at 8 years, *Kohs Block Design, Goldstein-Scheerer Stick Test,* and the *Bender Visual-Motor Gestalt Test,* Per performed at a 6-year level, but when these tests were administered again, nearly two years later and after a prolonged period of training, he showed a retardation of only one year. Is it possible that as body schema, posture, and directionality matured, space perception no longer was seriously deficient?

Growth of Perceptual Processes. For many months Per's progress was scarcely discernible. Then perhaps because of the stimulus of a new environment and the training program in other departments of the hospital school, Per began to show a slight advance in language learning. He seemed for the first time to want to communicate with others. Previously he had made speech attempts but they did not appear to relate to him. One had the impression that he was not participating as an individual in communication. Of course it must be remembered that Per was not accustomed to *participation,* to the give and take in dynamic communication.

We were eager to assess Per's advance in perceptual learning. Much earlier we had borrowed some sentences from standard psychological measures and made up others in order to explore his ability to categorize percepts by similarity or difference. Some familiar sentences were: *Ole is a little boy; Astrid is a little* _____; *In summer it is hot; in winter it is* _____; *A bird flies; a fish* _____. Whereas Per had been able to complete only 10 of the series of 25 sentences, now he completes 19. This time he did not make bizarre and nonessential contrasts or comparisons. The following day he brought in two sentences of his own making. We shifted then to a more difficult measure, to the game of *Twenty Questions,* another borrowed idea.[12] In this game he was to distinguish similarities and differences in birds, animals, or vehicles. Slowly Per was moving toward a procedure, a *system* of categorization. *Twenty Questions* remained his favorite game for a long time. We also wanted to appraise development of inner language but we had no suitable measuring stick. Inner language might be judged by his competence in marshalling concepts in a temporal sequence and in demonstrating inner logic in a short story. We devoted many sessions to this exercise. Unfortunately we could not understand much of what he recounted. We would have to wait until his speech became more intelligible.

[12] C. E. Renfrew, Spoken language in intellectually handicapped children. In C. Renfrew and K. Murphy, Eds., *The child who does not talk.* London: Heinemann, 1964. P. 138.

Grammar and Syntax. Per's ability to perceive grammatical and syntactical relationships is another measure of language comprehension and use. We constructed our own version of an auditory-vocal test which, however, we could not consider to be automatic.[13] We began with the use of plurals, continued with verb tense, voice, and pronouns, and ended with conjunctions and prepositions. The inflective relationships, *Where is your brother's friend?* and *Where is Astrid's sister's friend?* were too complex for him, even at 9 years.

Motor Speech. During the first year of Per's residence in the hospital school, no objective assessment of his speech was made. There was, in fact, little speech to assess, and what he said was largely unintelligible. Breathing was shallow, nonrhythmic; pitch, intensity, and quality were uncontrolled. Furthermore a course in physical therapy had been projected as a precedent to training in speech. Accordingly little was done in specific training of *motor* speech. All our time was devoted to the development of language. We were encouraged by his progress.

Educational Guidelines

Per's enrollment in the resident hospital school was his good fortune, for he was to have the unusual advantages of total *situational* education. It was our good fortune to be a part of an educational plan in cooperation with skilled workers from several areas. The team was made up of physical therapists, occupational therapists, language clinicians, classroom teachers, music and crafts teachers, and medical, psychological, and social counsellors. The experience demonstrated the imperative of team endeavor. The profile of Per underscores our belief that language training should not, cannot, be extracted from the total educational milieu. Insofar as it becomes an integral part of the child's education, it will be successful.

The team agreed that Per's education should proceed along these lines: 1. A program of perceptual-motor education employing the Bobath method should precede training in the oral use of language. The sequence is logical when one considers the alternatives. If tonic neck and labyrinthine reflexes, mass flexion and extension of reflexes, and the postural and righting reflexes are organized, even partially, correct postural and movement patterns should mature. (Although K. and B. Bobath use the term, *reflexes*, a more accurate term is reflexogenic, or automatic response–patterns.[14]) On the other hand, if abnormal reflexes are not trained to respond in an organized pattern, contractures and distortions

[13] See J. J. McCarthy and S. A. Kirk, *Examiners manual: Illinois test of psycho-linguistic abilities.* Urbana, Ill.: The University of Illinois Press, 1961. P. 31f.

[14] K. Bobath, and B. Bobath, A treatment of cerebral palsy based on the analysis of the patient's motor behaviour. *Brit J Phys Med* (May 1952), 15: 1–11.

of movement will continue to develop. If asymmetrical tonic neck reflexes are not inhibited, for example, every part of the speech apparatus—respiration, phonation, and articulation—will suffer. Should motor patterns of sucking, chewing, and swallowing remain infantile, development of articulatory patterns will be difficult. Feedback, serviceable to perceptual processes, should result from setting the sensory-motor system in order.

Although the team elected to employ the Bobath method, its general premise is also the basis of the Kabat-Knott resistance-traction technique [15] and Young's moto-kinesthetic system of education.[16] Since motor learning is directed and controlled by feedback, they conclude that distortions of motion can be corrected by changing the character of the message transmitted through the feedback monitor. And when inaccurate sensory-motor signals are eliminated, distortions of movement will be corrected, excess motion shut out, and useful patterns of posture and movement elaborated.

The Bobath method has as its specific rationale the interruption of gross automatic response-patterns of movement, to be followed by the facilitation of finer patterns of the speech musculature. The cerebral-palsied child must be freed from his primitive reflex patterns of movement so that he may use parts of these patterns, resynthesized and elaborated, for voluntary activities.[17] If the tonic reflexes, for example, can be inhibited, then the muscles may be placed in a proper status so that proprioceptive feedback will incite proper impulses in surrounding muscles before either stretch or relaxation is attempted. Favorable reflex-inhibiting postures (RIP) are those which induce optimum selective summation, adaptation, and reciprocal innervation of fine muscles. The Bobaths describe the method:

In order to effect reflex inhibition, the posture has to be changed in such a way that neither the flexion nor the extension reflex can operate. While the hips and knees remain in full flexion, the flexor spasticity of the trunk is counteracted by extending the spine. The arms are moved forward and placed on the support, with full extension of the elbows, wrists and fingers. In order to counteract inward rotation of the upper arms and pronation of the forearms, the palms should face each other. Lastly, the head is raised, and thus flexion ought to be counteracted, and extensor activity facilitated by a change of the position of the head in space (again affecting tonic labyrinthine reflexes).

[15] H. Kabat and M. Knott, Proprioceptive facilitation techniques for treatment of paralysis. *Phys Ther Rev* (February, 1953), 33: 53–64.

[16] E. H. Young and S. S. Hawk, *Moto-kinesthetic speech training*. Palo Alto, Calif.: Stanford Univer. Press, 1955.

[17] M. Crickmay, *Description and orientation of the Bobath method with reference to speech rehabilitation in cerebral palsy*. Chicago: National Society for Crippled Children and Adults, 1955.

The flexion pattern of the legs is broken up by placing the feet in plantar flexion and slight inversion.[18]

Appropriate positioning is basic to the reversal of tonic motor patterns. Hypertension of the neck and head, for example, which produces increased tension in the laryngeal area, will be reversed to one of reflexion by the forced assumption of the basic reflex-inhibiting posture in the child. At first, struggle may accompany the placement and maintenance of the child in the reflex-inhibiting posture. Gradually the child should adjust voluntarily to the new posture and be able to maintain the position by himself. At that juncture the speech mechanism presumably is in an optimum state; the neck and throat are relaxed, the jaw is in a proper resting position, and the stage is set for graded proprioceptive feedback that will shunt the excitation into previously inhibited muscles. Reciprocal innervation of fine muscles becomes operative in easy, relaxed phonation. Inhibition of these movement patterns, externally by the teacher, internally by the child, should induce finer and more mature movements to develop on the foundation of normal posture. The character of feedback messages presumably will be changed. The child now can "believe" proprioceptive information from the muscles and will be able to respond to the new sensory-motor patterns in a normal way. Eventually the child will extend individuation, synthesis, and elaboration to the fine movements of articulation. There will be setbacks in the process. Old automatic patterns under pressure may flare up and frustrations again will appear. Consistent and persistent training, however, should nullify temporary reversals. The team agreed that a training period of twelve to eighteen months in the Bobath method should precede Per's course in language skills.

2. Physical therapy designed to normalize posture and movement forms the broad base for perceptual-motor training. Its purpose is to develop and operate the organism as a unitary reaction system. Subtler perceptual-motor patterns must be developed, however, which depend not only upon haptic feedback but also upon visuomotor and auditory-motor circuits.

The language clinician begins a program in perceptual-motor skills of language while physical and occupational therapists *continue* perceptual-motor education in other behavioral responses. Our work cannot be boxed up in a self-contained cell of activity. Unless all parts of the program are closely coordinated we all fail. We may find, for example, that the physical therapist is better able than we are to train the child in breathing synergies essential for speech. We seek her assistance. The music teacher may reinforce our work in development of smooth synchronized patterns of phonation and articulation. Classroom teachers and house

[18] K. Bobath and B. Bobath, *op. cit.*

counsellors must provide opportunities for the exercise of Per's new competencies in speech. Constant intercommunication and mutual assistance are essential to the success of his education.

Speech production demands precise components: direction, force, sequence, and duration. These must be perceived before they can be executed; and the sequences of movement must be firmly imprinted in the central nervous system. Per's new postural and movement patterns are maturing, but they will need continuous reinforcement. We must anticipate occasional reversal to immature motor responses. Sudden tension in the sternocleidomastoid and platysma muscles will set off clavicular breathing; the position of the larynx may be altered momentarily by tension in the supra- and infrahyoid muscles which also will change the position of the hyoid bone. If training had modified completely oral-pharyngeal patterns of sucking, chewing, and swallowing, the velopharyngeal sphincter would not open suddenly and interrupt the speech synergy. As reinforcement of basic training continues our program in language learning is facilitated.

At this stage we will not stress precision in phonatory or articulatory patterns. For the present this goal is beyond Per's reach. We must be content with advances in the quantity and quality of expression which should reflect heightened perception of morphemic order, syntax, vocabulary, and the melody of speech.

3. Per one day should progress to intensive education of perceptual-motor processes associated with the *continuum of oral expression:* rapid and accurate sequencing of large linguistic units, aided by the development of vocabulary, grammar, syntax, prosodic qualities, and a measure of articulatory competence. The methods and materials of perceptual-motor training have been suggested in preceding chapters but they must be adapted to Per's needs. A language clinician proposed that at this stage we might use speech-reading (lip reading) as a technique for establishing visual-haptic coding, to be combined later with auditory reinforcement. Beginning with nonvocal mimetic tracking of stories told by the teacher, Per would go on to such exercises as reading stories aloud in concert with the teacher, demonstrating stories with pictures or actions, and finally repeating the same processes in conversational speech about school and community events. For aid in establishing rhythmic patterns of speech we would invite the cooperation of the music teacher. He had suggested at one time that if Per learned to play a tonette, basic breathing synergies would be improved. Now it should be tried, we thought. Rhythmic patterns also might be established through simple musical scores accompanied by action (tapping, rocking) or by sound sequences (*la-la-la; row, row, row your boat*). Action games and stories employing rhythmic repetitions of key sentences also would be useful.

Eventually Per must work toward a *measure* of competence in the use of the speech mechanism. The release of tension at the base of the tongue should ensure greater mobility of the tip. Control of the tongue by such haptic reinforcement as resistance or external pressure (rubber roller or tapper) might be tried. Our goal is not precision of speech skills. We would be satisfied if Per eventually could develop smooth, easy synergies of breathing and phonation, rolling sequences of tongue and lip movements, and simple rhythmic patterns.

Psychoemotional Development. The basis had been laid for a good adjustment by the combination of the new environment, help from counsellors, and a varied program of education. Social and physical isolation and undue parental solicitude undoubtedly had dulled Per's drive in his early years. There were frustrations and failures in physical and occupational therapy, to be sure, but they had been countered by an environment conducive to active learning. Per now exhibited drive and some control over his environment. He still reacts occasionally to situations of excitement and confusion either with fear or prolonged laughter but these episodes are much less frequent. Whereas before he was abnormally responsive to stimuli of his environment, reacting unselectively, passively, and without conscious intent, now he is a participant in his environment. Behavior, in other words, is a function, not of the external event alone, but of his *perception of it.* His greatest problems are to come in social life. Although he knows that he will always be regarded as a cerebral-palsied person, he wants to be accepted in a non-cerebral-palsied world. We hope to show him that such regard is a two-way street, that acceptance is based on mutual understanding. He must develop the sense of being a person, meeting others who also are real people in a knowable environment. We predict that he will achieve this goal.

The Profile of Karen: Language Disturbances of an Autistic Child

Karen is a pretty, curly-haired, slender child of 4.6 years who entered our Center on the recommendation of a psychiatrist. She skipped into the director's office ahead of her mother and raced around the room stopping for a second before each picture on the wall. She repeated *Hi* several times to no one in particular and then stood looking out of the window, completely oblivious to our request that she share the rocking chair with the teddy bear. She refused to remove her coat and cap but wandered into the adjoining playroom. There she found a doll, turned a large chair toward the window, away from the director and her mother in the next room, and began to hum in a high-pitched, nasal tone. The mother is attractive, modishly dressed, and reserved in mien and manner. She did not remove her gloves or dark glasses throughout the interview and apparently paid no attention to her daughter's action.

Family History.   There is nothing remarkable in the early history of Karen, except her position in the family. She was born fifteen years after her sister. The mother, 38 years of age, had had no intervening pregnancies. The mother proffered the information freely that she had not welcomed this child, probably because it had interfered with her well established and strenuous social schedule. The father, personnel director of several branches of a manufacturing firm, was at home only on weekends and in these brief intervals was absorbed in his own social interests. The sister, also an attractive, self-possessed girl, was busily engaged in high school activities and paid surprisingly little attention to her baby sister. The only significant notes in the family medical history pertained to migraine and endocrine disorders on the maternal side. The child was entrusted largely to the care of a prim housekeeper, introverted in personality and laconic in speech. Both the housekeeper and the mother maintained that Karen shunned any demonstration of affection, although there was precious little evidence of warmth in either person. As a staff member who made the home visit said, it was not strange that Karen permitted no one to fondle her; she was wise enough to realize that there would be little or no return in such an emotional investment. It was a home, the staff visitor reported, which was admirably suited to the needs and conveniences of adults, not children. The living room was formally but tastefully decorated. Karen's toys and play activities were confined to her own bedroom or to the back porch and patio. Toys and books were to be returned to the chests in her bedroom after play. When the mother was asked how the child played with the toys, she said that Karen generally took her doll or other objects, sat in a corner of her bedroom, back against the wall, and hummed as she rocked the doll or the object. In such episodes she did not respond to the mother's or housekeeper's call and seemed unaware of the presence of either in the room. The housekeeper gave other instances of the child's lack of interest in the purposeful use of toys. She often took a picture book, sat on the floor in her room, and turned the pages endlessly, swaying back and forth as she hummed but apparently taking no cognizance of the pictures. When a relative with her young son would come to call, Karen would retreat immediately into the closet of her bedroom and remain there until the relatives had left.

Developmental Data.   Some evidence of hyperactivity and retardation was noted in Karen's first year. According to the protocol in an outpatient clinic, the child sat alone at 7 months and walked at 2 years. She was late in walking, the pediatrician noted, because "the muscles of the legs were unbalanced." Karen did not gain voluntary control of the bladder or bowels until she was 3 years old. Her sleep pattern was regular but her food habits were idiosyncratic. She choked when semi-solid foods were presented and insisted upon having her bottle until she was 19 months old when the pediatrician instructed the mother to dispose of it. When Karen was 3 years old she ate only cream of wheat and orange juice for breakfast, egg sandwiches for lunch, and orange juice and toast for dinner. At 4 years she was still being assisted in eating by the housekeeper. She examined strange foods proffered her by smelling them, and then invariably refused to eat them. At 3 years she tried to dress herself but would not tolerate clothing that had to be put over her head. When such an attempt was made, her hostility and anxiety increased. At 4 years when she was admitted to the Speech Center she was under medical care for hyperactivity. Reserpine had been prescribed.

Language and Speech Development. The child began to say such words as *Daddy, Mommy,* and *moo-ka* (cow) when she was about 15 months old but at 3 years her speech was limited to these words and such phrases as *light on* and *get up.* If she wanted something, she would jump up and down, utter a bleating sound *n-n-n-n,* and take the hand of anyone who might assist her in procuring the object she wanted. Her early echolalic patterns, the mother said, were simple repetitions of syllables: *yuh, yuh, yuh* and *tee, tee, tee.* The humming pattern varied between *um-um-um* and *bum-bum-bum.* When asked if the child communicated in nonverbal ways with her, the mother said, "She never cries but she also never smiles or laughs, except to her dolls." We suggested to the mother that since these are responses to people, Karen would have no occasion to smile or laugh. The mother felt that speech had retrogressed after the first months of its development. When asked if she thought the child understood speech, the mother stiffened and said, "She hears what she wants to hear," but offered no proof of her statement.

Social Development. The observations of the mother and housekeeper are supported by reports from staff members in the first session of diagnostic teaching. The mother said that Karen does not know how to play with toys or with her peers. She finds herself rejected by the children in the neighborhood so she stays in her own yard. On rare occasions when children call to her, she disappears through the back door of her home. The mother says that Karen refuses to play with children. The staff would add that Karen no longer wishes to play purposively either with toys or her peers, that she has retreated from an environment with which she cannot cope.[19] Occasionally she may wish to reenter the real world; for a moment she may want to communicate with others. When this happens she becomes very tense, jumps up and down and bleats *n-n-n.* She does not persist long in this activity but retreats to

[19] B. F. Skinner, *Verbal behavior.* New York: Appleton-Century-Crofts, 1957. P. 439.

her own world. Even in that safe world she often ignores or destroys toys which she once enjoyed.

Mental Retardation and Infantile Autism. So much controversy has arisen over the interpretation of psychometric evaluations of the autistic child that it might be wiser to accept the results of a longitudinal study of progress rather than absolute IQ ratings. Better to ask, "How far has Karen come?" than to ask, "Is she feeble-minded?" We have the tentative estimates of Karen's mental age on the basis of objective measures taken over a period of years. The results support Bender's findings of retardation, not Kanner's belief that the autistic child is brilliant but appears to be retarded because his cognitive potentialities are masked by a basic affective disorder.[20] In the first year of diagnostic teaching the staff psychologist made two attempts to measure Karen's mental development through performance tests. The examiner's inability to establish a basal score on the *Ammons Picture Vocabulary Test* or on *Merrill-Palmer* performance items was not unexpected. Although the tests are nonverbal, they require comprehension of language, and Karen apparently was unable either to understand the directions or to react to language. In the *Leiter International Performance Scale* which requires no verbal direction, she was unable to match colors and shapes at 5.10 years (Leiter 4–0). One year later, when she was 6.10 years, she received a score of 84 (IQ) on the *Leiter Scale* and 73 on the *WISC*. At 7.7 years the *Stanford-Binet Test,* (Form L), was administered; on the basis of this test her intelligence quotient was 71.

Psychiatric Study of Mother and Child. The psychiatrist who had referred Karen to the Center continued his assistance to the family and to our staff. When Karen was 5 years old, the psychiatrist made his first detailed report on his findings. He described the mother as intelligent, highly motivated, and abnormally self-centered, possessing a tense, rigid, impatient personality "which she hides under a triple mask of super-cleanliness, emotional sterility, and intellectualism. The mask conceals but it does not eliminate underlying problems." With counselling the mask might be cracked, he thought, and the house made into a tolerably pleasant home. He had instructed her to scatter some of Karen's toys around the living room and library so that she might be enticed to play there. She was to place no restrictions on the child's motility or on eating habits. Karen was to eat when and what she wanted. No demand was to be made upon the child for socialization but when she smiled or "reached out" to them they were to reciprocate.

Karen, he reported, had been endowed with a weak ego which afforded her little protection against the impact of a very harsh reality. Great anxieties had developed which she could not control except as she

[20] S. L. Garfield, Abnormal behavior and mental deficiency. In N. R. Ellis, Ed., *Handbook of mental deficiency.* New York: McGraw-Hill, 1963. Pp. 578–579.

relinquished formidable reality for the world of fantasy. Fantasy provided her with a compulsive defense mechanism which removed her from contact with the sensory world. If she could cut off hearing, for example, she could prevent anxiety stimuli from overwhelming her defensive shell.[21] She would not have to accept the demands that auditory stimuli might impose upon her. We had observed closely her immunity to the noise of telephone, police sirens, and airplanes. She seemed not to hear them at all yet once when the telephone rang long and loud, it must have impinged for a second on her consciousness. Her eyelids fluttered, fingers waved and she began to mumble in a sing-song, "somebody, somebody, somebody." Did she mean to suggest that some one should answer the phone? If she were able to reject tactile and thermal sensations at the point of entry, she would further avoid reality. Consequently she did not like to be cuddled or caressed. She did not enjoy the feeling of warmth. Proof of the exclusion of haptic sensations was noted in the toneless muscles and bizarre body positions. Her favorite position for napping on the cot in the playroom was to lie, face up, with her head hanging over the end of the cot. The psychiatrist's report concludes:

Until Karen can acquire an autonomous existence as a person, I am afraid that she will live in an amorphous, boundless world, a kind of perceptual fog in which she identifies clearly neither her own self nor her environment. It is difficult to advise you how to break the ring of verbal fantasy which is your immediate concern. Verbal fantasy, whether overt or covert, is automatically reinforcing to the child as a listener.

In this report the psychiatrist has delineated three classic features of autism: (1) an unstable and indefinite self-concept; (2) a retreat from reality; and (3) an inability to make meaningful identifications. Since all three parameters are related directly to the language disturbance, we turn now to their exploration.

Exploration of an Unstable and Indefinite Concept of Self. Some workers in the field may question the role of language clinicians in psychoemotional education. It should be remembered, however, that the program was carried on with the close cooperation and material assistance of a psychiatrist. Following our first detailed report of the initial six-month period of evaluative teaching, the psychiatrist replied:

I have read the case summary of Karen with great interest and complete approval. Your staff is doing what we cannot do. Karen is too young for our type of psychotherapy, and speech therapy with "empathic" teachers *is* psychotherapy as far as I am concerned. I shall continue to counsel the mother but Karen is in your hands.

[21] S. M. Finch, *Fundamentals of child psychiatry*. New York: Norton, 1960. P. 182.

Karen had little sense of self-identity. This was evident from the first weeks of evaluative teaching. As one language clinician noted in Karen's records, "She knows her first name but she does not know *who* she is. Strange, isn't it, that she possesses as fuzzy a concept of herself as of other people? People scarcely exist in her world and sometimes I wonder if Karen thinks she does." The boundary between self and nonself, indeed, must be tenuous. Before one can have a sense of self-identity he must enjoy physical and emotional homeostasis, and there was little evidence that Karen could control the setting of either homeostat. The defense mechanisms which she exhibited undoubtedly were the result of tensions and anxieties, both organismic and psychologic. As a small child she must have suffered unusual anxiety in such a natural physical activity as eating. You will remember that she first refused, then regurgitated solid foods, and would take no food unless she had first smelled it. Whether the muscle imbalance attendant upon learning to walk was genuine or simply an avoidance mechanism we do not know. When she was on the playground at the Center (she was then 4.6 years of age) a group of children pushed her up the steps of the slide. The playground instructor was present and urged her on. She reached the top step and then fell forward onto the slide. Although she was not hurt, she vomited and had to be taken home. After this episode she refused even the helping hand of the teacher and eschewed the slide for sessions alone in the sandbox.

We could place little reliability in the results of the *Vineland Social Maturity Scale* administered to the mother, although every effort had been made to get her to lay aside her defenses and report accurately. Karen had no opportunity to discover herself in a house of disinterested adults; some measure of her serious social retardation must be attributed to this fact. The *Draw-a-Person Test* reinforced our belief that Karen's self-concept was most indefinite. The movements were vortical, frenetic scrolls but so small and compressed that the figure finally resembled a series of miniature buttons with freakishly thin legs and arms. Did not the drawing signify her dwarfed personality and a symptom complex of withdrawal? [22] When Karen was 7.6 years old, her teacher noted: "Karen can draw circles of different colors but she cannot make the body of a snowman without help."

Her bizarre movement patterns in other activities also manifest a lack of self-identity. When anxieties developed and she wanted to retreat from a situation she could not cope with, she would shake her head vigorously and continuously, flick her fingers rapidly in the air or on the table, and hum. It is doubtful if she had any concept of herself as a person in such episodes. The psychiatrist could not explain Karen's need

[22] A. Clawson, *The Bender Visual Motor Gestalt Test* as an index of emotional disturbance in children. *J Project Techn* (June 1959), 23: 198–206.

of possession of property. She would not remove her coat and scarf, for example, when she entered the Center. In fact for the first two weeks she could not be persuaded to part with them. Did they help to conceal her identity from others? To enclose and preserve what identity she had? Perhaps Bender's explanation is the most plausible: She wishes to consolidate her boundaries and body image by withdrawing and not taking a chance on growing up for fear of nonexistence.[23]

In order to accelerate Karen's sense of identity of self, we set up both immediate and long-term goals. Her immediate need was to have at least one adult who was need-satisfying to her. This person must stand *in loco parentis,* giving and receiving confidence according to Karen's wishes. In the language clinician, Mrs. Rony (Karen's name for her), she found a confidante and teacher. The establishment of emotional ties with Mrs. Rony had to precede the establishment of emotional relations with children and other adults. Once ties between Karen and Mrs. Rony, and Karen and the world, were "in process of concordance," anxieties should diminish and some contacts might be made. Then a broader attack on the problem of self-identification could be launched. The final implement of battle was language—its comprehension and use.

Retreat from Reality. Karen is addicted to stereotyped, repetitive movements highly characteristic of "ritualistic play." When she comes in each morning she clicks the light switch on and off many times and finally sits down at the table. Here she proceeds to smell everything on the table—pencil, paper, chalk, eraser, the picture books, the building blocks. Having completed this ritual she runs to the light switch again and, apparently oblivious of her language teacher or others in the room, repeats the routine. As Karen perseverates in purposeless motions, so she also persists in humming and in her play with one fractured teddy bear. Her activity with building blocks is equally stereotyped and perseverative. She makes the same design over and over again. She does not seek approval of her designs. Apparently she takes no notice of an intruder because at one point her teacher slipped a block out of a design and dropped it into her lap. Karen simply put another block in its place but did not recognize the teacher's action. Karen is indifferent to interpersonal or social play except as one takes her by the hand and leads her for a brief interval into the real world. In one session she found herself in a playroom with five children of her age. When one little boy approached to give her a toy, she turned, ran to the far corner of the room, crawled under a table and conducted a pantomimic session with an imaginary person. In the first term of diagnostic teaching, Karen resorted often to another retreat, particularly when other children were present. During the story-telling or "color-book" group sessions, she

[23] L. Bender, Childhood schizophrenia. *Amer J Orthopsychiat* (July 1956), 26: 499–506.

escaped to the piano and according to her teacher's report "spent long periods of time picking out a musical pattern. It was not random pounding. She finally learned to play *Three Blind Mice* and *Frère Jacques*." It was an avenue of which we would make use in subsequent periods. That her anxieties sometimes prompted her to "touch reality" rather than to retreat was evidenced in this episode: Toward the end of the first year of diagnostic teaching, the clinician with whom she was most comfortable was absent. The children had been told that her son was ill. On the first morning after the clinician's return, the group was engrossed in a classification game. "In this toyshop are a jumping jack, an electric train, a bunch of bananas, and a boat. Karen, what does not belong in this shop?" The child stared at the window, then said, "John sick?"

Language: Bridge to Reality. In no area is Karen's disjunction with reality more apparent than in language. We do not believe that the mother is correct in her assertion that the child "hears what she wants to hear." Instead of the mother's interpretation, we would hold that Karen rejects sensation at the point of entering because of a genetic inadequacy in drive which will not permit her to make the transition from inward orientation to outward drive. As a result, the verbal gestalt is completely plastic, formless.[24] Because the world of sight, sounds, colors, and motion is a threatening one, she has learned to exclude them all. Her sensitivity to all modalities is consistently at a low ebb. Words are noises, and she has learned to shut out all noise. In fact the threshold for all auditory and tactile-kinesthetic sequences pertaining to language is so high a hurdle that verbal signals rarely enter her perceptual field. And if they enter at all, they are not differentiated from the surround. Very occasionally there is a glimmer of recognition of verbal signals; it occurs generally at the very beginning of the daily session. She often is heard to repeat much later in the day something that was said in the preschool in the morning. As she played with blocks one afternoon she repeated in echolalic fashion, "that's very good, Karen," and "that's a good try, Karen,"—praise which she had received in the morning. She repeated the phrases, however, in a dull, meaningless intonation pattern and cluttered rhythm as if they were distant echoes of a real world. In terms of perception these echolalic phrases do not approach verbal communication yet they reflect the profound ambivalence towards the outside world that she has rejected yet not totally given up.[25] In a sense her echolalia is the precursor to the exchange of verbal communication for it represents some identification with the interlocutor. It was decided

[24] K. de Hirsch, The concept of plasticity and language disabilities. *Speech Path Ther* (April 1965), 8: 12–17.
[25] E. Stengel, Speech disorders and mental disorders. In A. V. S. de Reuck and M. O'Connor, Eds., *Disorders of language*. London: J. A. Churchill, 1964. P. 287.

to approach communication first by encouraging Karen to use facial and bodily gesture. If she could respond in this way, it would mean that she was forming emotional ties with others. She was to be taught to respond in action to verbal commands with gesture but no specific demands were to be placed upon her for vocal response. Eventually, we hoped to convert her echolalic responses into direct communication as an accompaniment to gesture.

Karen has developed certain destructive response patterns to ward off reality. Her group had set the table for a lemonade party. When the little girl across the table turned to ask Karen, "Would you like some lemonade?" Karen pulled the cloth, upset the glasses, and ran out of the room. In another session the teacher succeeded in gaining the attention of Karen with the pictures of the *Clark Phonetic Inventory*. But when she no longer was permitted to shuffle the picture cards, and her attention was directed to one card (picture of a puppy) which the teacher would talk about, Karen quickly stood up, picked up a crayon, and defaced the picture. She was told quietly, *Sit down, Karen.* She obeyed but immediately began to hum, her signal of retreat.

The child firmly resists the attempts of others to approach her through language. Why? Probably because language is the most direct bridge to the world of real people. If she developed the medium of communication, it might bring her into confrontation with a society of adults, and her ego could not tolerate this. She must not allow this bridge, for noncommunication is her last line of defense against a hostile environment.

The First Year of Diagnostic Teaching Ends. At midpoint in the first year of diagnostic teaching, the staff met to take a long look down Karen's way. The basic question was this: How could we determine the extent to which the child might be taught to comprehend and use language? Obviously we would be unsuccessful if the child did not form some emotional or feeling ties with children and adults, for without these ties she would have no use for verbal symbols. We turned these subsidiary questions over to her need-satisfying clinical teacher, Mrs. Rony, for answers to these questions: (1) Is the child aware that you are speaking to her? (2) When Karen is confronted by the teacher giving directions, does she follow them? (3) Can she be forced to attend by emotional shifts in the tone of voice? (4) Will she respond to specific commands for activity that she enjoys? (5) Will she respond to commands to engage in activity that she does not enjoy? (6) Will she perform action in imitation of the teacher? (7) Does she recognize names of people, actions? At the end of the first year several staff sessions were devoted to the answers. They were qualified and guarded. Karen's awareness of the speech of others varies with time, place, and her mental set. Monday is her worst day; she hums constantly as if to shut out all remembrance of the Sunday world and also to obviate the necessity of responding to the present regimen. There often is no way to stop her incessant clicking of light switches except to give a quiet but very determined command. Karen apparently recognized the firmness in the voice for she would quickly return to her work table. Although she likes to hop, skip, and run, she often does not recognize the name of the specific action. When her teacher said, "Hop, Karen," she might run or skip. If the teacher illustrated the activity, however, Karen very quickly followed suit. Some activities she disliked and therefore sedulously avoided. Finger painting was one; she would not soil her hands in this manner. The preschool teacher made a disheartening report to the language clinician, Mrs. Rony:

> Karen has not entered yet into games or table activities. At story-telling time we sit on the floor but as soon as the story is begun, I notice that Karen swivels around, faces the wall and begins a head-bobbing or foot-thumping rhythm. When we get out the fingerpaints and aprons, she disappears. She remains in the washroom until we go for her.

Actions, both pictured and real, were quite regularly and grossly misinterpreted. The hat on a snowman's head was a "bunny rabbit"; a snow ball was an egg. A Christmas party Karen interpreted as a birthday party so she began to blow out imaginary candles, counting *1-2-2-2* as she did so. On the plus side, Mrs. Rony reports that Karen does recognize the names of several staff members who work with her. Her greeting has become a by-word in the Center. "Mrs. Rony here?" It was never, "Are *you* here?"

   Language at 6.6 Years: Crossing the Bridge. Sometimes Karen would find herself communicating with other children or even with her favorite teacher. But before she had finished the excursion over the bridge, she would suddenly and perceptibly grow tense, jargon would flow, and she would retreat into silence. In one language exercise, large, colored story-pictures were presented. Mrs. Rony was in charge so Karen was not reticent at first in carrying on a soliloquy about the picture in her own way. The teacher noted that the commentary always was identifying rather than descriptive; it was also perseverative. A *cow* was a *donkey* but a *horse, tiger,* and *elephant* were *cows*. A *teddy bear, boy,* and *snowman* all were *clowns*. When she saw a hat on a snowman's head, the voice became tense and she shouted, "Rabbit; see the bunny hop, hop, hop." Then she enumerated many more animals, not pictured, increasing her rate and tension as she proceeded. Finally her recital tapered off into mumbled remarks and silence. The game was over for the day. No further responses could be elicited. We believe that this kind of perseverative repetition occurs in part because she is unable to make meaningful identification, and in part because the initial response is reverberative; she cannot break neuronal circuits and thus shift her attention. In a subsequent session Karen was restless, shuffling her feet and tapping on the table. In an effort to get her attention, her teacher prompted an interpretation of the picture with the question: "What did the girl put in the refrigerator?" Karen replied, "Feet in figerator." (Could she have meant *food* just as she may have intended to say, *the hen says cluck, cluck* but said, *the hat says cluck, cluck?*)

The language clinician also commented on Karen's disability in grammar and syntax. She omitted words, inverted the word order, and telescoped sentences until her speech became a word-salad. She used few pronouns. Her need-satisfying teacher [26] was always *Mrs. Rony*: "Mrs. Rony sick; Mrs. Rony open door." She could not form sentences spontaneously so personal pronouns were repeated just as heard. Hence Karen often referred to herself as *you*. "Do you want some orange juice?" asked the teacher. "Ya, you want juice," the child responded. [27] Echolalia was much less frequent in the second year of teaching, occurring chiefly with questions of *who, when, where,* and then the teacher thought the child did not comprehend the questions. Such reverberative and irrelevant phrases as *Hi, Karen; Where's Billy?; Nan don't go;* and *The mouse ran up the clock* still were present but they were less frequent. To be sure she made few direct remarks giving information, except to imaginary people and to her dolls, yet she was beginning to take steps over the bridge to reality. The cross-over is slow but it is definite. At 6.6 years her vocabulary age is slightly over the 3-year level; her use of proper grammatical and syntactical forms parallels that of a child, 2.6–3.0 years old. Word order remains disturbed and confusing. Under tension, clutter patterns appear. The perseverative compulsion has been broken but it has not disappeared. She may or may not look at the children as she speaks to them; she carefully avoids all eye contact with adults. The road is long with many a turning but Karen has made the first one, we think.

Language Training: Karen at 7.6 Years. In the third year of teaching, Karen's teachers found an approach which reduced markedly the child's echolalic and perseverative behavior: They allowed her little opportunity to make these responses. Let us quote from the record:

We have embarked on a highly-structured language program. The picture which is to be the basis for her verbal responses is interpreted for her. Then the questions to be asked are printed on the board and repeated orally although Karen cannot always read them. Each question is asked in order and she is encouraged to respond immediately. No time must intervene between question

[26] B. Bettelheim, Schizophrenia as a reaction to extreme situations. *Amer J Orthopsychiat* (July 1956), 26: 507–518.

[27] M. A. Cunningham and C. Dixon, A study of the language of an autistic child. *J Child Psychol Psychiat* (November 1961), 2: 193–202.

and answer. As a result, she has less opportunity to introduce extraneous material, and word order, on which she has been drilled, is more successful. It is a tightly structured, formal approach but it has succeeded whereas "free-wheeling sessions" generally end in echolalia or jargon.

Training in Meaningful Identification. Karen's teachers made systematic approaches to other facets of language development, notably sensory-motor training and systematic exercise in discrimination and classification. Their plan of tactile-kinesthetic and auditory training did not seem entirely logical yet it worked. Sounds were not amplified; in fact the teacher generally employed a very quiet tone. But she did prolong, accentuate, and repeat the sentence. The units of speech were small with a regular word order: subject, verb, object. The tempo was slow. Karen was taught to watch the speaker's face and to mimic the articulatory and facial movements. The scheme did not seem entirely sound for two reasons. We feared that the stress on mimesis might negate efforts to reduce echolalic speech, and emphasis on measured, slow speech could logically intensify Karen's demand for sameness and endless repetition. Karen enjoyed routine; she was meticulous in detail—which often was the wrong detail—to the point that she lost sight of the whole. Her whole behavior, in short, was governed by an obsessive desire for the maintenance of a sameness that no one but the child might interrupt. Her insistence on sameness was exemplified in color matching. An orange red or flamingo red was not a red color to Karen. Having lost the red scarf which matched her coat, she was forced to wear a scarf somewhat brighter in hue than the coat. She hid the scarf; it could not be found when it was time for her to go home.

Our fears may have been logical; in terms of achievement they were groundless. As training in discrimination and classification continued, Mrs. Rony shifted from the matching of colors to the assembly of objects which belonged together. Karen learned to furnish properly every room in the doll house, assembled the correct clothing for dolls of all sizes, and learned the appropriate food for breakfast and dinner. The things which belonged in a toy shop were more difficult; frequently the bananas reposed between a train and a sailboat. Then she moved on to materials from the Leiter kit (*Leiter International Performance Scale*), materials which called for the matching of genus, of ages (e.g., grandmother with grandfather, little boy with little girl), and of the typical position of objects (e.g., tea kettle on the stove; milk bottles in the refrigerator). Pictured pieces representing semi-abstract phenomena presented a more complex task in discrimination. Phenomena associated with *day*—blue sky, dog romping on green grass with a small boy, sun—must be selected and put together. "Putting the night together" was even harder. Finally moon, stars, and a lighted house made up the picture of night on the flannel-board. Karen, however, must have been making steady gains in comprehension because reports from other departments of the program —crafts and preschool—indicated that the child was listening and following directions. She might absent herself from some parts of the program, noted the preschool teacher, but "she always joined directed activities during listening time and was particularly happy to hear the continued story of the puppet, *Porky Pig*." Because Karen had made so many mistakes in visual interpretations, Mrs. Rony prepared a giant scrapbook containing pictures of significant parts of the story which Karen followed as she told it.

The child experienced particular difficulty when she was asked to enlarge the scope of the relations of object with object. Milk was only to be drunk; it could not be used in the preparation of ice cream or other foods. "What can you do with an apple, Karen?" the instructor asked. "Eat it,"—and Karen demonstrated. "Could I bake it in a pie?" "No." "Could I make apple sauce?" "No, you eat it, like this," Karen persisted. Apparently she could not differentiate relations associated with a common object and then regroup these relations in one nucleus—the food uses of an apple. Her teacher proceeded to show her how to build up relations, first with one object in terms of use, then to recognize relations between objects, with and without overt experimentation. The progress was slow at first. At a birthday luncheon party, she put chocolate syrup on her salad. When we explained that tropical fish do not eat nuts, that the nuts had been saved for the squirrels, she was puzzled. The next day she surreptitiously dropped more nuts into the tank. Karen was nearly 8 years old before she consciously attempted to relate objects and to make inferences without overt experimentation. Arduous though this task of learning was, it had to be attacked, for as Strauss and Kephart have said, "If the child had to build up concretely all the possible combinations with which he will be required to deal, a lifetime would be too short to even approximate an adequate experience." [28]

Gains in Speaking and Reading. On the *Peabody Picture Vocabulary Test* she exceeded the expectations of the staff when she obtained a vocabulary age of 4 years (CA 7.6). Her comprehension of language had improved markedly, an indication of increased participation in the real world and of firmer emotional ties with people. Generally she responded at once to such directions as, *Put the egg-beater in the sink* or *Push your chair up to the table.* Occasionally and inexplicably her threshold of excitability for incoming verbal stimuli was so high that the command had to be repeated.

Karen was learning to read (CA 8 years) so her teachers capitalized on the use of preprimer tests of simple, two-line stories about a picture. Before each page was turned Karen was to predict what happened next.

[28] A. A. Strauss and N. D. Kephart, *Psychopathology and education of the brain-injured child.* New York: Grune & Stratton, 1955. II: 121.

Here they were trying to educate the child's expectancies, the ability to predict, a necessary adjunct to all learning. The teachers attempted to counter the development of rigid, unalterable concepts by adding to the possibilities before the page was turned. If new percepts were to be developed, the basic percept must be clear and definite; it, in turn, must be recombined so that new schemata of ideas result. The ability to combine and recombine elements was definitely hampered by her compulsion to hang on to an identification although it was not correct. In the *Blacky Pictures* used in this exercise of discrimination (a purpose for which they were not devised), Karen persisted in repeating her original identification although she had been corrected. She was unable to relinquish perseveration as a response pattern. An association that was firmly established also might interfere with new associations. For example, when Karen was shown a picture of a policeman holding up his hand (to signal *stop*), and was asked "What is the policeman doing? Why is he holding up his hand?" she answered, "Five soldiers." In a finger play she had learned, "Five little soldiers standing in a row," she was taught to hold up her hand in the same manner as the policeman. Only after considerable discussion did she abandon her first association.

Language at 9 Years. In this last term of instruction in the Center, Karen was making valiant efforts to use language in order to bind herself to reality. It was not speech appropriate to her age but it was communication. Syntactic and grammatic relations still were somewhat bizarre. She made many mistakes, particularly in the use of personal pronouns but she was using them. Large gaps remained in her vocabulary but we could not assess an exact vocabulary age because at this stage we were more concerned with the *quality* of her vocabulary than its variety. In terms of the number of different words used, it is reported that in the vocabulary of a child 2.6 years old, 51 percent of the words are different words whereas in a 7-year-old autistic child, the number of different words is 35 percent.[29] At 9 years, Karen's vocabulary, judged qualitatively, approached that of a child of 5 years.

Even more disturbing than paucity of vocabulary was the dysrhythmic, nonfluent character of her speech. It was usually cluttered and explosive, the result, we thought, of continued disturbances in perception of grammar, syntax, and in the perception of the normal sequence of speech units. She had little feeling for rightness in word order or phraseology. This was particularly true when she found herself with a new group of children and under pressure to respond verbally to questions involving inner logic. Under these circumstances repetitions and dysrhythmia blocked her speech, her hands would flutter, and communication involving verbal concepts would break down.

[29] M. A. Cunningham and C. Dixon, A study of the language of an autistic child. *J Child Psychol Psychiat* (November 1961), 2: 193–202.

In the final staff conference, her teachers in the Center noted many positive and identifiable gains. Karen had learned to use purposive speech. She rarely retreated from her peers; she backed off from adults occasionally but only for short periods. Perception was improving although she still made verbal sorties which ended in a "squirrel track up a tree," or in that inevitable echo-finale, "That's O.K.; see ya 'morrow," although the session might be far from over. She could be stopped now in such a side excursion and brought back into the Center again. Echolalic indulgence, irrelevant echo remarks, and humming as retreat mechanisms were much less frequent. Facial expression, although not animated, was not limited to a mask broken by fleeting anxieties. She communicated by facial and bodily gesture both with her peers and adults. Karen has advanced through the stages of egocentric speech: echolalia, monologue, and finally collective monologue (i.e., the presence of another who serves only as a stimulus but who is not an interlocutor). She has come into the clearing of social language. She has yet to master the use of language as an instrument of ideation and learning.

Appendix A   Chapter 6

Appraising the Use of Language

Rules for Classification of Words and Sentences *

A. Rules for Counting Number of Words
   1. Contractions of subject and predicate like "it's" and "we're" are counted as two words.
   2. Contractions of the verb and the negative such as "can't" are counted as one word.
   3. Each part of a verbal combination is counted as a separate word: thus "have been playing" is counted as three words.
   4. Hyphenated and compound nouns are one word.
   5. Expressions which function as a unit in the child's understanding were counted as one word. Thus "oh boy," "all right," etc. were counted as one word, while "Christmas tree" was counted as two words.

B. Classification of Sentence Structure

   1. Complete sentences.
      a. Functionally complete but structurally incomplete. This includes naming; answers in which omitted words are implied because they were expressed in the question; expletives; and other remarks, incomplete in themselves, which are clearly a continuation of the preceding remark.
      b. Simple sentence without phrase.

* M. Templin, *Certain language skills in children*. Minneapolis: University of Minnesota Press, 1957. Pp. 160–161.

c. Simple sentence containing (1) phrase used as adjective or adverb in apposition, (2) compound subject or predicate, (3) compound predicate.

d. Complex sentence (one main clause, one subordinate clause) with (1) noun clause used (a) as subject, (b) as object, (c) in apposition, (d) as predicate nominative, (e) as objective complement; (2) adjective clause (a) restrictive, (b) nonrestrictive; (3) adverbial clauses of (a) time, (b) place, (c) manner, (d) comparison, (e) condition, (f) concession, (g) cause, (h) purpose, (i) result; (4) infinitive.

e. Compound sentence (two independent clauses).

f. Elaborated sentence; (1) simple sentence with two or more phrases, or compound subject, or predicate and phrase; (2) complex sentence with more than one subordinate clause, or with a phrase or phrases; (3) compound sentence with more than two independent clauses, or with a subordinate clause or phrases.

2. Incomplete sentences.

a. Fragmentary or incomprehensible. Example: "Well—not this, but—."

b. (1) Verb omitted completely, (2) auxiliary omitted, verb or participle expressed, (3) verb or participle omitted, auxiliary expressed.

c. Subject omitted, either from main or subordinate clause.

d. Introductory "there" omitted.

e. Pronoun other than subject of verb omitted.

f. Preposition (usually needed sign of infinitive) omitted.

g. Verb and subject omitted.

h. Main clause incomplete, subordinate clause or second clause of compound sentence complete.

i. Main clause complete, subordinate or second clause incomplete. Example: "I know why."

j. Omissions from both main and subordinate clauses.

k. Essential words present, but sentence loosely constructed because of (1) omission of conjunction, (2) insertion of parenthetical clause, (3) changes in form halfway in sentence. Example: "We have—my brother has a motorcycle."

l. (1) Definite, (2) indefinite article omitted.

m. Object omitted from either main clause or prepositional phrase.

n. Sentence left dangling.

Table A-1. Increase in size of vocabulary with age.

Age Years-Months	N	Average IQ	Number of Words	Words Gained
8	13		0	
10	17		1	1
1-0	52		3	2
1-3	19		19	16
1-6	14		22	3
1-9	14		118	96
2-0	25		272	154
2-6	14		446	174
3-0	20	109	896	450
3-6	26	106	1222	326
4-0	26	109	1540	318
4-6	32	109	1870	330
5-0	20	108	2072	202
5-6	27	110	2289	217
6-0	9	108	2562	273

SOURCE: M. Smith, *Vocabulary in young children.* Iowa City: Iowa Studies Child Welfare (1962), 3 (5).

Table A-2. Mean complexity score for remarks of boys and girls, upper and lower socioeconomic status groups, and total subsamples, by age.

C.A.	Boys (N=30)		Girls (N=30)		USES (N=18)		LSES (N=42)		Total Subsamples (N=60)	
	Mean	SD	Mean	SD	Mean	SD	Mean	SD	Mean	SD
3	36.4	19.7	32.2	16.5	40.6	20.4	31.4	16.6	34.3	18.3
3.5	38.1	17.3	43.2	18.2	49.2	19.1	36.9	16.1	40.6	17.9
4	48.0	18.8	54.9	20.7	50.6	14.2	51.8	22.1	51.6	20.1
4.5	50.9	24.0	52.9	16.6	61.8	16.3	47.7	20.9	50.4	24.1
5	50.6	18.8	63.2	23.5	55.6	19.4	57.4	22.3	56.9	21.5
6	71.5	22.1	68.7	17.4	70.5	16.0	69.9	21.4	70.1	22.7
7	69.7	20.0	73.9	16.6	70.0	16.5	72.6	19.2	71.8	18.5
8	74.4	18.7	79.2	28.7	91.0	23.5	71.9	21.3	77.7	33.8

SOURCE: M. Templin, *Certain language skills in children.* Minneapolis: University of Minneapolis Press. P. 82.

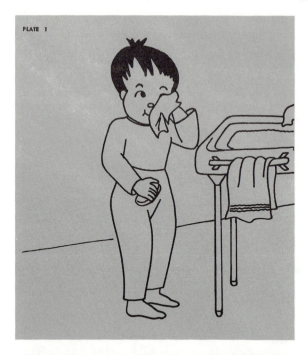

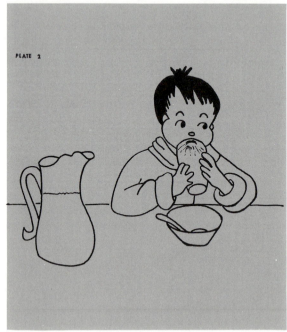

Figure A-1. Picture story language test.

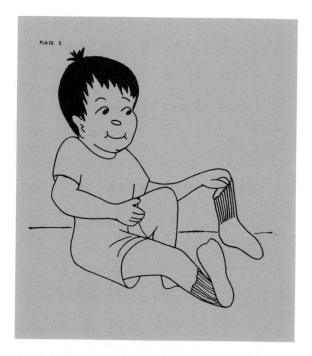

PLATE 3

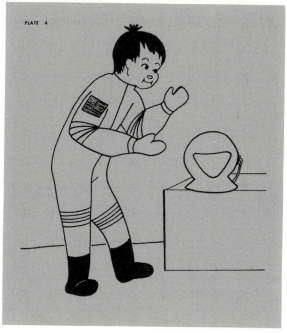

PLATE 4

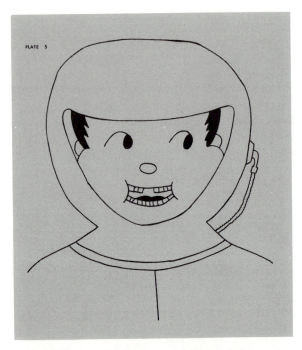

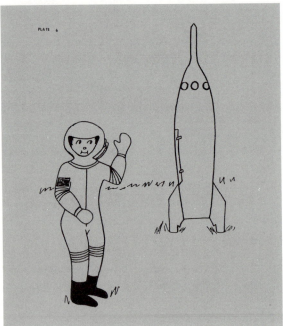

Figure A-1. Picture story language test (continued).

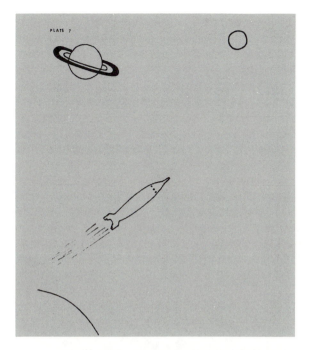

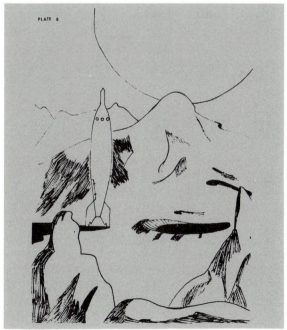

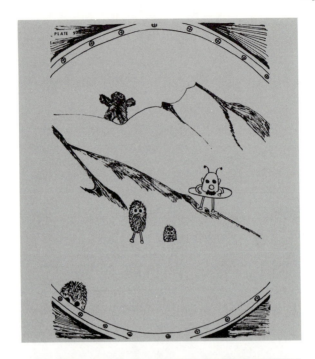

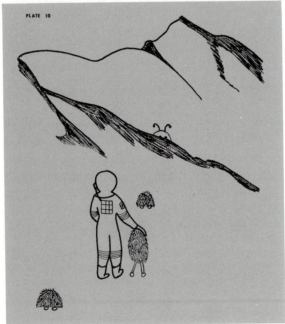

Figure A-1. Picture story language test (continued).

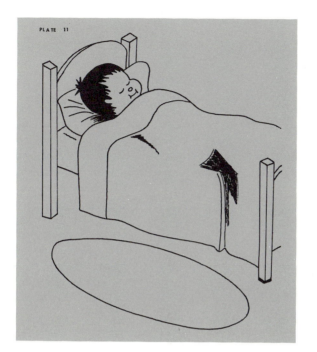

PLATE 11

Appendix B   Chapter 7

Utah Test of Language Development, Score Sheet, 1–8 Years

1–2 Years
1. Responds to name and "no-no."
2. Follows simple instructions.
3. Marks with pencil or crayon.
4. Recognizes names of common objects.
5. Recognizes parts of body when named (3 or more parts).
6. Recognizes parts of body when named. (4 or more parts).
7. Identifies common pictures when named.
8. Word combinations of two or more.

2–3 Years
9. Names common pictures (2 or more).
10. Names common pictures (8 or more).
11. Repeats two digits.
12. Responds to simple commands.
13. Identifies action in pictures.
14. Names one color.
15. Receptive vocabulary.

3–4 Years
16. Repeats three digits.
17. Says full name.

18. Names common pictures.
19. Says at least one nursery rhyme.
20. Copies a cross.

4–5 Years
21. Names colors.
22. Repeats four digits.
23. Carries out three commissions.
24. Repeats a twelve syllable sentence.
25. Draws with pencil or crayon.

5–6 Years
26. Copies a square.
27. Prints simple words.
28. Receptive vocabulary.

6–7 Years
29. Names penny, nickel, and dime.
30. Writes numbers to the thirties.
31. Tells a familiar story.
32. Reads words on preprimer level.
33. Recites numbers from one to fifty.
34. Copies a diamond.

7–8 Years
35. Receptive vocabulary.
36. Names quarter, half-dollar, and dollar.
37. Repeats five digits.
38. Names the days of the week.[1]

[1] *Utah Test of Language Development.* Copyright 1967 by M. J. Mecham, J. L. Jex, and J. D. Jones. Box 11012, Salt Lake City, Utah: Communication Research Associates.

Developmental Language Items Classified According to Linguistic
Processes, Utah Test of Language Development

Semantic Decoding	Age	N
Responds to name and "no-no"	0-9	496
Recognizes names of objects	1-6	496
Recognizes names of 3 body parts	1-7	3,187
Identifies names of pictures	1-10	496
Identifies action in pictures	2-8	496
Receptive vocabulary	2-11	3,187
Receptive vocabulary	5-10	3,187
Reads words in preprimer	6-6	393
Receptive vocabulary	7-1	3,187
Receptive vocabulary	9-11	3,187
Receptive vocabulary	12-7	3,187
Receptive vocabulary	15-4	3,187

Semantic Decoding	Age	N
Marks with pencil or crayon	1-4	883
Names common pictures	2-2	496
Names common pictures	2-3	496
Names a color	2-9	496
Names common pictures	3-5	496
Names primary colors	4-1	496
Draws with pencil or crayon	5-0	883
Prints simple words	5-6	883
Names penny, nickle, dime	6-1	393
Names quarter, $\frac{1}{2}$ dol., dollar	7-3	393
Can rhyme words	9-0	3,187

Sequential Decoding	Age	N
Responds to simple instructions	1-1	883
Can repeat 2 digits	2-5	3,187
Responds to simple commands	2-6	3,187
Can repeat 3 digits	3-1	3,187
Can repeat 4 digits	4-4	3,187
Carries out 3 commissions	4-7	3,187
Can repeat 12 syll. sentence	4-9	3,187
Can repeat 5 digits	7-7	3,187
Can repeat 16 syll. sentence	8-3	3,187
Can repeat 4 digits reversed	9-5	3,187
Can repeat 6 digits	10-5	3,187
Can repeat 20 syll. sentence	10-11	3,187
Can repeat 5 digits reversed	12-0	3,187
Can repeat 5 1-syll. words	13-5	3,187
Can repeat difficult sentence	14-6	3,187
Follows directional sequences	16-0	3,187

Sequential Encoding	Age	N
Word combinations of two or more	2-0	496
Says full name	3-3	496
Says a nursery rhyme	3-8	496
Copies a cross	3-10	3,187
Copies a square	5-3	3,187
Writes numbers to thirties	6-3	393
Tells a familiar story	6-5	393
Counts by ones to fifty	6-8	393
Copies a diamond	6-11	3,187
Names the days of the week	7-11	3,187
Writes cursively	8-8	883

SOURCE: M. J. Mecham, Differential evaluation of verbal language disabilities in children. Paper read at *Amer. Speech Hear. Assoc.* Annual Convention. Chicago, 1967.

Scoring Sheet: The Houston Test for Language Development

Name _____ Birthdate _____ Sex _____

Parents _____ Address _____

Date of Test _____ Examiner _____

Referred By _____ Reason for Referral _____

Items	Age in Months					
	6	12	18	24	30	36
Smiles	X					
Vocalizes back vowels	X					
"Talks" to inanimate objects	X					
Attends to voice	X					
Blows bubbles	X					
Laughs out loud	X					
Controls volume	X					
Squeals	X					
Uses vocal grunt	X					
Holds out arms to be taken		X				
Vocalizes syllables		X				
Repeats syllables		X				
Imitates sounds		X				
Uses reflexive jargon		X				
Responds to "bye, bye"		X				
Uses 2–3 words		X				
Will pat-a-cake		X				
Understands inhibitions		X				
Converses in jargon			X			
Points to indicate wants			X			

Houston Test (continued)

Age in Months

Items	6	12	18	24	30	36
Uses 10 or more words			X			
Identifies parts of doll			3	5		
Obeys prepositions				1	2	3
Names pictures			1	8	11	16
Points to pictures			5	10	15	19
Articulates labials				X		
Articulates dentals					X	
Articulates velars						X
Uses three-word sentence				X		
Verbalizes action					X	
Uses pronoun I					X	
Gives four lines from memory						X
Tells what happened						X
Names his sex						X
Gives full name						X
Announces his action						X
Protests inaccuracies						X

Scoring Summary

Age in Months	Item Value	No. Items Passed		Score
6	.666		=	
12	.666		=	
18	1		=	
24	1		=	
30	1		=	
36	.6		=	
		TOTAL SCORE	=	

Basal Age (Age at which all items were passed) =

Upper Age (Highest age at which any item is passed) =

Language Age (Total Score from Score Summary) =

SOURCE: M. Crabtree, Ed.D., The Houston Test for Language Development, Part I. The Houston Test Company, P. O. Box 35152, Houston, Texas.

The Age Group at Which 60 Percent of Children Comprehend Each Linguistic Item Tested (Carrow)

Form Classes and Function words	3-0	3-6	4-0	4-6	5-0	5-6	6-0	6-6	7-0
Nouns coat, glass, ball, car, tree, chair, dog, bicycle, baby, table, man, plane, pencil, farm, box, mother, sheep, boy, paint, spoon, bird, shoe, book, hand, cat, fish, girl	X								
half								X	
pair			X						
Verbs jump, run, eat	X								
hit		X							
catch			X						
give				X					
Adjectives Qualitative contrasts little/big, fast/slow, big/little	X								
tall/short		X							
alike/different							X		
Color red, brown, blue	X								
orange, black, green, yellow		X							
Number or relative quantity two			X						
some, many, middle					X				
more, four						X			
few, fourth							X		
Direction or space relations left/right							X		
Adverbs Direction or space relations up/down	X								
Demonstratives these/those					X				
that/this					X				
Interrogatives who/what	X								
when/where			X						
Prepositions on, under, in	X								
by, between		X							
in front of			X						

Linguistic Comprehension by Age Groups (continued)

Morphological Constructions	3-0	3-6	4-0	4-6	5-0	5-6	6-0	6-6	7-0
Noun/Noun + Derivational Suffix "er" farm/farmer				X					
paint/painter				X					
Verb/Verb + Derivational Suffix "er" catch/catcher						X			
Adjective/Adjective + Derivational Suffix "er": tall/taller					X				
Noun/Noun + Derivational Suffix "ist" piano/pianist									→
bicycle/bicyclist									→
Grammatical Categories									
Gender and Number, Pronoun masculine, singular/feminine, singular and neuter plural of third person, nominative case: he/she, they		X							
feminine, singular/masculine, singular and neuter plural of third person, nominative case: she/he, they						X			
plural/singular, third person, nominative case: they/he, she	X								
feminine, singular/masculine, singular and neuter plural of third person, objective case: her/him, them		X							
masculine, singular/feminine, singular and neuter plural of third person, possessive case: his/her, their			X						
Number, Noun singular/plural, marked by inflection: ball/balls, chair/chairs			X						
plural/singular, marked by inflection: coats/coat, tables/table					X				
Number, Verb singular/plural: is/are			X						
plural/singular: are/is								X	
Tense, Verb present progressive/past, future: Is riding/rode, will ride	X								
past/present, future: painted/paints, will paint			X						
future/present, past: will jump/jumps, jumped				X					
present perfect/present progressive, future: has eaten/is eating, will eat							X		
Voice, Verb doer/receiver, active voice: The car bumps the train/The train bumps the car; The boy pushes the girl/The girl pushes the boy	X								

Grammatical Categories (continued)	3-0	3-6	4-0	4-6	5-0	5-6	6-0	6-6	7-0
receiver/doer, passive voice: The man is hit by the boy/ The boy is hit by the man							X		
The boy is chased by the dog/ The dog is chased by the boy						X			
Status, Verb affirmative/negative: The baby is crying/The baby is not crying	X								
negative/affirmative: The girl is not riding/The girl is riding	X								
negative/affirmative: The girl isn't running/The girl is running		X							
negative/affirmative: Neither the boy nor the girl is jumping/ The boy and the girl are jumping									X
Mood, Verb Imperative	X								
Syntactic Structure									
Predication, Noun-verb, Number agreement The cat plays	X								
The boys jump					X				
Complementation direct/indirect object: Show me the ball	X								
She showed the girl the boy				X					
Modification noun phrase with single adjective modifier: a big cat/a small cat	X								
noun phrase with two adjective modifiers: a large blue ball/a large red ball, a small blue ball				X					
simple imperative sentence: Stand up	X								
complex sentence with independent clause and dependent adjectival clause: Bring me the car that is on the chair	X								
complex imperative sentence with conditional clause: If you are a (girl, boy) show me the car; if not, show me the ball						X			
When I clap my hands stand up			X						
Coordination compound imperative sentence using *and*: Put the car under the table and bring me the book				X					
compound imperative sentence using *either . . .or*": Either open the door or show me the pencil				X					

SOURCE: M. A. Carrow, The development of auditory comprehension of language structure in children. *J Speech Hearing Dis* (May 1968), 33: 105–108.

388

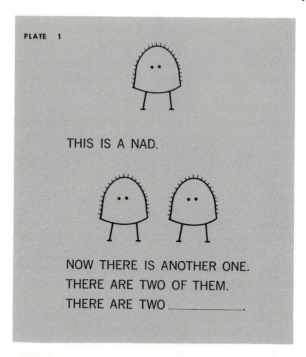

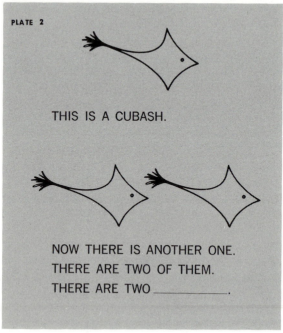

Figure B-2. Exploratory test of grammar (Berry and Talbott).

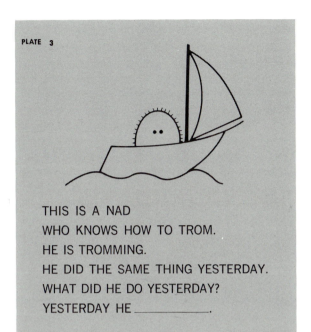

PLATE 3

THIS IS A NAD
WHO KNOWS HOW TO TROM.
HE IS TROMMING.
HE DID THE SAME THING YESTERDAY.
WHAT DID HE DO YESTERDAY?
YESTERDAY HE _____.

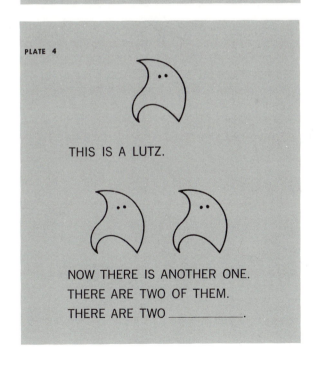

PLATE 4

THIS IS A LUTZ.

NOW THERE IS ANOTHER ONE.
THERE ARE TWO OF THEM.
THERE ARE TWO _____.

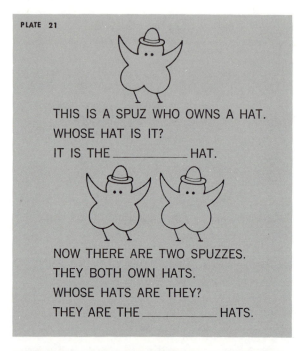

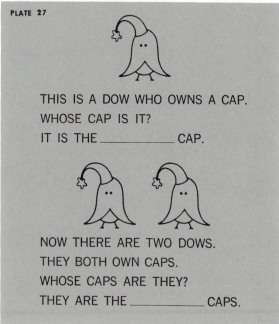

Figure B-2. Exploratory test of grammar (continued).

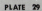

PLATE 29

THIS TASS HAS LIGS ON HIM.

THIS TASS HAS MORE LIGS ON HIM.

AND THIS TASS HAS

    EVEN MORE LIGS ON HIM.

THIS TASS IS LIGGY.

THIS TASS IS _____ .

AND THIS TASS IS THE _____ .

PLATE 30

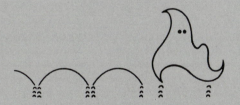

THIS IS A LUTZ

WHO KNOWS HOW TO BINE.

WHAT IS IT DOING?

IT IS _____ .

WHAT WOULD YOU CALL A LUTZ

    WHOSE JOB IT IS TO BINE?

IT IS A _____ .

Record Form: Exploratory Test of Grammar (Berry-Talbott)

NAME: _____

PARENT'S NAME: _____   ADDRESS: _____

BIRTHDATE: _____   AGE: _____

ENTERED LANGUAGE CENTER: _____

PLATE	TRIAL I	TRIAL II	TRIAL III
I			
II			
III			
IV			
V			
VI			
VII			
VIII			
IX			
X			
XI			
XII			
XIII			
XIV			
XV			
XVI			
XVII			
XVIII			
XIX			
XX			
XXI			
XXII			
XXIII			
XXIV			
XXV			
XXVI			
XXVII			
XVIII			
XXIX			
XXX			

COMPOSITE SCORES NUMBER CORRECT — TRIAL	I	II	III
PLURAL NOUN (PLATES I II IV VII IX X XII XIII XVI XVII)			
PAST TENSE (PLATES III V XI XIV XVIII XX XXII XXVI)			
THIRD PERSON SINGULAR (PLATES XV XIX)			
POSSESSIVE SINGULAR — PLURAL (PLATES XXI XXIII)			
DERIVED ADJECTIVE (PLATES VIII XXVIII)			
ADJECTIVE: COMPARATIVE — SUPERLATIVE (PLATES XXIV XXIX)			
DIMINUTIVE — DERIVED WORD (PLATE VI)			
PROGRESSIVE — DERIVED WORD (PLATES XXV XXX)			

Full-range Picture Vocabulary Test, Ammons, Form A: Selected Word List

1. pie (1.7)
2. window (1.7)
3. seed (6.5)
4. sill (6.7)
5. athletes (8.6)
6. counter (4.0)
7. pump (4.4)
8. clerk (6.4)
9. sport (7.6)
10. recreation (10.8)
11. shrubbery (9.8)
12. horse (1.5)
13. wagon (2.3)
14. insect (6.7)
15. transportation (8.6)
16. discussion (7.7)
17. firecracker (2.7)
18. clothes (3.0)
19. explosion (4.9)
20. clean (5.5)
21. farm (4.1)
22. furniture (4.4)
23. steel (6.0)
24. refreshment (6.2)
25. liquid (7.3)
26. container (9.5)
27. clock (1.6)
28. locket (3.0)
29. numbers (3.4)
30. engraving (9.8)
31. hot (5.2)
32. fear (7.4)
33. nutrition (10.4)
34. telephone (2.1)
35. crying (2.9)
36. accident (3.0)
37. vehicles (9.5)
38. destruction (10.0)
39. portrait (10.2)
40. communication (10.6)
41. bed (1.6)
42. newspaper (2.5)
43. propellers (3.7)
44. harbor (8.1)
45. locomotive (8.2)
46. danger (5.6) [2]

[2] R. Ammons and H. Ammons, *Full-range Picture Vocabulary Test.* Copyright, 1948 by Robert B. Ammons. Missoula, Montana: Psychological Test Specialists, 1958.

Instructions

1. Point to the ball.

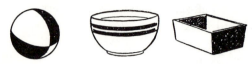

2. Put your finger on the smallest book.

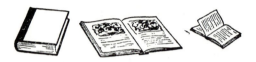

3. Here are some things to eat. Put your finger on the bowl of fruit.

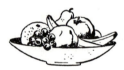

4. Here are 3 children playing a game. One is hitting, one is standing, and one is running. Put your finger on the one that is hitting.

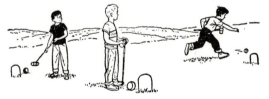

Figure B-3. Test of comprehension span.

SOURCE: G. Rochford and M. Williams, The measurement of language disorders. *Speech Path Ther* (April 1964), 7: (1) 6–7.

5. Here are 3 things which you might see outside in the country. Two of them are animals. Show me the one that has both roots' and leaves, and grows in the ground.

6. At different times of the year we have different sports. One of these men is climbing a mountain and, as you see, he is warmly dressed to keep out the cold. Draw a circle with your finger around the man's hat.

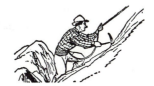

7. When this man leaves his room, he likes to make sure that he has put all his things away. That is why there is nothing lying on either the chair or the chest of drawers. Draw a line with your finger from the chair to the man.

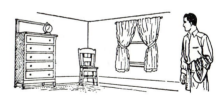

8. Here are the faces of 5 members of a family, and if you look carefully at them you will see that 2 of them are young boys. They are the sons of the first 2 people and it is their grandfather whom you see in the middle. Put your finger on all of these faces one after the other.

Appraising Closure by Completion Sentences, 4–8 Years

1. A lemon is sour; sugar is _____. (sweet)
2. A mile is long; an inch is _____. (short)
3. Please pass the salt and _____. (pepper)
4. When it rains, we must wear our _____. (coats, raincoats, boots, rubbers)
5. Apples are _____. (red, yellow)
6. Santa Claus comes on _____. (Christmas, sleigh, sled, Christmas Eve)
7. Snow is _____. (cold, white, water, wet, or made of rain)
8. Sister is a girl; brother is a _____. (boy)
9. I like ice cream and _____. (cake, cookies)
10. I like bread and _____. (butter, jam, jelly, peanut butter)
11. By each plate, please put a knife, _____ and _____. (fork and spoon)
12. In school we learn to read and _____. (write, numbers)
13. For breakfast I like bacon and _____. (eggs)
14. On my cereal I always put milk and _____. (sugar)
15. We smile when we are happy; we cry when we are _____. (sad, unhappy, feel bad)
16. We work in the daytime; we sleep at _____. (night)
17. A chair is made of wood; a window is made of _____. (glass, plastic)
18. A car goes on the ground; an airplane goes in the _____. (sky, air)
19. I listen both with my eyes and my _____. (ears)
20. May I have a glass of _____. (water, milk)
21. Daddy smokes a _____. (pipe, cigar, cigarette)
22. If you play with matches you may get _____. (burned)
23. First I put on my socks, then my _____. (shoes)
24. Here comes the postman with the _____. (letters, mail)
25. An elephant is big; a mouse is _____. (little, tiny)

Table B-1. Mean scores on 176-item Diagnostic Test of Articulation by age for boys, girls, sexes combined, and upper and lower socioeconomic groups.

C.A.	Girls (N=30)*		Boys (N=30)		Both Sexes (N=60)		Upper SE** (N=18)		Lower SE** (N=42)	
	M	SD	M	SD	M	SD	M	SD	M	SD
3	88.2	31.8	98.3	35.0	93.3	33.8	97.6	33.1	91.5	34.0
3½	118.2	31.0	105.5	37.6	111.9	35.0	115.9	31.1	110.1	36.5
4	125.5	26.7	127.2	31.6	126.4	29.3	136.1	18.9	122.2	31.8
4½	131.2	29.5	127.2	32.2	129.2	31.0	141.7	29.8	123.8	29.9
5	141.8	33.9	128.8	38.1	135.3	36.7	146.9	26.8	130.3	39.1
6	156.9	21.8	143.7	33.8	150.3	29.2	154.5	28.6	140.4	42.7
7	166.4	10.8	157.3	21.7	161.9	17.7	167.8	11.4	151.4	38.9
8	166.6	13.2	167.6	8.6	167.1	11.1	169.7	7.3	166.0	12.3

*N represents number of subjects at each of the eight age levels.
**Upper SE subjects are in classes I, II and III, and lower SE subjects are in classes V, VI and VII according to the Minnesota Scale of Paternal Occupations.

SOURCE: M. Templin and F. Darley, *The Templin-Darley Tests of Articulation.* Iowa City, Iowa: Bureau of Educational Research, The University of Iowa, 1960. P. 18.

Scoring Form: Developmental Articulation Test

Name: _____ Age: ____ Grade: ____ Date I: _____ Date II: _____

Age	Sound	Initial	Test I	Test II		Test I	Test II	Final	Test I	Test II	Is:I	Is:II
3.6	p	pie			apple			cap				
3.6	b	bear			rabbit			bathtub				
3.6	m	milk			camera			ice cream				
3.6	w	window			sidewalk							
3.6	h	house										
4.6	t	table			potatoes			cat				
4.6	d	dog			saddle			bed				
4.6	n	nose			banana			crown				
4.6	g	girl			eggs			dog				
4.6	k	cat			cooking			milk				
4.6	ŋ				swings			ding dong				
4.6	j	yellow			onion							
5.6	f	fish			telephone			leaf				
6.6	v	valentine			leaves			glove				
6.6	ð	this/ that			mother							
6.6	ʒ				measure							
6.6	l	lamp			jello			ball				
6.6	ʃ	shirt			dishes			fish				
7.6	θ	thumb			bathtub			teeth				
7.6	z	zipper			scissors			cheese				
7.6	s	soup			pencil			glass				
7.6	tʃ	cheese			matches			peach				
7.6	dʒ	jeans			engine			bridge				
7.6	r	running			iron			bear				
7.6	l	flag			airplane			clown				
7.6	s	spoon			slide			snowman				
7.6	r	train			frog			brush				

SOURCE: Hejna, R. *Developmental Articulation Test.* Storrs, Conn: Hejna, 1955.

Instructions: Within the brackets write the phonetic symbol for the sound deep tested, e.g., [s]. Use the symbols you prefer to indicate whether the sound was articulated correctly or the nature of the incorrect articulation (substitution, omission, or distortion) for each of the indicated phonetic contexts. Not all phonetic contexts can be tested. To determine the percent of correct articulations, divide the number of *correct* responses by the number of phonemes tested and multiply the quotient by 100.

INDIVIDUAL RECORD SHEET for a DEEP TEST OF ARTICULATION

Name _____ Age _____ Grade _____ Date _____

Address or School _____ Test used: _____

Tester _____

Sentence   Picture

[ ]   [ ]   [ ]   [ ]

*

p — 1 — p	p — 1 — p	p — 1 — p	p — 1 — p
b — 2 — b	b — 2 — b	b — 2 — b	b — 2 — b
t — 3 — t	t — 3 — t	t — 3 — t	t — 3 — t
d — 4 — d	d — 4 — d	d — 4 — d	d — 4 — d
k — 5 — k	k — 5 — k	k — 5 — k	k — 5 — k
g — 6 — g	g — 6 — g	g — 6 — g	g — 6 — g
m — 7 — m	m — 7 — m	m — 7 — m	m — 7 — m
n — 8 — n	n — 8 — n	n — 8 — n	n — 8 — n
f — 9 — f	f — 9 — f	f — 9 — f	f — 9 — f
v — 10 — v	v — 10 — v	v — 10 — v	v — 10 — v
θ — 11 — θ	θ — 11 — θ	θ — 11 — θ	θ — 11 — θ
ð — 12 — ð	ð — 12 — ð	ð — 12 — ð	ð — 12 — ð
s — 13 — s	s — 13 — s	s — 13 — s	s — 13 — s
z — 14 — z	z — 14 — z	z — 14 — z	z — 14 — z
ʃ — 15 — ʃ	ʃ — 15 — ʃ	ʃ — 15 — ʃ	ʃ — 15 — ʃ
tʃ — 16 — tʃ	tʃ — 16 — tʃ	tʃ — 16 — tʃ	tʃ — 16 — tʃ
dʒ — 17 — dʒ	dʒ — 17 — dʒ	dʒ — 17 — dʒ	dʒ — 17 — dʒ
l — 18 — l	l — 18 — l	l — 18 — l	l — 18 — l
r — 19 — r	r — 19 — r	r — 19 — r	r — 19 — r
j — 20 — j	j — 20 — j	j — 20 — j	j — 20 — j
w — 21 — w	w — 21 — w	w — 21 — w	w — 21 — w
h — 22 — h	h — 22 — h	h — 22 — h	h — 22 — h
ŋ — 23 — ŋ	ŋ — 23 — ŋ	ŋ — 23 — ŋ	ŋ — 23 — ŋ
i — 24 — i	i — 24 — i	i — 24 — i	i — 24 — i
ɪ — 25 — ɪ	ɪ — 25 — ɪ	ɪ — 25 — ɪ	ɪ — 25 — ɪ
ɛ — 26 — ɛ	ɛ — 26 — ɛ	ɛ — 26 — ɛ	ɛ — 26 — ɛ
æ — 27 — æ	æ — 27 — æ	æ — 27 — æ	æ — 27 — æ
ʌ — 28 — ʌ	ʌ — 28 — ʌ	ʌ — 28 — ʌ	ʌ — 28 — ʌ
u — 29 — u	u — 29 — u	u — 29 — u	u — 29 — u
ɔ — 30 — ɔ	ɔ — 30 — ɔ	ɔ — 30 — ɔ	ɔ — 30 — ɔ
%Correct	%Correct	%Correct	%Correct
___	___	___	___
Date Tested	Date Tested	Date Tested	Date Tested
___	___	___	___

*The numbers correspond to the sentence number or picture number in The Deep Test of Articulation

Ⓒ Stanwix House 1964

Figure B-4. Individual record sheet: A deep test of articulation.

SOURCE: E. McDonald, *A deep test of articulation.* Pittsburgh: Stanwix House, 1964.

Appendix C   Chapter 8

General Classification Scales

Selected Items from the California First-Year Mental Scale

1. Postural adjustment
2. Lateral head movements
3. Momentary regard of ring
4. Responds to sound
5. Prolonged regard
6. Responds to voice
7. Arm and leg thrusts
8. Social smile
9. Vocalizations
10. Eyes follow pencil
11. Manipulates ring
12. Reaches for ring
13. Blinks at visual stimulus
14. Vocalizes to social stimulus
15. Fingers hand in play
16. Carries ring to mouth
17. Aware of strange situation
18. Anticipatory adjustment to lifting
19. Plays with rattle
20. Inspects hand
21. Turns head to sound
22. Beginning thumb opposition
23. Active table manipulation
24. Reaches for cube
25. Partial thumb opposition
26. Picks up cube
27. Recovers rattle
28. Discriminates strangers
29. Vocalizes eagerness
30. Lifts cup
31. Accepts second cube
32. Vocalizes pleasure
33. Vocalizes displeasure
34. Turns after fallen spoon
35. Says several syllables
36. Bangs in play
37. Unilateral reaching
38. Vocalizes satisfaction
39. Lifts cup with the handle
40. Rotates wrist
41. Smiles at mirror image
42. Manipulates bell: interest in details
43. Looks for fallen spoon
44. Likes frolic play
45. Vocalizes recognition
46. Interest in sound production
47. Complete thumb opposition
48. Vocal interjections
49. Attends scribbling
50. Listens to familiar words
51. Says "da-da" or equivalent

52. Explores form board holes
53. Attempts to secure 3 cubes
54. Interest in throwing
55. Playful response to mirror
56. Differentiates words
57. Rings bell purposively
58. Puts cube in cup on command
59. Attempts to scribble imitatively
60. Holds crayon adaptively
61. Inhibits on command
62. Repeats performance laughed at
63. Strikes doll in imitation
64. Imitates words
65. Stirs with spoon in imitation
66. Holds cup to drink from
67. Says two words
68. Spontaneous scribble
69. Uses expressive jargon
70. Builds tower of 2 cubes
71. Round block in reversed Gesell board
72. Looks at pictures in book
73. Throws a ball
74. Builds a tower of 3 cubes
75. Turns pages
76. Square or triangle in Gesell board
77. Names one object (ball, pencil, cup, watch, scissors)
78. Puts cover on box on command [1]

Goodenough-Harris Drawing Test
Short Scoring Guide: Woman Point Scale *

1. Head present
2. Neck present
3. Neck, two dimensions
4. Eyes present
5. Eye detail: brow or lashes
6. Eye detail: pupil
7. Eye detail: proportion
8. Cheeks
9. Nose present
10. Nose, two dimensions
11. Bridge of nose
12. Nostrils shown
13. Mouth present
14. Lips, two dimensions
15. "Cosmetic lips"
16. Both nose and lips in two dimensions
17. Both chin and forehead shown
18. Line of jaw indicated
19. Hair I
20. Hair II
21. Hair III
22. Hair IV
23. Necklace or earrings
24. Arms present
25. Shoulders
26. Arms at side (or engaged in activity or behind back)
27. Elbow joint shown
28. Fingers present
29. Correct number of fingers shown
30. Detail of fingers correct
31. Opposition of thumb shown
32. Hands present
33. Legs present
34. Hip
35. Feet I: any indication
36. Feet II: proportion
37. Feet III: detail
38. Shoe I: "feminine"
39. Shoe II: style
40. Placement of feet appropriate to figure
41. Attachment of arms and legs I
42. Attachment of arms and legs II
43. Clothing indicated

[1] N. Bayley, *The California First-year Mental Scale*. Berkeley: University of California, Syllabus Series, 1933, No. 243.
* For use only after the scoring requirements have been mastered.

44. Sleeve I
45. Sleeve II
46. Neckline I
47. Neckline II: collar
48. Waist I
49. Waist II
50. Skirt "modeled" to indicate pleats or draping
51. No transparencies in the figure
52. Garb feminine
53. Garb complete, without incongruities
54. Garb a definite "type"
55. Trunk present
56. Trunk in proportion, two dimensions
57. Head-trunk proportion
58. Head: proportion
59. Limbs: proportion
60. Arms in proportion to trunk
61. Location of waist
62. Dress area
63. Motor coordination: junctures
64. Motor coordination: lines
65. Superior motor coordination
66. Directed lines and form: head outline
67. Directed lines and form: breast
68. Directed lines and form: hip contour
69. Directed lines and form: arms taper
70. Directed lines and form: calf of leg
71. Directed lines and form: facial features [2]

[2] D. B. Harris, *Goodenough-Harris Drawing Test Manual.* New York: Harcourt Brace & World, 1963. P. 292.

Norms for the Board Form of the Progressive Matrices Test

Table C-1. Normal score composition.

Total Score		10	11	12	13	14	15	16	17	18	19	20	21	22	23	24	25	26	27	28	29	30	31
Expected	A	6	6	6	7	7	8	8	8	9	9	9	9	9	9	9	10	10	10	10	11	11	11	11
Score On	Ab	2	3	3	3	4	4	4	5	5	5	6	7	7	8	8	8	9	9	9	10	10	10
Each Set	B	2	2	3	3	3	3	4	4	4	5	5	5	6	6	6	7	7	8	8	8	9	10

Table C-2. Working percentile points estimated from the scores obtained by 291 Dumfries School children over 5 and under 10 years of age.

Percentile Points	Chronological Age in Years								
	5½	6	6½	7	7½	8	8½	9	9½
95	21	23	24	25	26	27	29	30	31
90	19	21	22	23	24	25	27	28	29
75	15	17	18	20	21	23	24	25	26
50	12	14	16	17	18	20	21	22	23
25	10	11	13	14	16	17	18	19	20
10	—	10	11	12	13	14	15	16	17
5	—	—	10	11	12	13	14	15	16

Although carefully selected for the purpose of an experimental survey, the sample of 291 children was too small to estimate percentile points for the general population at all accurately.

SOURCE: J. C. Raven, *Guide to using the coloured progressive matrices* (sets A, Ab, B). London: H. K. Lewis, 1960. P. 35.

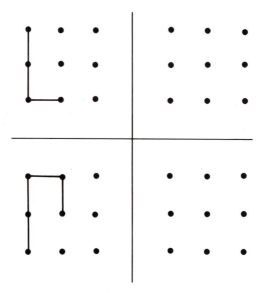

*Figure C-1.   Frostig developmental test of visual perception,
subtest Vb.*

SOURCE: M. Frostig, *et al.* Reproduced by special permission from *The developmental
test of visual perception: Administration and scoring manual.* Copyright 1964 by
Marianne Frostig.

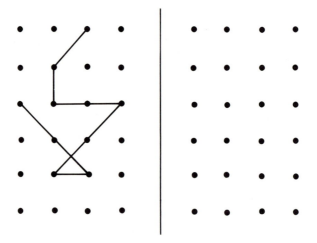

*Figure C-2.   Frostig developmental test of visual perception, subtest
Vd, first grade and up only.*

SOURCE: M. Frostig, *et al.* Reproduced by special permission from *The developmental
test of visual perception: Administration and scoring manual.* Copyright 1964 by
Marianne Frostig.

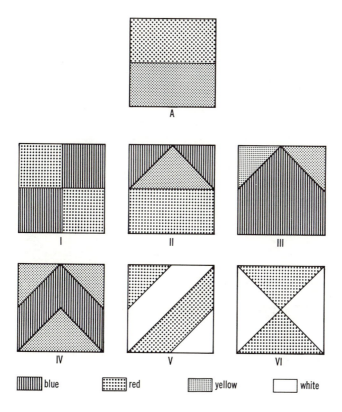

Figure C-3. *Kohs block designs.*

SOURCE: S. C. Kohs, *Intelligence measurement.* New York: Macmillan, 1923. Pp. 66–67.

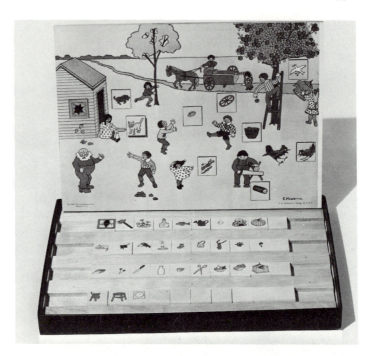

Figure C-4. Healy picture completion test I.
SOURCE: *Pinter-Paterson performance scale.* Chicago: C. H. Stoelting, 1917.

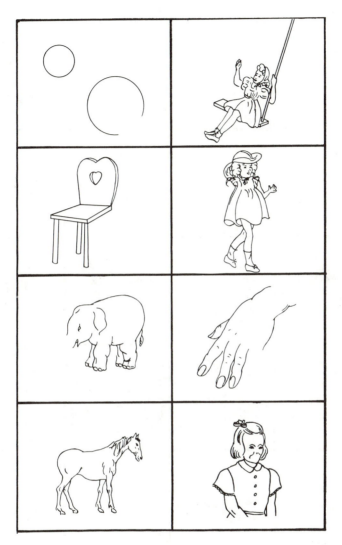

Figure C-5.   Completion of drawings, test of closure.

SOURCE: M. S. Hiskey, *Hiskey-Nebraska test of learning aptitude*. Lincoln, Nebr.: University of Nebraska, 1966.

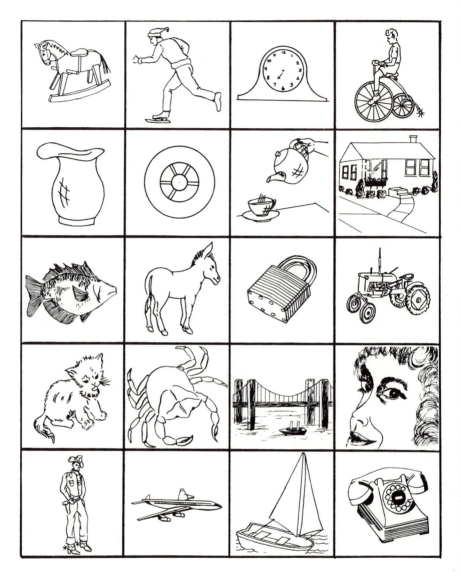

Figure C-5.   Completion of drawings, test of closure (continued).

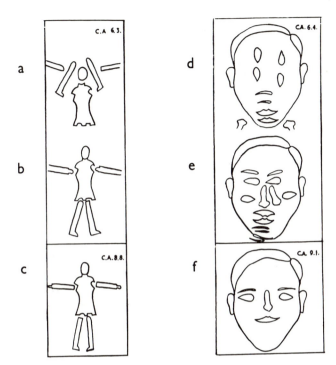

Figure C-6. Results of object assembly test. Parts (a), (b), and (c) are attempts made by a spastic child, I.Q. 89, to assemble a mannikin; (a) was done at age 6 years, 3 months, and (b) shows improvement after demonstration. At age 8 years, 8 months (c), he is able to get roughly the same result without demonstration, but the fit is still not good. Parts (d), (e), and (f) are attempts made by a spastic child of I.Q. 68 to assemble a face; the outline of the head is provided, and a double set of eyes, eyebrows, nose, and mouth. At age 6 years, 4 months (d), he is unable to place the parts correctly, but after being shown how to do so, (e) he makes a better attempt but spoils it by using both sets of parts. At age 9 years, 1 month (f), however, he can make the face correctly.

SOURCE: K. Wedell, Follow-up study of perceptual ability in children with hemiplegia, *Hemiplegic cerebral palsy in children and adults: Little Club Clinics in developmental medicine No. 4.* London: Heinemann, 1961. Pp. 76–85.

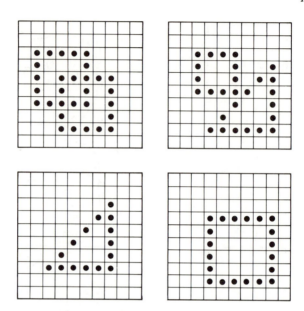

Figure C-7.   Marble-board test designs.

SOURCE: A. Strauss and H. Kephart, *Psychopathology and education of the brain-injured child*, Vol. II. New York: Grune & Stratton, 1955. P. 216.

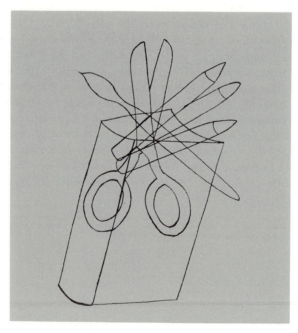

Figure C-8.   Mixed figure test I.

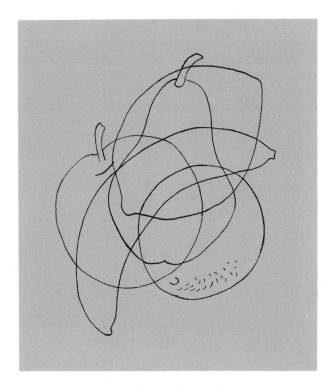

Figure C-9.   Mixed figure test III.

SOURCE (Figures C-8 to C-11): Adapted from tests by H-L. Teuber and R. Rudel, Behaviour after cerebral lesions in children and adults. *Devel Med Child Neurol* (February 1962), 4: 3–20.

Exploratory Tests of Figure-Ground

Marble Board Test.[3] The children are given two similar boards in which there are holes, spaced irregularly so as to make a background design. In addition to the background pattern, a design of marbles is placed on one board. The child is asked to make a similar design on the empty board.

The Mixed Figure Test illustrated here is adapted from the work of Teuber and Rudel [4] and is the result of their work with children who have suffered "brain injury." The child is asked to select one figure from overlapping figures.

[3] A. Strauss and N. Kephart, *Psychopathology and education of the brain-injured child, Vol. II.* New York: Grune & Stratton, 1955. P. 216.
[4] H. Teuber and R. Rudel, Behaviour after cerebral lesions in children and adults *Develop Med Child Neurol* (February 1962), 4: 3–20.

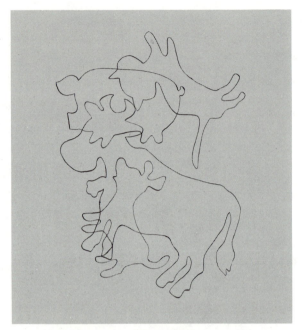

Figure C-10.   Mixed figure test IV.

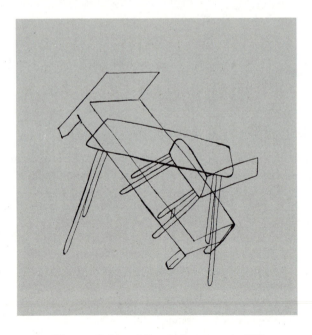

Figure C-11.   Mixed figure test VII.

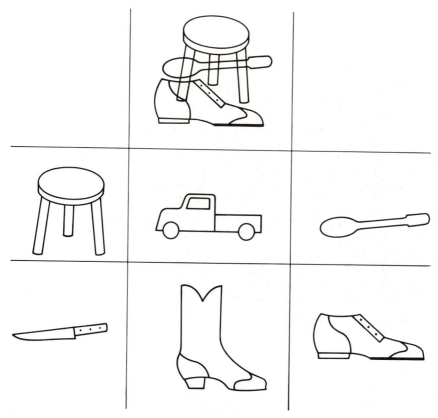

Figure C-12. Southern California figure-ground visual perception test, test trial plates 1A-1B.

SOURCE: A. J. Ayres, Ph.D., *Southern California figure-ground visual perception test.* Los Angeles: Western Psychological Services, 1966.

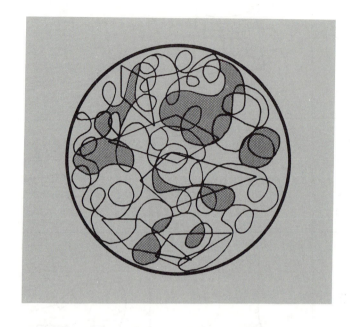

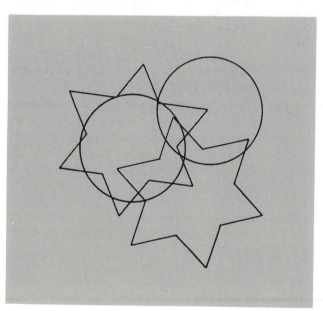

Figure C-13. Two items from the figure-ground test of the Frostig developmental test of visual perception (subtest II B). The child is asked to outline the two stars and the "kites."

SOURCE: M. Frostig, et al. Reproduced by special permission from *The developmental test of visual perception: Administration and scoring manual.* Copyright 1964 by Marianne Frostig.

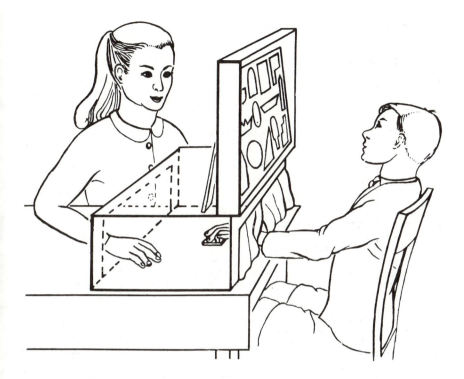

Figure C-14.   Cross-modality matching.   Child feels a cut shape in a "shadow box" which prevents his seeing it, and chooses a figure which matches it from a visual array.

SOURCE: M. L. J. Abercrombie, *Perceptual visuo-motor disorders in cerebral palsy.* London: Heinemann, 1964. P. 53.

Test of Cross-Modality Matching

Abercrombie uses the form board and a shadow box in testing cerebral palsied children in cross-modality matching. You will note in the illustration (Figure C-14) that the flat shapes are felt but not seen. The child indicates the hole into which the shape should fit.

Tests of Motor Development and Skills

Some Test Items from *A Scale of Motor Development*

Age Placement in Months	Test Items	Scores		
		Test 1	Test 2	Test 3
.5	Postural adjustment when held to shoulder			
.6	Lateral head movements			
2.6	Dorsal suspension—lifts head			
3.5	Prone—elevates self by arms			
3.6	Holds head steady			
5.0	Turns from back to side			
5.7	Simultaneous flexion and thumb opposition			
6.7	Rotates wrist			
8.5	Sits alone with good coordination			
9.2	Prewalking progression			
10.6	Stands up			
12.5	Stands alone			
16.9	Walks backward			
24.3	Walks upstairs alone; marks time			
29.3	Stands on right foot alone			
31.3	Walks on line; general direction			
35.5	Walks upstairs, alternating forward foot			
41.5	Jumps over rope less than 20 cm. high			
50.0	Walks downstairs, alternating forward foot			
54.5	Hops on left foot, less than two meters			

SOURCE: N. Bayley, The development of motor abilities during the first three years. *Monog Soc Res Child Develop*, 1935, 1 (1): 1-25.

Score Sheet. *The Lincoln-Oseretsky Motor Development Scale*

Item	Description	R-L	Trials	Pts.	Notes
1	Walking backwards, 6 ft.		2		
2	Crouching on tiptoe		2		
3	Standing on one foot	R/L	2/2	/	
4	Touching nose		1		
5	Touching fingertips	R/L	2/2	/	
6	Tapping rhythmically with feet and fingers		1		
7	Jumping over a rope		1		
8	Finger movement		3		
9	Standing heel to toe		2		
10	Close and open hands alternately		3		
11	Making dots		2		
12	Catching a ball	R/L	5/5	/	
13	Making a ball	R/L	2/2	/	
14	Winding thread	R/L	1/1	/	
15	Balancing a rod crosswise	R/L	3/3	/	
16	Describing circles in the air		1		
17	Tapping (15″)	R/L	2/2	/	
18	Placing coins and matchsticks		1		
19	Jump and turn about		1		
20	Putting matchsticks in a box		1		
21	Winding thread while walking	R/L	1/1	/	
22	Throwing a ball	R/L	5/5	/	
23	Sorting matchsticks	R/L	1/1	/	
24	Drawing lines	R/L	2/2	/	
25	Cutting a circle	R/L	1/1	/	
26	Putting coins in box (15″)	R/L	1/1	/	
27	Tracing mazes	R/L	1/1	/	
28	Balancing on tiptoe		1		
29	Tapping with feet and fingers		1		
30	Jump, touch heels		1		
31	Tap feet and describe circles		1		
32	Stand on one foot	R/L	1/1	/	
33	Jumping and clapping		1		
34	Balancing on tiptoe	R/L	1/1	/	
35	Opening and closing hands		1		
36	Balancing a rod vertically	R/L	3/3	/	

SOURCE: W. Sloan, The Lincoln-Oseretsky Motor Development Scale. *Gen Psychol Monog* (1955) 51:247.

Iowa Performance Test of Selected Manual Activities

Scoring. The purpose of this test is to determine a person's dextrality quotient (percentage of right-handedness) on the basis of observation of 64 operations in the performance of 32 activities. The dextrality quotient for each subject can be found by means of the formula

$$DQ = \frac{R - (B/2)}{N}, \text{ in which R and B represent}$$

the number of operations performed by the right hand and by both hands (neither hand predominating), respectively, and N represents the total number of operations performed.

Materials. The materials needed for the test are: A room with a window having a shade which can be easily manipulated by a seven-year-old child; a desk of the type from which articles are taken with equal ease from both sides, i.e., the open shelf type, and in which the articles to be removed are not observed; a pencil; a small pencil sharpener of the type held in one hand; a tablet of paper of customary school size; a pencil with eraser attached; a box of crayons; scissors in which the finger holes are the same on both sides; five regular flash cards; a blackboard; a piece of chalk; eight 1¼″ cubes; . . . and a large picture book with pages which can be readily handled.

Procedure. Before calling the child, the tablet, pencil, pencil sharpener, and crayons are placed in the desk. As soon as the child enters the room the following directions are given:

"Will you please *pull down the curtain* a little? That is fine, but will you please *pull it down* a trifle more?" See that the child has taken his hand from the curtain before being instructed to make the second adjustment. Also, be sure that he approaches the shade so that it can be as readily pulled with one hand as with the other.

"Now will you please *take the articles out of the desk* one at a time and place them on the top of the desk?" The first two responses are recorded for this item. The tester picks up the articles and places only the tablet in front of the child, and says, "Please *tear out* one sheet of paper and *turn over* the paper."

The tester then puts the pencil and pencil sharpener in front of the child, and says, "Please *sharpen the pencil.*" The activity is scored by recording the hand that does the actual turning.

The tester next places the pencil directly in front of the child and continues, "*Write your name* at the top of the paper. No, please *erase it,* and *write it* at the bottom of the sheet. Now will you please *draw* a picture; and when you are finished, *put the pencil in the desk.*"

Then a box of crayons is placed directly in front of the child by the tester who says, "Now *color* the picture." Note which hand is used in *taking out each crayon* (score the first two), in *coloring,* in *placing each crayon* in the box (score the first two), and in *closing the box.* In case the child does not voluntarily use more than one color, the tester may say, "Let's use another color for this part of the picture." As soon as the child is through and no longer has his hands on the box, say: "Let's look in the box to see if we have all the crayons in it." This gives a second score for *closing the box.*

Next the scissors are placed directly in front of the child. *"Cut off the bottom line,* please." Note the hand used in *picking up the scissors.* "Now *put the scissors in the desk."*

The tester next arranges the blocks in a straight line from one side of the table to the other, the middle block being directly before the child, and says, *"Point to A; point to G,"* etc. Be sure to see that the child is relaxed and ready to start with neither hand favored before the second letter is named. The first two letters, the only ones scored, are called off in a definite order, the sixth from the left being called first and the third from the left next. "Now pile the blocks one on top of the other to make a pile eight blocks high, being sure to *pick up* only one block at a time." Note the hand used in *picking up,* as well as in *placing,* the second and fourth blocks. The blocks are again put on the desk, and the tester instructs the child by saying, "Please carry these over to that desk one at a time." If there is not a second desk handy, some other surface may be substituted. Record the hand used in *picking up* first and third blocks. Do not record the hand used in carrying the blocks.

Next the tester places five flash cards on the top of the desk and says, "Please *point* to the cards as I name them." Call first for the second from the left and then for the fourth from the left. "Now please *pick them up* one at a time and now *lay them down* one at a time." (For these last two items, record the first two responses in each case.)

Now a tablet is placed directly in front of the child, and the tester says, "Please *tear out* another sheet of paper; *turn over the sheet of paper;* and *fold it* in the middle." The hand which actually creases the folded edge is the one recorded.

Next the pencil sharpener and pencil are again presented in the midline, and the child is instructed to *sharpen the pencil.*

Following this activity, the picture book is presented in the middle of the desk, and the tester says, "Please *turn* to the picture of Casper Carrot." Any picture will do so long as two or more pages are turned. Record the hand used in turning each of the first two pages. Then after the pencil is again presented directly in front of the child, the examiner says, "Now *draw* the picture, and when you are through *put the pencil in the desk."*

Next the book is removed and the scissors are placed directly in front of the child, and the tester says, "Please cut out your picture, and then *put the scissors in the desk."* Also, the hand used in *picking up* the scissors is recorded.

. . . .

The last two activities are concerned with the blackboard. The child is directed to stand squarely in front of it where the chalk can be as easily reached with one hand as with the other. The tester says, "Please write your name." Score the hand used in *picking up the chalk,* as well as in *writing.* Lastly, the tester asks the child, "Will you please *print* your name?" This also gives the second score for *picking up the chalk.* This concludes the test.

Any remarks by the child or further directions by the tester, in case there is difficulty in grasping the directions, need not be curtailed, provided they do not influence hand preference. Total test time: 20–25 minutes.

NORMS: In Table C-3, the lowest and highest percentiles, respectively, represent the lowest and highest D.Q. in each group. Suppose a six-year-old child scores a D.Q. of .86. By referring to this table it is to be found that he falls at the 70th percentile for his age group. This means that he is more right-handed than 70 percent and less right-handed than 30 percent of the six-year-olds tested by Johnson and Duke. In such terms any child's score may be evaluated. It must be kept in mind, of course, that these norms are only for the age levels indicated in the table. The score of a child at some other age level is to be evaluated by reference to the table only by taking into account the difference in age. This can be done only with a limited degree of accuracy, of course, and evaluations should be tempered accordingly. However, it will be noted that differences between high-school-age subjects and the two groups of younger subjects are not great. Since the activities involved in this test were originally selected by observing actual school-room activities of six-year-old children, it would seem reasonable to conclude that the hand which an individual has come to use consistently for a given activity at the age of seven years or so is the hand he will use for the same activity eight or ten years later.[5]

Blau's Objective Test of Laterality

1. *Cutting Test.* This requires a single type of scissors with fingerhold, made so as not to discriminate against the use of the left hand. The child is asked to cut out circles drawn on a piece of paper, first with one hand and then the other. In all probability, the child will not be able to manipulate the scissors with each hand. If he does, the relative dexterity of each hand can be seen. Record the more expert hand.

2. *Batting Test.* Require the child to hold a bat as if ready to strike a ball to be pitched by the examiner. Record the upper hand which is nearer the batting end.

3. *Crossing Thumb Test.* Ask the child to clasp his hands in front of his body. The examiner may demonstrate what is wanted. Record the hand with the thumb on top. Folding the arms may also be tried.

4. *Sighting Eye Test.* Ask the child to sight a distant object through a small hole in a large piece of paper or cardboard held at arm's length in front of the face. Without moving the paper, the left eye is closed while the right is open; if the object is still visible, the child is right-eyed, if not, he is left-eyed. The observer can usually check this by observing which eye is being used.

5. *Nose and Finger Near-Seeing Test.* Have the child hold his finger in a vertical position about a foot in front of the nose. With both eyes looking at the finger, have the child bring the finger toward his face. Observe whether the finger moves toward the right or left eye. The eye toward which the finger moves is the dominant eye for near-seeing.

[5] W. Johnson, F. Darley and D. Spriestersbach, *Diagnostic methods in speech pathology.* New York: Harper and Row, 1963. Pp. 303–305.

Table C-3. Scores on Iowa Performance Test of Selected Manual Activities, by percentiles, for 6-year-old, 7-year-old, and high-school age subjects.

Percentile	6-Year-Olds[a] N=50	7-Year-Olds[b] N=100	High-School-Age[c] (13-19 years) N=100
0	.07	.12	.01
10	.52	.63	.43
20	.65	.71	.64
30	.74	.78	.69
40	.80	.81	.74
50	.82	.83	.79
60	.84	.85	.84
70	.86	.88	.87
80	.90	.92	.91
90	.94	.95	.95
100	1.00	1.00	.97

[a]W. Johnson and D. Duke, Revised Iowa hand usage dextrality quotients of six-year-olds. *J Educ Psychol,* Vol. 31, No. 1 (1940), 45-52.
[b]W. Johnson and D. Davis, Dextrality quotients of seven-year-olds in terms of hand usage. *J Educ Psychol,* Vol. 28, No. 5 (1937), pp. 346-354.
[c]W. Johnson and V. L. Bissell, Iowa hand usage dextrality quotients of one hundred high-school students. *J Educ Psychol,* Vol. 31, No. 2 (1940), pp. 148-152.

SOURCE: W. Johnson, F. Darley, and D. Spriestersbach, *Diagnostic methods in speech pathology.* New York: Harper & Row, 1963. P. 321. Form 20.

6. *Kicking Test.* Ask the child to kick, as if at a football. Record the kicking leg.
7. *Crossing Legs Test.* Ask the child to cross his legs while seated. Record the upper leg.
8. *Hopping Test.* Ask the child to hop on one leg. Record the leg used.[6]

Harris Tests of Lateral Dominance

Harris includes in his complete test of *hand dominance* the following subtests: Hand preference, simultaneous writing, handwriting, tapping, dealing cards, and strength of grip. We include here some items from the test:

Hand Dominance.

1. Hand preference. Right _____% Left _____%
   a. Turn the door knob.　　　　　e. Comb hair.
   b. Wind a watch.　　　　　　　　f. Erase the board.
   c. Hammer a nail.　　　　　　　　g. Cut with knife.
   d. Brush teeth.　　　　　　　　　h. Screw jar top.

[6] A. Blau, Objective test of laterality. Reprinted in H. Bakwin and R. Bakwin, *Clinical management of behavior disorders in children.* Philadelphia: Saunders, 1953. P. 297.

2. Simultaneous bimanual writing. "Take the pencil on your left in your left
hand. Take the pencil on your right in your right hand. Now write the
numbers 1 through 12 going down on this paper with both hands at the
same time. Write as fast as you can." Repeat with vision screened.

    Number of inversions: R _____; L _____
    Number of reversals: R _____; L _____
    Comparative legibility: R _____; L _____

3. Pencil-paper test. The child is given a small motorcar. The teacher draws
a wide line, one-half inch in diameter, with a brush pen, representing
a road and sketching at one end a line drawing of a garage; at the other end
a grocery. Direct the child to run the car on the road from the garage to the
grocery being careful not to get off the road. He has five trials with each
hand. (The right hand may take the car from the garage to the grocery, the
left from the grocery to the garage.) Judge the comparative skill of the hands
in *direction, smoothness,* and *accuracy.* Ask the child to drive the car with the
hand he prefers.

    Record: Better hand in (a) direction _____.
                         (b) smoothness _____.
                         (c) accuracy _____.

4. Dealing cards. (Three trials with right hand; three with left.)
    Record:

    Average total elapsed time: R _____; R _____; R _____
    Average total elapsed time: L _____; L _____; L _____
    Faster hand: R _____; L _____

Foot Dominance. Right _____% Left _____%

1. Tapping (*E* taps on desk with hand; *S* taps the same way with foot; three
trials with each foot). Record better foot in following pattern.
2. Kicking football to set goal.
    a. Five trials; no instruction as to foot.
       Record preferred foot.
    b. Four trials, two with R foot; two with L foot.
       Record: Better foot (strength, direction, accuracy)

          Right _____; Left _____

3. Halt spinning top. (Three trials.) (*E* says: I am going to spin this top.
When it is spinning, reach out and touch it with your toe.)

    Record: Preferred foot: R _____; L _____ [7]

[7] A. J. Harris, *Harris tests of lateral dominance.* New York, The Psychological
Corporation, 1955. Pp. 12–13.

Tests of Social Maturity and Adjustment, Birth to 9 Years

VINELAND SOCIAL MATURITY SCALE

Date: _____

Directions

The scale provides a definite outline of detailed performances in respect to which children show a progressive capacity for looking after themselves and for participating in those activities which lead toward ultimate independence as adults. The items of the Scale are now arranged in order of increasing average difficulty, and represent progressive maturation in self-help, self-direction, locomotion, occupation, communication and social relations. This maturation in social independence may be taken as a measure of progressive development in social competence.

The Scale. The revised scale is printed herewith. Each item of the Scale has been given a categorical designation (See first two paragraphs, *Manual of Directions* E. A. Doll, p. 8) which is indicated by the following letters:

S H G—self-help general   O—occupation
S H E—self-help eating   C—communication
S H D—self-help dressing   L—locomotion
S D—self-direction   S—socialization

The recorder, retaining the scoring sheet himself and not supplying one to the informant, begins by questioning the informant well below the anticipated final score in each serial group of items, as assumed from age and general presumption of the subject's ability.

It is important to avoid asking whether the *S* can do so-and-so, but rather does he usually or habitually do so. These answers are then checked by detailed questioning until the examiner is able to score the item as a whole. It is also important to avoid leading questions and to follow up all general answers with detailed questions. Thus the examiner asks to what extent does the *S* feed himself, or how much does the *S* do for himself in dressing, or in what ways does the *S* help around the house, or what kind of work does the *S* perform. In this way the examiner may score several items at once in the same category on the basis of the degree of accomplishment in a series of related items. There is no substitute for finding out just what the *S* actually and habitually does in respect to each item.

Scoring: To score, consult Vineland Social Maturity Scale, *Manual of Directions,* E. A. Doll, pp. 12–18.

VINELAND SOCIAL MATURITY SCALE

Name _____ Sex _____ Grade _____ Date _____

Residence _____ Descent _____ Born _____

M.A. or   I.Q. or
M.G.U. _____ P.A. _____ Test Used _____ When _____ Age _____

Occupation _____ Class _____ Yrs. Exp. _____ Schooling _____

Father's Occupation _____ Class _____ Yrs. Exp. _____ Schooling _____

Mother's Occupation _____ Class _____ Yrs. Exp. _____ Schooling _____

Informant _____ Relationship _____ Recorder _____

Informant _____ Basal Score _____

Additional Pts. _____

Total Score _____

Age Equivalent _____

Social Quotient _____

Categories	Items	Age Levels
		0–1
C	1.	"Crows"; laughs.
S H G	2.	Balances head
S H G	3.	Grasps objects within reach
S	4.	Reaches for familiar persons
S H G	5.	Rolls over
S H G	6.	Reaches for nearby objects
O	7.	Occupies self unattended
S H G	8.	Sits unsupported
S H G	9.	Pulls self upright
C	10.	"Talks"; imitates sounds
S H E	11.	Drinks from cup or glass assisted
L	12.	Moves about on floor
S. H G	13.	Grasps with thumb and finger
S	14.	Demands personal attention
S H G	15.	Stands alone
S H E	16.	Does not drool
C	17.	Follows simple instructions

I–II

		L	18.	Walks about room unattended
		O	19.	Marks with pencil or crayon
S H	E		20.	Masticates food
S H	D		21.	Pulls off socks
		O	22.	Transfers objects
S H	G		23.	Overcomes simple obstacles
		O	24.	Fetches or carries familiar objects
S H	E		25.	Drinks from cup or glass unassisted
S H	G		26.	Gives up baby carriage
		S	27.	Plays with other children
S H	E		28.	Eats with spoon
		L	29.	Goes about house or yard
S H	E		30.	Discriminates edible substances
		C	31.	Uses names of familiar objects
		L	32.	Walks upstairs unassisted
S H	E		33.	Unwraps candy
		C	34.	Talks in short sentences

II–III

S H	G	35.	Asks to go to toilet
	O	36.	Initiates own play activities
S H	D	37.	Removes coat or dress
S H	E	38.	Eats with fork
S H	E	39.	Gets drink unassisted
S H	D	40.	Dries own hands
S H	G	41.	Avoids simple hazards
S H	D	42.	Puts on coat or dress unassisted
	O	43.	Cuts with scissors
	C	44.	Relates experiences

III–IV

	L	45.	Walks downstairs one step per tread
	S	46.	Plays cooperatively at kindergarten level
S H	D	47.	Buttons coat or dress
	O	48.	Helps at little household tasks
	S	49.	"Performs" for others
S H	D	50.	Washes hands unaided

IV–V

S H	G	51.	Cares for self at toilet
S H	D	52.	Washes face unassisted
	L	53.	Goes about neighborhood unattended

Vineland Social Maturity Scale (continued)

IV–V (continued)

S H D	54.	Dresses self except for tying
O	55.	Uses pencil or crayon for drawing
S	56.	Plays competitive exercise games

V–VI

O	57.	Uses skates, sled, wagon
C	58.	Prints simple words
S	59.	Plays simple games
S D	60.	Is trusted with money
L	61.	Goes to school unattended

VI–VII

S H E	62.	Uses table knife for spreading
C	63.	Uses pencil for writing
S H D	64.	Bathes self unassisted
S H D	65.	Goes to bed unassisted

VII–VIII

S H G	66.	Tells time to quarter hour
S H E	67.	Uses table knife for cutting
S	68.	Disavows literal Santa Claus
S	69.	Participates in pre-adolescent play
S H D	70.	Combs or brushes hair

VIII–IX

O	71.	Uses tools or utensils
O	72.	Does routine household tasks
C	73.	Reads on own initiative
S H D	74.	Bathes self unaided

IX–X

S H E	75.	Cares for self at table
S D	76.	Makes minor purchases
L	77.	Goes about home town freely

SOURCE: E. A. Doll, *Vineland Social Maturity Scale,* Minneapolis: American Guidance Service, 1936. The complete scale extends from birth to 25 years. Section presented above covers age group treated in this text.

Short Form Bellak *CAT* Blank: Analysis Sheet

	Story 1	Story 2	Summary

1. *Main theme (diagnostic level):* If descriptive and interpretative level are desired, use a scratch sheet.

2. *Main hero:* age _____ sex _____ vocation _____ abilities _____ interests _____ traits _____ body image _____ adequacy _____ and/or self image
_____

3. *Main needs of hero:*
   a. behavioral needs of hero (as in story):
   _____
   b. figures, objects, or circumstances *introduced:* _____
   c. figures, objects or circumstances *omitted:* _____
      implying need for or to: _____
      _____

1-3. Unconscious structure and drives of subject (based on variable 1-3)

4. *Conception of environment (world) as:*
   _____

4. Conception of world: eye for eye, tooth for tooth

5. a. Parental figures (m _____ ; f _____) are seen as _____
      and subject's reaction to *a* is _____
      _____

   b. Contemp. figures (m _____ , f _____) are seen as _____
      and subject's reaction to *b* is _____
      _____

   c. Junior figures (m _____ , f _____) are seen as
      _____
      and subject's reaction to *c* is _____
      _____

5. Relationship to others (as described in 1-3):

6. *Significant conflicts:* _____
   _____

6. Significant conflicts: How to meet aggression—with counter aggression, guilt, occasional compliance. Meets feeling of smallness and passivity and need for counter-action by wishful thinking.

7. *Nature of anxieties:*
   of physical harm and/or punishment _____
   of disapproval _____
   of lack or loss of love _____
   of illness or injury _____
   of being deserted _____
   of deprivation _____
   of being overpowered and helpless _____
   of being devoured _____ other _____

7. Nature of anxieties:

8. *Main defenses against conflicts and fears:*
   repression _____ reaction-formation _____
   regression _____ denial _____
   introjection _____ isolation _____
   undoing _____ rationalization _____
   other _____

8. Main defenses used: showing off, fantasy (lying), denial, aggressive acting-out

Short Form Bellak *CAT* Blank (continued)

	Story 1	Story 2

9. *Severity of superego as manifested by:*
punishment for "crime" _____
immediate _____ just _____
too severe _____ delayed _____
unjust _____ too lenient _____
delayed initial response or pauses
_____ stammer _____

10. *Integration of the ego, manifesting itself in:*
_____
Hero: adequate ___ inadequate _____
outcome: happy ___ unhappy _____
realistic _____ unrealistic _____
drive control _____
Thought processes as revealed by plot being:
_____
stereotyped _____ original _____
appropriate _____ inappropriate _____
complete _____ incomplete _____
syncretic _____ concrete _____
contaminated _____
Intelligence _____
Maturational level _____

Summary

9. Superego structure: uninte-grated superego—in many ways too weak for appropriate control, and then again primitively retaliatory, probably more so than appropriate for his age.

10. Integration and strength of ego: good intelligence, inventive, perceptive, and with a good structure of thought processes —except where they are in the service of making himself bigger. Then it leads to acting out and fanciful and wishful distortions.

SOURCE: L. Bellak and S. Bellak, Children's Apperception Test, rev. ed.: *Manual.* C.P.S. Inc., P. O. Box 83, Larchmont, N. Y. 10538. Reproduced with permission of C.P.S. Inc. and Leopold Bellak, M.D.

The exemplary interpretations in the *Summary* column are from a case study reported in L. Bellak and C. Adelman, The children's apperception test. In A. Rabin and M. Haworth, Eds., *Projective techniques with children.* New York: Grune & Stratton, 1960. P. 79.

Glossary

aberrant. Deviating from the usual course, as for example, aberrant fibers of the pyramidal tract.

acetylcholine. Chemical substance found at synaptic junctions, thought to be an effective inhibiting agent in neural transmission and integration.

acoustic nerve. *See* **Nerve.**

action potential. Changes in electrical potential at the surface of a nerve or muscle occurring at the moment of excitation; the potential is exhibited by momentary negativity (spike potential) followed by a period of secondary oscillations in potential.

affricates. [tʃ] [dʒ]. Phonemes transcribed as digraphs but which, in reality, are distinct phonemes, both linguistically and physiologically. They are characterized by an initial stop with a fricative release instead of plosion of the breath stream.

agnosia. Disturbance of recognition of objects, persons, or events in one's environment so that they are not readily compared with previously observed objects, persons, or events.

alalia. Literally, *without speech.* A general term for speech disorders characterized by complete disability to articulate meaningful speech. *See also* **dyslalia.**

allophone. Phonetic term referring to the sounds that are classified as belonging to a particular phoneme, despite the differences among them detectable by the human ear.

alpha wave. Dominant electrical rhythm of the post-central cortex maintained in the resting state. In infants, the wave is 3 Hz; in adults it varies from 10–12 Hz. The alpha rhythm is relatively low in frequency and high in voltage.

amygdaloid nucleus. *See* **Nucleus.**

analog computer. Computer that solves a given problem by using physical analogues, as electric voltages or shaft rotations of the numerical variables occurring in the problem.

anlage. Rudiment; embryonic cells or tissue from which an organ or part develops.

anoxemia. Deficiency of oxygen content of blood.

anterior pituitary gland. Master gland of the endocrine system. Secretes thyrotropin, growth hormone, adrenocorticotropin, follicle-stimulating hormone, luteinizing hormone, prolactin, and other hormones.

Aphasia:

adult aphasia. General language deficit that crosses all language modalities (perception, speaking, reading, and writing) and may or may not be complicated by such other sequelae of brain damage as impaired auditory, visual, and sensorimotor processes not associated with verbal disturbance.

developmental aphasia. Developmental language delay. Syndrome of behavior occurring in children with deficient or disturbed sensorimotor organization and manifested in disturbance of language function which is more marked than other adaptive inadequacies.

apraxia. Sensorimotor disorder characterized by confused perception of the sequential pattern of movements required for the act, or by inability to carry out the movement patterns although perception of the sequence is adequate. Gesture and pantomime accompanying speech are markedly affected. Synonym: *ideokinetic apraxia.*

ataxia. Marked loss of motor coordination and appearance of intention tremor caused by lesions of cortex, brain stem, or cerebellum.

athetosis. *See* **Cerebral Palsy.**

attention. Selective activity producing a focus on a stimulus, object, situation, or idea. Its neurological correlate is *set-to-attend* or *perceptual set.*

attention span. Consistent level of extensity with respect to stimuli. The largest number of objects that can be reported after limited display of them.

Audition:

auditory acuity. Sensitivity of the human ear to auditory stimuli.

auditory agnosia. *See* **dysacusis.**

auditory feedback. The auditory "return" of one's own speech; hearing oneself talk. Because the distance between mouth and ears is constant one hears one's own speech as being more sonorous than it really is.

auditory perception. *See* **Perception.**

delayed auditory feedback. Delay, usually experimentally produced, in returning one's speech output to auditory input.

direct auditory system. Classical neural route of auditory coding via ventral and dorsal cochlear nuclei, lateral lemniscus, and internal capsule to temporoparietal cortex.

indirect auditory system. Neural route of auditory coding employing reticular networks associated with nuclei in olive, midbrain, and metathalamus. Antonym: *direct auditory* or *classical system.*

autism, infantile. Child psychosis reflected in inability to identify or communicate with others and with the environment; behavior is frequently bizarre, compulsive, repetitive, and nonpurposive.

axone. Process of a neurone along which a nerve impulse passes away from the cell body.

basal nuclei. *See* **Nucleus.**

beta wave. Cortical rhythm, 20–30 Hz, which can be recorded electrically in the resting state in frontal areas. The wave is generally associated with the attention state and motor projection in the cortex.

bilingual. Having two native languages.

binary digit. Unit of measurement of quantities of *selective information* as used in communication theory. Broadly, one digit of a scale-of-two notation. Abbreviation: *bit.* Synonym: *binit.*

bit. *See* **binary digit.**

Bobath method. *See* **Cerebral palsy.**

brachium conjunctivum. Superior cerebellar peduncle, composed of nuclei and tracts connecting the cerebellum with the brainstem.

brachium pontis. Middle cerebellar peduncle, composed of nuclei and tracts, connecting cerebellum with the brainstem.

Broca's area. Inferior frontal gyrus in the left (major) cerebral hemisphere, identified by Broca in 1861 as the cortical organizing center for motor speech. Now thought to be only *one* of the areas associated with motor speech. Synonym: *Brodmann's area 44.*

Brodmann's area 4. Precentral gyrus containing Betz cells that give rise to voluntary motor fibers. Kinesthetic fibers also are found here.

Brodmann's area 41. Transverse temporal gyri and angular gyrus in parietal-temporal area associated with auditory perception.

Brodmann's area 44. *See* **Broca's area.**

CAT. Children's Apperception Test; a projective test of personality.

caudate nucleus. *See* **Nucleus.**

central nervous system (CNS). That part of the nervous system comprising the brain and spinal cord.

cerebellum. Inferior part of the brain lying below the cerebrum and above the pons and medulla. It consists of the lateral lobes; cerebellar hemispheres; and a middle lobe, the flocculus; probably assists in coding temporospatial patterns of balance, rhythm, and movement.

cerebral cortex. *See* **Cerebrum.**

cerebral dominance. *See* **Cerebrum.**

Cerebral Lobes:

  cerebral lobes. Five pairs of lobes, one of each pair comprising each of the two cerebral hemispheres.

  frontal lobe. Part of the cerebral hemispheres, located in front of the central sulcus (Fissure of Rolando) and above the lateral cerebral fissure (Fissure of Sylvius).

  limbic lobe. Part of the medial aspect of the cerebral hemisphere; c-curved structure encircling thalamus; includes cingulate and hippocampal gyri.

  occipital lobe. Part of the cerebral hemispheres, located posterior to the occipitoparietal fissure; triangular area at the occipital extremity.

  parietal lobe. Cerebral lobe above the lateral cerebral fissure (Fissure of Sylvius) and behind the central sulcus (Fissure of Rolando).

  temporal lobe. Part of the cerebral hemispheres below the lateral cerebral fissure (Fissure of Sylvius) and continuous posteriorly with the occipital lobe.

Cerebral Palsy:

  cerebral palsy. Neurological disorder caused by lesions of CNS; although motor manifestations of spasticity or athetosis predominate, perceptual losses have also been demonstrated. Injury to the CNS may be imperceptible or extensive in the behavior of the individual.

  athetosis. Recurring series of slow shifts in motor activity from agonist to antagonist in skeletal muscles, most frequently seen in writhing movements, marked in upper extremities, neck, and face of the cerebral-palsied.

  Bobath method. System of neuromuscular rehabilitation of the cerebral-palsied whereby proper muscle synergies for basic postures are established by external techniques of manipulation; the resulting proprioceptive feedback tends to incite proper impulses in surrounding muscles before either stretch or relaxation is attempted. Thus, righting reflexes and equilibrium reactions are kinesthetically stimulated, while undesired tonic reflex activity is simultaneously inhibited.

  choreoathetosis. Slow writhing movement of athetosis which is accompanied by a quick component.

clonus. A series of movements characterized by rapid alternating flexions and extensions; clonic spasm caused by irregular contraction of muscles when stretched suddenly.

Kabat-Knott method. System of neuromuscular training of the cerebral-palsied inducing proper proprioceptive stimulation and feedback in muscle synergies by maximal resistance, stretch, pressure, and traction.

Young-Stinchfield method. *See* **motokinesthetic training.**

cerebral peduncles. Two large bands of sensorimotor fiber tracts which form the ventral part of the midbrain. Made up, in part, of the pyramidal tracts.

Cerebrum:

cerebrum. Anterior part of the brain overlying the rest of the brain; consists of the cerebral hemispheres, basal nuclei, and connecting structures. Hypothesized to mediate final steps in coding perception, retention, inner speech, and expression. *See also* **Cerebral Lobes.**

cerebral cortex. The convoluted layer of gray substance that covers each cerebral hemisphere. *See also* **Cerebral Lobes.**

cerebral dominance. Genetically determined characteristic of neural activity in which the left cerebral hemisphere (even in left-handed individuals) is the major hemisphere in sensorimotor processes concerned with perception, ideation, memory, and language. Synonym: *cortical lateralization.*

corpus callosum. Great band of white matter at the base of the cerebrum joining the cerebral hemispheres. The callosum probably contains nearly two hundred million fibers. The extent to which learning is impaired by destruction of the callosum is not known. In young children the impairment seems to be minimal.

classical conditioning. *See* **Conditioning.**

closure. Principle of *gestalt* psychology describing the process by which percepts attain stability, *viz.,* the subjective closing of gaps, or completion of incomplete forms, so as to constitute wholes. The frame of expectation in which the phrase, clause, or sentence occurs.

cluttering. Temporal disorder of oral language characterized by dysrhythmic, rapid speech and faulty articulation. Synonym: *tachyphemia.*

cochlea. Cavity of the inner ear resembling a snail shell. It describes 2½ turns about a central core or modiolus, and contains the Organ of Corti or sensory end organs of hearing. The spiral canal around the modiolus is about 1½ inches in length.

cochlear nerve. *See* **Nerve.**

code. Agreed *transformation* or set of unambiguous rules, whereby information is converted from one representation to another. Set of physical events that is part of the communication system of a homeostat.

cognate. Words in two languages from the same original source. (English: *cold;* German: *kalt*).

cognition. General term to denote the act or process of knowing; discrimination. The *cognitive* function is often contrasted with the *affective* (feeling) function. *See also* **Perception.**

colliculi, inferior. Posterior pair of rounded eminences arising from dorsal portion of midbrain. The nuclei with their reticular connections assist in integration of auditory information chiefly via the indirect auditory route. Synonym: *inferior quadrigeminal body.*

colliculi, superior. Anterior pair of rounded eminences arising from dorsal portion of the midbrain. The nuclei with their reticular connections assist in integration of visual information chiefly via the indirect visual route. Synonym: *superior quadrigeminal body.*

comprehension span. Greatest number of events, things and processes of human experience which an individual can perceive (judged by response) in a spatial-temporal sequence of stimuli.

Conditioning:

    classical conditioning. Process by which a response comes to be elicited by constant association with a stimulus, object, or situation that normally or naturally could not produce the response. Synonym: *respondent conditioning.*

    operant conditioning. Process by which new patterns of learning are acquired by associating them with systematically applied rewards and punishment. Whereas the distinctive character of classically conditioned behavior is that it is in response to stimuli, the characteristic of operant behavior is that it operates on the environment. Synonyms: *instrumental conditioning; operant learning.*

corpora quadrigemina. Rounded eminences of the dorsal section of midbrain. *See also* **colliculi, inferior** *and* **colliculi, superior.**

cortex. *See* **Cerebrum.**

cybernetics. Study of human control functions and of mechanical and electrical systems designed to replace them. The application of statistical mechanics to communication engineering. The study of the interaction between situations and individuals in terms of communication.

decussation. Crossing of nerve tracts over the midline in the CNS.

delta rhythm. Projected cortical rhythm, 1–4 Hz, thought to occur during deep sleep in infants and in organic brain disease in adults.

dendrite. Process of a neurone, varying in length and number of branches; it presumably mediates nerve impulses in the direction of the cell body.

dendritic-glial layer. Arborescent neuronal endings embedded in the neuroglial or "connective tissue" substance of the cerebrum.

deoxyribonucleic acid. *See* **DNA.**

diadokokinesis. Performance of repetitive movements in discrete muscle synergies reflecting alternation of neural inhibition and facilitation. Repetitive movements of mandible, lips, and fingers are used as tests of this function.

diencephalon. Part of the brain between the telencephalon (cerebral cortex, olfactory lobes, and corpus striatum) and mesencephalon (midbrain). *See also* **thalamus.**

digital computer. Computer that processes information in digital form (use of numerical digits expressed in a scale of notation to represent all variables occurring in a problem).

diphthong. [eɪ] [aɪ] [aʊ] [oʊ] [ɔɪ] [ju]. Unsegmentable, gliding speech sound, varying continuously in phonetic quality but held to be a single phoneme.

diplacusis. Hearing a tone differently in each ear, as if it were two tones of different pitch.

discrimination. *See* **Perception.**

DNA (deoxyribonucleic acid). Any of the class of nucleic acids that contain deoxyribose, found chiefly in the nucleus of cells, and which functions in the transference of genetic characteristics and in the synthesis of protein.

dysacusis. Impairment of auditory perception of speech, resulting not from a loss of acuity, but from dysfunction of cochlea and/or auditory circuits of CNS. Sometimes called *auditory agnosia.*

dysarthria(s). Complex sensorimotor syndromes characterized by interruption of patterning of phasic and subphasic movements of speech. Except in Parkinson's syndrome repetitive movements of articulation are slow. The injury or deficit in the nervous system may be either peripheral or central.

dyslalia. Defective articulation of speech.

dyslexia. Neurological disorder characterized by visuomotor disturbances in reading.

dysphonia. Any defect of phonation.

electroencephalograph (EEG). Electronic instrument for graphically recording electrical currents (brain waves) developed during active states in the cerebral cortex.

encephalitis.   Infection of the brain and/or meningeal membranes enclosing it.

endocrine system.   A group of interacting ductless glands under the control of the master gland, the *anterior pituitary section* of the *hypophysis.* Other glands in the endocrine ring are pancreas, parathyroid, thyroid, thymus, adrenal, and secondary sex glands (testicular and ovarian).

engram.   Hypothesized memory trace in CNS produced by permanently altered condition of neural tissue as a result of activity; basis of physiological memory.

epithalamus.   Upper and dorsal portion of the diencephalon including the habenula, pineal gland, and the posterior commissure.

extrapyramidal system.   Formerly thought to be a distinct system associated with neural activity of frontal cortex and basal nuclei and governing fine motor coordination; its functions now have been merged with those of the pyramidal system.

facial nerve.   *See* **Nerve.**

facilitation and inhibition.   Ability of CNS to reduce asynergies, incoordination, response times, and perceptual errors by increasing potential of certain sensorimotor circuits and reducing potential of others that would retard efficiency in coding. Synonym: *gating.*

fastigium.   Portion of the cerebellum which forms an angle in the roof of the fourth ventricle.

Feedback (Speech):

  feedback.   (1) The aspect of speech whereby one responds tactile-kinesthetically and auditorially to his own speech. Some authorities refer to five types of feedback: (*a*) auditory; (*b*) vibratory (bone conduction felt by the speaker or in the event of hearing loss by placing fingers on speaker's face); (*c*) kinesthetic (the proprioceptive response to phonatory and articulatory movements); (*d*) tactile (the peripheral touch response to articulatory contacts); (*e*) intention (deep psychological response, whereby one knows his own intention in speech).

  (2) Perceptual reaction of a person to his own response, a process by which direct responses are controlled and corrected.

  delayed auditory feedback.   Probably temporal decorrelation of a critical subset of the total pattern of sensory feedback being utilized for the organization and control of sensorimotor processes of speech.

  experimentally delayed auditory feedback.   Experimental delay, 180–200 msec., in the "return" of one's speech, which generally results in complete disorganization of temporal patterning of speech. Speech under these conditions is characterized by articulatory disturbances and wide fluctuations in intensity and pitch.

feedback loop. Functional unit of nervous system replacing reflex arc.

figure-ground. Organization of a salient central feature or figure, which is part of, but separate and distinct from its surround.

Fissure of Sylvius. Deep fissure of the brain extending to lateral surface of the hemisphere and consisting of a short vertical and long horizontal branch, the latter separating the temporal from the frontal and parietal lobes. Also called *lateral cerebral fissure.*

fixation mechanism. Retention by nervous system of a relationship among neuronal assemblies that have responded together in earlier time-space events and may be reproduced when needed. Process whereby organized time-space events are carried forward in time. Synonym: *memory.*

flocculus. One of two fundamental lobes of the cerebellum, the first to appear both phylogenetically and ontogenetically.

formant. (1) One of the regions of concentration of energy, prominent on a sound spectrogram, which collectively constitute the frequency spectrum of a speech sound.

(2) in the spectrum, a region where pitch is indicated by the spacing between the harmonics of the formant, and the timbre or quality is indicated by the number of formants that occur.

fornix. Paired structure at base of cerebrum comprised of nerve fibers connecting the hippocampus with the mammillary bodies, habenula, and preoptic areas.

fourth ventricle. One of the four cerebral vesicles bounded by the pons, upper medulla, and the cerebellum.

fricative. [s], [z], [ʃ], [ʒ], [f], [v], [θ], [ð], and [h]. Consonantal sound which in English speech is made by directing the breath stream with adequate pressure against one or more surfaces, principally the hard palate, gum ridge behind the upper teeth, teeth, and lips. The breath stream is continuously flowing but constricted.

frontal lobes. *See* **Cerebrum** *and* **Cerebral Lobes.**

gamma spindle. Peripheral nerve fibers in muscle spindles equipped with both sensory and motor endings, thus providing motor control of muscle afferents. A self-regulative or feedback mechanism of muscle activity. Single system of neural input-output.

Ganglia:

    ganglion. Massed group of cell bodies or nerve cells outside the CNS.

    basal ganglia. *See* **Nucleus.**

    spiral ganglia. Collection of cells of the cochlear nerve lodged in spiral canal of modiolus in the inner ear.

gating. *See* **facilitation and inhibition.**

geniculate bodies. *See* **lateral geniculate body, medial geniculate body,** *and* **metathalamus.**

glia.   General term for the fibrous and cellular supporting elements of the nervous system. Synonym: *neuroglia*.

glide.   [r], [w], [j], [hw]. Speech sound which consists primarily of the movement of an articulator, in contrast to sounds produced with the articulators held in a relatively static position. Nonsyllabic vocoid.

glossopharyngeal nerve.   *See* **Nerve.**

grammar.   Study of the system underlying such formal features of a language as morphemes, words, and sentences.

gyrus.   Convolution on the surface of the cerebral hemisphere.

haptic feedback.   A collective term denoting tactile and kinesthetic feedback. *See also* **Feedback.**

haptic perception.   *See* **Perception.**

haptic sensation.   Dual experience of touch and kinesthesis which are combined, for instance, in taking an object in one's hand and feeling it totally while moving a finger over it to experience its shape.

Heschl's gyri.   Two or three gyri which transversely cross the upper surface of the superior temporal gyrus. Synonym: *transverse temporal gyri*.

hippocampus.   Curved elevation in the under part of the cerebrum, consisting largely of gray matter in the floor of the inferior horn of the lateral ventricle. It has been included by some authorities in the limbic system.

holophrastic dictionary.   Memory of the word in all contextual cues.

homeostasis.   Tendency of a system, especially the physiological system of primates, to maintain internal stability, owing to the response of the neuroendocrine system to any stimulus or situation tending to disturb its normal condition or function. State of physiological equilibrium, maintained in part, by reticular, limbic, and endocrine systems. Synonym: *Controlled lability*.

hypoglossal nerve.   *See* **Nerve.**

hypothalamus.   Region of the forebrain below, and the underpart of, the thalamus, including the mamillary bodies, optic chiasma, and hypophysis. Neuro-endocrine in function, it is involved in emotional and visceral regulative processes.

Hz (Hertz).   A unit of frequency equal to one cycle per second.

idiopathic language retardation.   Delay in development of language for which no physiological cause is known.

inferior colliculi.   *See* **colliculi, inferior.**

inferior olivary nucleus.   *See* **Nucleus.**

inhibition. *See* **facilitation and inhibition.**

inner language. Perceptual response to verbal stimuli which may or may not result in overt speech. A subliminal response to verbal stimuli; inner speech "gone underground." Synonym: *implicit speech.*

input modalities. Sensory impulses of audition, taction, vision, and kinesthesis entering the CNS.

instrumental conditioning. *See* **conditioning.**

insula. Portion of cortex overlying the corpus striatum; in the adult brain it lies buried within the Sylvian fissure.

internal auditory meatus. Canal beginning on the posterior surface of the petrous bone which gives passage to the acoustic and facial nerves and the internal auditory artery.

internal capsule. Great band of nerve fibers on the outer side of the thalamus and between the caudate and lenticular nuclei. It is continuous with the cerebral peduncles and consists of fibers to and from the cortex.

internuncial pool. Masses of nerve cells providing functional connections for several tracts.

intonational contour. Component of prosody or melody of speech which is distinguished chiefly by pattern of pitch and duration denoting meaning. A sequence of levels of pitch or stress typically extending over several successive words in the utterance.

kinesthesis. Sense of perception of movement, weight, resistance, and position mediated through sensations in muscles resulting from stimulation of tendons and joints. Sometimes static sensations from semicircular canals of the inner ear are included in kinesthesis. Synonym: *proprioception. See also* **Perception.**

Language:

    language. Structured system of arbitrary vocal sounds and sequences of sounds which is used in interpersonal communication and which rather exhaustively catalogs the things, events, and processes of human experience. The system inherent in a language derives essentially and primarily from the sequence of articulated, heard sounds in *spoken* utterances or messages.

    egocentric language. Early stage in child's linguistic development characterized by the initial inability to decenter, to shift the given cognitive or mental perspective in social and other relationships in which language plays a part. Closed cycle in which the child vocalizes his perceptual processes.

lateral geniculate bodies. Pair of oval, flattened bodies on posterior inferior aspect of the thalamus whose nuclei receive optic impulses from optic tracts and relay them to other neuronal assemblies, including the occipital cortex. *See also* **metathalamus.**

lateral sound. A phonetic term used to designate speech sounds in which the breath stream escapes over the sides of the tongue. English speech has but one lateral sound: [l].

Lemniscus:

    lemniscus. Pathway of CNS composed of sensory fibers that usually have decussated and terminate around nuclei in the upper brainstem, thalamus, or cortex.

    lateral lemniscus. Auditory fibers arising in the cochlear nuclei and ascending in the brainstem; some fibers synapse with nuclei in the inferior colliculi and the medial geniculate body, others synapse with nuclei in the cortex.

    medial lemniscus. Bands of neural fibers arising in the nucleus gracilis and nucleus cuneatus in the medulla, crossing immediately to opposite side of brainstem and terminating in the cerebellum, upper brainstem, thalamus, and somesthetic cortex. It contributes chiefly proprioceptive information (body posture, muscle tone) to neural networks.

lenticular nucleus. *See* **Nucleus.**

lexical. Relating to words, word formatives, and vocabulary as distinct from grammatical forms and constructions.

limbic lobe. *See* **Cerebrum** *and* **Cerebral Lobes.**

limbic system. Functionally integrated system predominantly concerned with motivation, attention, and emotionally determined functions that pertain to the preservation of the self or of the species. Nuclear structures associated with the limbic system include hypothalamus, gyrus cinguli, hippocampus, septum, amygdala, certain thalamic nuclei, parts of basal nuclei (corpus striatum), and possibly some brainstem nuclei.

longitudinal study. Evaluative study covering comprehensive time period.

mammillary bodies. Two small, spherical masses of gray matter in the hypothalamus. Formerly thought to be associated with olfaction; now considered a part of the limbic system.

medial geniculate bodies. Pair of oval, flattened bodies on the posterior and inferior aspect of the thalamus. Together with the *lateral* geniculate bodies, they constitute the metathalamus. The medial geniculate nuclei are associated both with cortical and brainstem coding of auditory impulses via the indirect, reticular route. Some authorities ascribe discrimination of frequency and intensity of sound to these bodies. *See also* **metathalamus.**

medial lemniscus. *See* **Lemniscus.**

medulla. Lowest part of the brainstem extending from the pons to the spinal cord and truly representing an extension of the latter. All except four cranial nerves exit from the medulla. Among its many activities is the regulation of respiration and circulation.

memory. *See* **fixation mechanism.**

meninges. Three coverings investing the brain and spinal cord.

mesencephalon. *See* **midbrain.**

metathalamus. Nuclear masses adjacent to the thalamus, containing the lateral and medial geniculate bodies.

midbrain. Part of the brain stem developed from the middle cerebral vesicle of the embryo; it includes the cerebral peduncles and the corpora quadrigemina (superior and inferior colliculi). Synonym: *mesencephalon.*

modality. Qualitative aspect of sense experience as belonging to an order of stimuli; two sensations are said to differ in modality when it is impossible to pass by gradations of quality from one to the other, as for example, the *color, red* and the *tonal frequency, 256 Hz.*

molar. Pertaining to body of matter as a whole, as contrasted with *molecular* and *atomic.*

Moro reflex. Concussion reaction, elicited by a sudden sharp noise or by upsetting the equilibrium, normally observed only in newborn infants. In normal response of neonates, both legs are drawn up and the arms brought up as in an embrace.

Morpheme:

morpheme. Minimal unit of speech that is recurrent and meaningful. The syllable is generally regarded as the minimal unit.

bound morpheme. Syllable that cannot be used by itself.

free morpheme. Minimal unit that can stand alone.

Motivation:

motivation. Phenomena involved in the operation of incentives or drives.

primary motivation. Incentive derived from basic genetic drive.

secondary motivation. Incentive derived from external forces.

motokinesthetic training, Young-Stinchfield method. Method of speech habilitation employing stimulation of articulatory patterning by external tactile-kinesthetic cues. The teacher directs tongue, jaw, and lip movements by touch and manipulation.

multimodal neurones. Neurones that have the capacity to receive and transmit information from several sensory modalities.

Muscle:

infrahyoid muscles. Small, flat muscles below the hyoid bone, including sternohyoid, omohyoid, sternothyroid, and thyrohyoid muscles.

platysma muscle. Subcutaneous muscle in the neck, extending from the face to the clavicle.

sternocleidomastoid muscle. Muscle extending from sternum to the clavicle and to the mastoid process; muscle of inhalation and of head movement.

suprahyoid muscles. Group of muscles attached to the upper part of the hyoid bone, including stylohyoid, mylohyoid, and geniohyoid muscles.

nasal sound. [m], [n], [ŋ]. Phonetic term used to designate the phones (in English) which have a dominant nasal resonance.

Nerve:

acoustic nerve. VIIIth cranial nerve, having two roots, the vestibular branch originating in the vestibule and the semicircular canals, and the cochlear branch originating in the cochlea. Nerve mediating hearing and equilibration.

cochlear nerve. Section of acoustic nerve (C-VIII) which enters CNS at mid-pons. Its first cell bodies make up the spiral ganglion of the cochlea; second-level neurones are ventral and dorsal cochlear nuclei.

facial nerve. VIIth cranial nerve, sensory (proprioceptive) and motor in function, innervating certain extrinsic muscles of the tongue and the muscles of facial expression.

glossopharyngeal nerve. IXth cranial nerve, sensory fibers of which are distributed to the middle ear, pharynx, and tongue. Sensorimotor fibers go to muscles of soft palate and pharynx.

hypoglossal nerve. XIIth cranial nerve providing both sensory (proprioceptive) and motor innervation to intrinsic muscles of the tongue.

oculomotor nerve. IIIrd cranial nerve, sensorimotor in function, innervating all extrinsic eye muscles except lateral rectus and superior oblique.

trigeminal nerve. Vth cranial nerve; its ophthalmic and maxillary branches are primarily sensory to the face; its mandibular branch provides sensorimotor innervation to the mandible.

trochlear nerve. IVth cranial nerve that innervates the superior oblique muscle of the eye.

vagus nerve. Xth cranial nerve; sensory and motor components are distributed to larynx, lungs, esophagus, heart, and abdominal viscera.

neural plasticity. Genetically determined differential in variability and strength of synaptic potentials.

neural wave front. Neurones in parallel mediating same or similar impulse.

neurone. Basic unit of structure of the CNS, consisting of a cell body with its processes. *See also* **plurivalent neurone.**

Nucleus:

ambiguous nucleus. Nucleus in the reticular formation of the medulla and pons whose cells give origin to sensorimotor fibers of glossophyarngeal and vagus nerves. An important nuclear complex associated with innervation of respiration, phonation, resonation, and articulation.

amygdaloid nuclei. Gray matter continuous with the cortex of the hippocampal gyrus and lying at the tip of the inferior horn of the lateral ventricle. It may function as a part of the limbic system.

basal nuclei. Nuclear masses and fibers at the base of both cerebral hemispheres, lying adjacent to the anterior horns of the lateral ventricles, and consisting of caudate, lenticular (putamen, globus pallidus) and amygdaloid nuclei, and the internal capsule that separates them. Presumably they are a part of cortical and brainstem circular networks operative in final stages of coding oral expression. Synonyms: *striate bodies; basal ganglia.*

caudate nuclei. Part of the corpus striatum; arched gray nuclear masses projecting into and forming part of the lateral wall of the lateral ventricle. Intimately associated with the cortex in the final stages of sensorimotor coding.

dentate nuclei. Largest and most laterally placed nuclear mass of cerebellum. Its bipolar nuclei have bidirectional connections with basal nuclei and cortex and with the brain stem via the reticular system.

dorsal lateral nuclei. Part of the lateral nuclei of thalamus. Continuous with the pulvinar, they receive fibers from other thalamic nuclei, and connect with the cortex of the parietal lobe.

facial nuclei. Collection of nerve cells in the lateral portion of the reticular formation of the pons, giving origin to some sensorimotor components of the facial nerve.

fastigial nuclei. Nuclei in midline position in that part of the cerebellum overlying roof of fourth ventricle.

globose nuclei. Nuclei in the cerebellum which have been linked directly with the red nucleus and the reticular organizing system.

globus pallidus (Pallidum). Inner and lighter part of the lenticular section of the corpus striatum.

gracile and cuneate nuclei. Nuclear masses in lower medulla from which fiber tracts, largely proprioceptive in function, emanate to make up a part of the medial lemniscus.

hypoglossal nuclei. Nuclei near midline throughout the medulla whose cells give origin to the sensorimotor fibers of the hypoglossal nerve which innervate the tongue.

inferior olivary nucleus. Great nuclear complex in medulla which distributes fibers to all parts of cerebellum and receives fibers from reticular and basal nuclei. Function is largely concerned with patterned movement.

lenticular nuclei. Nuclear mass in striate bodies consisting of two parts: globus pallidus and putamen.

motor nucleus of the trigeminal nerve. Collection of cells in the reticular formation of the pons giving origin to sensorimotor fibers innervating muscles of the mandible.

nuclei ruber. *See* **red nuclei.**

putamen nuclei. The outer, darker part of the lenticular section of the corpus striatum.

red nuclei. Large oval nuclei situated in the midbrain and thalamus ventral to the cerebral aqueduct. An important part of the reticular system. Synonym: *nuclei ruber.*

reticular nuclei. Diffuse cell groups in the reticular formation associated with bidirectional tracts connecting all levels of the brain stem with the cortex.

superior olivary nuclei. A nuclear complex in the pons which has multiple connections with the indirect auditory system and with motor nuclei of trigeminal and facial nerves.

ventral and dorsal cochlear nuclei. Nuclear masses, dorsal and ventral respectively, to the restiform body, mediating the first synaptic connections of the cochlear nerve in the brainstem.

occipital lobe. *See* **Cerebral Lobes.**

operant conditioning. *See* **Conditioning.**

organ of Corti. Sensory part of the cochlea of the inner ear; end organ of hearing.

ossicles. Three small bones in the tympanic cavity: *malleus, incus* and *stapes;* part of the conductive mechanism of the middle ear.

otitis media. Inflammation of the middle ear. Called *suppurative otitis media* when accompanied over a prolonged period by production of pus.

paradigm. Model; standard.

parietal lobe. *See* **Cerebral Lobes.**

Parkinsonian dysarthria. Condition characterized by rigid, mumbling, nonprosodic speech.

Parkinson's syndrome. Complex of symptoms stemming from lesions of the corpus striatum (basal nuclei) and possibly the thalamus. The syndrome is identified by four major behavioral manifestations: rigidity, tremor, akinesia, and loss of spontaneous and automatic movement.

Perception:

> **perception.** Act of meaningful awareness and affective appreciation of stimulus, object, or situation; the result of multisensory integration with the integration of ideational patterns of memory. Both a cognitive and an affective phenomenon. Synonym: *discrimination;* partial synonym: *cognition.*

> **auditory perception.** Act of meaningfully interpreting (or discriminating) sounds and sound sequences employed in oral communication. Synonyms: *auditory discrimination; auding.*

> **haptic perception.** Meaningful awareness of stimulus, object, or situation produced by sensations of taction and kinesthesis; presumably both modalities contribute to a single effect. Synonym: *tactile-kinesthetic perception.*

> **kinesthetic perception.** Feedback from motor pathways producing awareness of sensations in muscles resulting from stimulation of tendons and joints. Synonym: *proprioception. See also* **haptic perception.**

> **perceptual set.** Selective focusing by CNS upon sensorimotor patterns, determined by antecedent conditions of recency and frequency.

> **proprioception.** *See* **kinesthetic perception.**

> **visual perception.** Meaningful awareness and appreciation of visual stimuli.

> **visuomotor perception.** Act of reproducing sequence of visual stimuli from memory.

perinatal. Around or about the time of birth.

phasic movement. State of synchronous muscle activity in which agonists and antagonists work in even or rhythmic alternation.

phone. Any speech sound, considered as a physical event; it may or may not fit into the structure of a given language.

phoneme. Minimal unit of distinctive sound features. A finite set of mutually exclusive classes of speech sounds.

phonemic sequence. Linguistic unit which possesses a characteristic distribution and interrelationship.

phonology. Study of phonemic and prosodic patterns of speech. Covering term for the general description of the speech event.

pituitary body. Body in hypothalamic region of the brain; partially endocrine, partially nervous in function. A common anatomic division is anterior pituitary, posterior pituitary, and pars intermedia. Synonym: *hypophysis cerebri. See also* **anterior pituitary gland.**

plosive. Consonantal sound which is produced in English by a complete blocking of the breath stream at some point, followed by a sudden release and explosion of the breath stream.

plurivalent neurone. Neurone that is not specific for one modality.

pons. Convex white eminence situated above the medulla and below the midbrain. It consists of great nuclear masses and fiber tracts and has direct connections through its peduncles with the cerebellum.

postcentral gyrus. Cerebral convolution lying immediately posterior to the fissure of Rolando (central sulcus). Sensorimotor areas of bodily organization and control. Function of this area formerly was considered to be exclusively somesthetic.

posterior pituitary body. Neuro-endocrine body secreting antidiuretic hormone and oxytocin; the latter stimulates contraction of smooth muscles of the uterus.

postsynaptic membrane. Neural tissue subjacent to the synaptic knob, which becomes depolarized and thus permits synaptic transmission.

postsynaptic potential (PSP). Initially rising phase in strength of neural impulse after synapse, produced by brief depolarization and then spreading decrementally over whole postsynaptic membrane.

pragmatics. Relation of signs to people who use them.

precentral gyrus. Cerebral convolution lying immediately anterior to the fissure of Rolando (central sulcus). Motor-sensory region of bodily organization and control, principally of skeletal musculature. Formerly only primary motor function was assigned to this area. *See also* **Brodmann's area 4.**

presynaptic potential. The building up of a rhythmic discharge of impulses in centrally directed fibers by means of a continuous depolarizing process before synapse with motor nuclei.

projective tests. A type of mental test employed to determine *personality traits* through the completion of sentences, interpretation of inkblots (Rorschach test), interpretation of pictures, and making of designs. In projective tests there is no right or wrong answer; the individual is left free to follow his own inclinations and imagination.

proprioception (kinesthesis). *See* **perception.**

prosody. Melody of speech determined primarily by modifications of pitch, quality, strength, and duration, perceived primarily as stress and intonational patterns.

Purkinje cells. Cells of the cerebellar cortex whose axones end in central cerebellar nuclei.

pyramids. Two columns, embracing both sensory and motor tracts, which lie on either side of the median fissure making up the central region of the medulla.

red nucleus. *See* **Nucleus.**

reflex inhibiting postures (RIP). System of training (Bobath method), aim of which is to establish inhibitory postures in the cerebral-palsied as a method of control of abnormal infantile reflex mechanisms. Tonic neck reflexes are most notable in producing abnormal postural and righting responses.

restiform body. Inferior cerebellar peduncle, composed of bands of nuclei and fibers, connecting cerebellum with brainstem.

retention and recall. Persisting trace left behind as an after-effect of a response or excitation and which may alter subsequent responses or excitations; the basis of learning or memory. Neurological correlate: *fixation mechanism.*

reticular system. Activating and integrating system promoting arousal, motivation, attention, and facilitation-inhibition in coding. A region of polysensory and motor convergence which "filters" all sensorimotor impulses by means of feedback circuits. Origin: Reticular formation of lower brainstem at crossroads of sensorimotor tracts from which it receives collaterals; may include part of cerebellum. Extends through upper brain stem, parts of thalamus, striate bodies; it effects reciprocal influence on neocortex through widespread corticofugal connections.

Rh factor. One or more hereditary antigens that occur in the red blood cells of about 85% of the population (*Rh positive*) and that on repeated transfusion into a person lacking it (*Rh negative*) cause severe hemolysis of the erythrocytes; when transferred to an Rh-negative mother by an Rh-positive fetus and returned to subsequent fetuses, *erythroblastosis fetalis* results.

ribonucleic acid. *See* **RNA.**

RNA (ribonucleic acid). Any of the class of nucleic acids containing ribose that is found in all living cells, especially as a component of cell-nucleus proteins. Found at synaptic junctions and thought to be the effective agent in neural transmission, integration, and in retention of learning. An intermediate of DNA.

Rolandic rhythm. Basic rhythm of the sensorimotor fields of the cortex around the fissure of Rolando.

salience. Psychological prominence of a speech unit in the speaker's mind.

semantics. The study of meaning in language, including the relations between language, thought, and behavior; a science dealing with the relations between *referents* and *referends* and with the historical changes in the meanings of words and forms. Relation of signs to meaning.

semology. Perception of linguistic information; it bears the same relation to *semantics* as does phonemics to phonetics. Semantics is the hyphenated discipline that relates semology to percepts. Synonym: *sememics.*

sensorimotor patterns. Circular networks of neural activity or events that occur along the time dimension, sometimes in closer proximity to the behavioral response than to stimulus; patterns that in a strict sense are not linked exclusively with stimulus or response.

set-to-attend. Neurological mechanism that increases the potential in appropriate cortical and subcortical areas and decreases excitation in adjacent areas, thus permitting cognition of one group of stimuli and excluding others.

SIR arc. Simple reflex circuit of stimulation, integration, and response.

spasticity. Increased tonus or tension of a muscle which is associated with exaggeration of deep reflexes, and frequently with clonus and partial or complete loss of voluntary control.

striate bodies (basal ganglia). *See* **basal nuclei.**

substantia nigra. Broad thick plate of large pigmented cells extending through the midbrain into the hypothalamus. Probably associated in function with reticular activating and organizing systems.

sulcus. Linear depression on the cerebral hemispheres separating convolutions or gyri.

superior colliculi. *See* **colliculi, superior.**

superior olivary nucleus. *See* **Nucleus.**

synapse. The point at which *functional* connection is made between the axone of one neurone and the dendrite or cell body of another.

synaptic knobs. Small swellings at the end of a nerve fiber or along its course which together with the subsynaptic membrane make up the synapse.

syncretism. Understanding of the whole before the parts are analyzed. Perception of the whole and nothing first.

syndrome. A group of symptoms and signs, which, when considered together, characterize a disease or lesion.

synkinesis. Mirror movement patterns of right and left sides of body.

syntactic structure. Significant unit denoting word order and relationship; determiner of morphological building blocks of language.

syntactics. Relation of signs to signs.

syntax. Study and science of sentence construction; relation of signs to signs.

tachyphemia. *See* **cluttering.**

taction. *See* **haptic.**

temporal lobe. *See* **Cerebrum** *and* **Cortical Lobes.**

temporal-spatial pattern. Theory that perceptual ability is based on recognition of temporal and spatial differences in neural wave patterns. The more basic dimension in auditory discrimination is temporal resolving power; in visual discrimination, spatial resolving power.

thalamus. Mass of gray matter situated at the base of the cerebrum, projecting into and bound by the third ventricle. Considered by some authorities as a part of reticular activating and organizing systems; by others a part of the limbic system controlling emotion. Often referred to as *thalamus proper,* thus distinguishing it from hypothalamus, metathalamus, and epithalamus.

theta wave. Rhythmic activity, 4–7 Hz, recorded from temporal and central areas of cortex *of the child* during early stage of sleep.

Tracts:

corticobulbar tract. Network of proprioceptive and motor fibers which pass through the internal capsule and terminate in nuclei in the brainstem. They are concerned in finely coordinated voluntary movement mediated by cranial nerves.

corticofugal tract. Neural pathway making up circular network between cerebral cortex and subcortical nuclear masses.

corticospinal tract. A circular network containing both proprioceptive and motor fibers. Fibers originating in the cortex undergo incomplete decussation in the medulla to form the lateral and ventral corticospinal tracts. They are concerned in finely coordinated voluntary movement.

limbic-subcortical tract. Bidirectional pathways from pyramidal cells of hippocampus via the fornix, which connect anterior nuclei of thalamus, epithalamus and basal nuclei with affectoceptor and affectomotor areas of the limbic system.

pyramidal tract. Great trunks of sensory (proprioceptive) and motor fibers that synapse with nuclei at all levels of the CNS.

olivocochlear tract. Band of fibers running from superior olive to cochlea, which presumably suppresses activity of the auditory nerve; a feedback mechanism.

reticulocerebellar tract. Nerve fibers which arise in the reticular formation and end in the cerebellum.

reticulocortical tract. Pathways linking the cortex with the reticular activating and organizing systems.

striocortical tract. Nerve fibers which arise in the putamen (of the lenticular nucleus) and caudate nucleus and connect these bodies with the cortex.

thalamocortical tract. Bidirectional fiber tracts between thalamus and cortex.

transverse temporal gyri. *See* **Heschl's gyri.**

trapezoid body. Transverse decussating fibers in the central tegmental part of the pons, which connect the cochlear nuclei of one side with the lateral lemniscus of the other side.

trigeminal nerve. *See* **Nerve.**

trochlear nerve. *See* **Nerve.**

vagus nerve. *See* **Nerve.**

velopharyngeal sphincter. Purse-string closure of the nasopharyngeal airway by means of combined action of superior constrictor, levator palati, and palatopharyngeus muscles.

vestibule. Part of the bony labyrinth of the inner ear, between the cochlea and the semicircular canals, containing the utricle and the saccule.

visuomotor perception.   *See* **Perception.**

Wernicke's area.   Area in the first and second convolutions of the temporal lobe, usually of the left hemisphere, ascribed by Wernicke to be a center for auditory comprehension of oral language.

Word Classes:

    functional classes.   Words having grammatical rather than lexical meaning, used primarily to show relationship: prepositions, auxiliary verbs, conjunctions, articles, and interjections.

    lexical classes.   Words or vocabulary of a language, especially as contrasted with its grammatical and syntactical aspects; nouns, verbs, adjectives, adverbs, pronouns.

Young-Stinchfield method.   *See* **motokinesthetic training.**

List of Journal Abbreviations

Acta Neurol Belg: Acta Neurologica et Psychiatrica Belgica (Bruxelles)

Acta Neurol Scand: Acta Neurologica Scandinavica (København)

Acta Otolaryng (Stockholm): Acta Oto-laryngologica (Stockholm)

Acta Physiol Scand: Acta Physiologica Scandinavica (København)

Acta Psychiat Neurol: Acta Psychiatrica et Neurologica (København)

Amer J Orthopsychiat: American Journal of Orthopsychiatry (New York)

Amer J Psychiat: American Journal of Psychiatry (Hanover, N. H.)

Amer J Psychol: American Journal of Psychology (Austin)

Amer Sci: American Scientist (New Haven)

Ann Otol: Annals of Otology, Rhinology and Laryngology (St. Louis)

Ann Rev Physiol: Annual Review of Physiology (Stanford)

Ann Rev Psychol: Annual Review of Psychology (Stanford)

Arch Neurol (Chicago): Archives of Neurology (Chicago)

Arch Psychiat Nervenkr: Archiv fur Psychiatrie und Nervenkrankheiten vereingt mit Zeitschrift fur die Gesamte Neurologie und Psychiatrie (Berlin)

Arch Psychol: Archives de Psychologie (Genève)

Asha: Journal of the American Speech and Hearing Association (Washington)

Brain: Brain, Journal of Neurology (London)

Brit J Phys Med: British Journal of Physical Medicine (London)

Brit J Psychiat: British Journal of Psychiatry (London)

Brit Med J: British Medical Journal (London)

Child Develop: Child Development (Lafayette, Ind.)

Children: Children (Washington)

Clin Sympos: Clinical Symposia (Summit, N. J.)

Confin Neurol: Confinia Neurologica (Basel)

Cortex: Cortex (Milano)

Develop Med Child Neurol: Developmental Medicine and Child Neurology (London)

Electroenceph Clin Neurophysiol: Electroencephalography and Clinical Neurophysiology (Amsterdam)

Exceptional Child: Exceptional Children (Washington)

Exp Neurol: Experimental Neurology (New York)

Fed Proc: Federation Proceedings (Baltimore)

Fiziol Zh SSSR Sechenov: Fiziologicheskii Zhurnal SSSR imeni I. M. Sechenova (Moskva)

Folia Phoniat (Basel): Folia Phoniatrica (Basel)

Gen Semantics Bull: General Semantics Bulletin (Lakeville, Conn.)

Genet Psychol Monogr: Genetic Psychology Monographs (Provincetown)

Hum Biol: Human Biology (Detroit)

Izv Akad Nauk SSSR [Med]: Izvestiia Akademii Nauk SSSR; Seria Meditsina (Moskva)

J Abnorm Psychol: Journal of Abnormal Psychology (Washington), formerly Journal of Abnormal and Social Psychology (Washington)

J Abnorm Soc Psychol: Journal of Abnormal and Social Psychology (Washington), *see J Abnorm Psychol*

J Acoust Soc Amer: Journal of the Acoustical Society of America (New York)

J Appl Psychol: Journal of Applied Psychology (Washington)

J Child Psychol Psychiat: Journal of Child Psychology and Psychiatry and Allied Disciplines (London)

J Educ Psychol: Journal of Educational Psychology (Baltimore)

J Exp Educ: Journal of Experimental Education (Madison, Wisc.)

J Nerv Ment Dis: Journal of Nervous and Mental Disease (Baltimore)

J Neurophysiol: Journal of Neurophysiology (Springfield, Ill.)

J Neurosurg: Journal of Neurosurgery (Chicago)

J Ontario Speech Hearing Ass: Journal of the Ontario Speech and Hearing Association (Ontario)

J Pediat: Journal of Pediatrics (St. Louis)

J Physiol (London): Journal of Physiology (London)

J Project Techn: Journal of Projective Techniques and Personality Assessment (Glendale)

J S Afr Logoped Soc: Journal of the South African Logopedic Society (Johannesburg)

J Sch Health: Journal of School Health (Columbus)

J Speech Hearing Dis: Journal of Speech and Hearing Disorders (Washington)

J Speech Hearing Res: Journal of Speech and Hearing Research (Washington)

J Verbal Learn Verbal Behav: Journal of Verbal Learning and Verbal Behavior (New York)

J Wash Acad Sci: Journal of the Washington Academy of Science (Seattle)

Laryngoscope: Laryngoscope (St. Louis)

Med Times: Medical Times (Manhasset)

Monogr Soc Res Child Devel: Monographs of the Society for Research in Child Development (Lafayette, Ind.)

Nat Geog Mag: National Geographic Magazine (Washington)

Neurology (Minneap): Neurology (Minneapolis)

New York Acad Sci: New York Academy of Science (New York)

Percept Motor Skills: Perceptual and Motor Skills (Missoula)

Phys Ther: Physical Therapy; Journal of the American Physical Therapy Association (New York) formerly *Phys Ther Rev*

Phys Ther Rev: Physical Therapy Review (New York); now *Phys Ther*

Physiol Rev: Physiological Reviews (Washington)

Plast Reconstr Surg: Plastic and Reconstructive Surgery (Baltimore)

Psychiat Res Rep Amer Psychiat Ass: Psychiatric Research Reports of the American Psychiatric Association (Washington)

Psychol Bull: Psychological Bulletin (Washington)

Psychol Monogr: Psychological Monographs: General and Applied (Washington)

Psychol Rev: Psychological Review (Washington)

Psychosom Med: Psychosomatic Medicine (New York)

Quart J Exp Psychol: Quarterly Journal of Experimental Psychology (Cambridge)

Quart J Speech: Quarterly Journal of Speech (New York)

Res Publ Ass Res Nerv Ment Dis: Research Publications of the Association for Research in Nervous and Mental Disease (Baltimore)

Rev Laryng (Bordeaux): Revue de Laryngologie, Otologie, Rhinologie (Bordeaux)

Sci Amer: Scientific American (New York)

Science: Science (Washington)

Southern Speech J: Southern Speech Journal (Tampa)

Speech Monogr: Speech Monographs (New York)

Speech Path Ther: Speech Pathology and Therapy (London) (*now* Disorders of Communication)

Technol Rev: The Technological Review (Cambridge, Mass.)

US Office of Educ Coop Res Program Monogr: U. S. Office of Education Cooperative Research Program Monograph (Washington)

Index

Italic page numbers identify charts, tables, figures, and complete directions or materials for administration of tests.

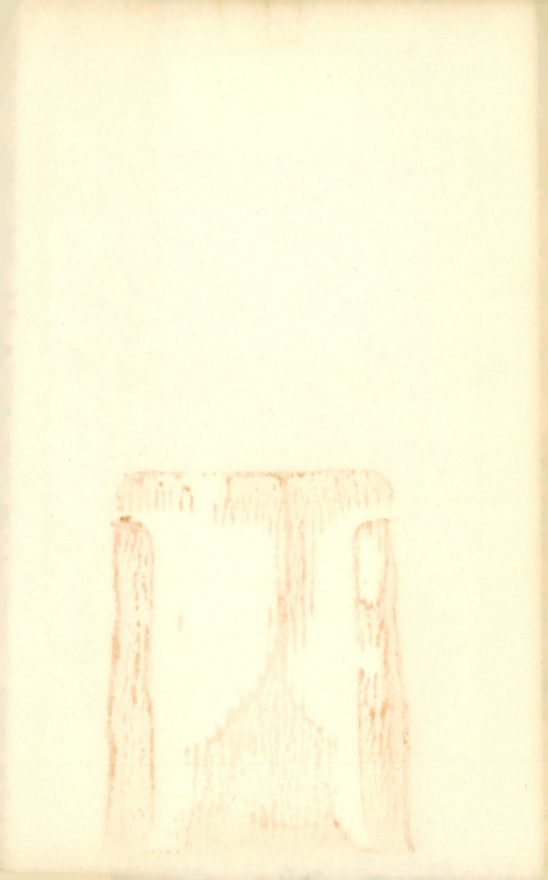

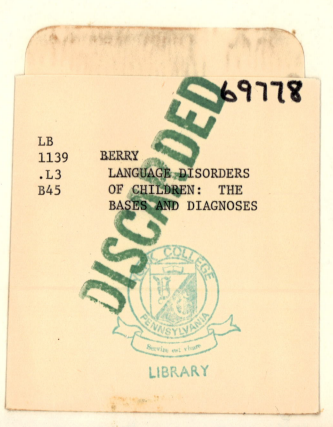